ALZHEIMER'S DISEASE

Forget Antioxidants & Supplements

Plus,
An Addendum of 90 Studies
Showing Antioxidant Ineffectiveness.

By
Author : Dr. Randolph M. Howes, M.D., Ph.D.

ISBN-10: 1466457414

ISBN-13: 978-1466457416

ALZHEIMER'S DISEASE:

*Forget Antioxidants
&
Supplements*

By
Prof. Hon. Randolph M. Howes, M.D., Ph.D.

Physician, Surgeon and Scientist (Biochemist)

Adjunct Assistant Professor of Plastic Surgery,
The Johns Hopkins Hospital, Baltimore, MD USA

Espaldon Professor of Plastic and Reconstructive Surgery,
University of Santo Tomas, Manila, Philippines

Adjunct Professor of Biological Sciences,
Southeastern Louisiana University

Founder, Director and Chairman of the Scientific Advisory Board;
U.S. Medical Scientific Research Foundation, Inc.

ALZHEIMER'S DISEASE:

Forget About Antioxidants
&
Supplements

Contemplating
Antioxidant Failures

A Selective Review for
medical scientists, physicians and
informed consumers

By
Prof. Hon. Randolph M. Howes, M.D., Ph.D.

Physician, Surgeon and Scientist (Biochemist)

By Dr. Randolph "HealR" Howes: The "PHENOM"

NOTICE TO USERS:

The information given herein is not intended as medical advice. Always consult with your doctor for underlying illness. Before beginning dietary investigation, consult a dietician or a physician with an interest in nutrition. Information is drawn from the scientific literature, web research, and personal enquiry; while all care is taken, information is not warranted as accurate and the author cannot be held liable for any errors and omissions.

Financial disclosure:

Dr. Howes has no financial conflicts of interest and is not involved in the sale of dietary supplements or fitness equipment. The author holds no stocks or interests in companies in the food additive or antioxidant supplement business.

ACKNOWLEDGEMENTS

Special thanks Don Neale Piatt, Sr. for proof reading.
Also, special thanks to Michael R. Root, M.S. for his unwavering encouragement.

The story of antioxidants, as they relate to disease
prevention, cure, and antiaging is the story of ....
FAILURE!

R. M. Howes, M.D., Ph.D.
6/2/11

ABOUT THE AUTHOR
Dr. Randolph M. Howes M.D., Ph.D.

Biographical sketch:

As a champion of the people, Dr. Howes anticipates and hopes for the active involvement of all connected parties (patients, caregivers, healthcare professionals, etc.) as an integral approach to educating consumers and the public about the potential dangers of excessive antioxidant-containing supplements.

Some people are born with a silver spoon in their mouth but Dr. Howes had to earn his. Even as a child, Dr. Howes could think with adult clarity. He could envision his future but it would require "decades of dedication" to make it a reality. From childhood, Dr. Howes was motivated to become a medical doctor and scientist. Assuredly, having been born on a small strawberry farm in rural Louisiana, his journey to the top has proved to be arduous and demanding.

However, he was fortunate to acquire the confidence of Sister Elizabeth at St. Joseph's school and went on to gain the support of his high school speech teacher, Mrs. Iris Brann, who also had strong beliefs in his abilities and potential. Ultimately, with the help of his guitar and his singing ability, he defeated the star quarter back of the high school football team to become the president of the student body. With the aid of a $25 dollar legislative scholarship, he went on to Southeastern Louisiana College (SLC).

At SLC, he was selected for honors chemistry, made the Dean's list, worked at the Psychology Research Lab forty hours a week, maintained a premed study load, and was elected president of the Junior Class and the Interfraternity Council. To earn badly needed funds, he played music on weekends in a small combo, The Three Blind Mice. Next, he matriculated to Tulane University School of Medicine.

His initial dream was to try to combine both medicine and science. In that regard, he began work as a technician with Dr. Andrew Schally at the Endocrine Polypeptide Lab in the isolation of thyrotropin releasing factor. This work led to a Nobel Prize for Dr. Schally. Dr. Howes had been highly impressed with the enthusiasm of biochemist, Dr. Richard H. Steele, who accepted him as a doctoral candidate under his tutelage. Dr. Howes graduated in the top 10 of his class, won the Louisiana Pathology Association Award, was elected to the Sigma Xi honor fraternity and was the first in the history of Tulane to become a Doctor of Medicine and a Ph.D. in biochemistry concurrently. Next, he was selected to pursue a career in surgery at the prestigious Johns Hopkins Hospital.

Unbelievably, at Dr. Howes' urging, he was allowed to operate his own research lab during his surgical internship and residency training. He worked hand in hand with the greats in American medicine and surgery. Independently, he garnered grants, trained lab techs, wrote papers, slept on the cold floor, proudly served as a Captain in the U.S. Army Reserves Medical Corp and finished with board eligibility in both general and plastic surgery in an unheard of six year period. In another first, he was appointed as an Adjunct Assistant Professor of Plastic Surgery at Johns Hopkins Hospital. For decades, Dr. Howes gave unselfishly to pro bono medical missions in the Philippines and he holds the Ernesto Espaldon Chair as Professor of Plastic Surgery at the University of Santo Tomas. Upon retirement from a career in cosmetic plastic surgery, he is living his dream of trying to revolutionize the treatment of cancer, heart disease, HIV/AIDS and malaria, with his in depth knowledge of the arcane biochemistry of oxygen metabolism. He is a work in progress! Dedicated and passionate, he is on a mission for mankind.

Dr. Howes was the first in the history of Tulane School of Medicine to be awarded a Doctorate of Medicine degree and a Ph.D. in Biochemistry at the same time. He was trained as a General surgeon and a Plastic surgeon at the prestigious Johns Hopkins Hospital, in Baltimore, Maryland. He was the first in the history of Johns Hopkins Hospital to obtain board eligibility in both general and plastic surgery in a six year period.

Dr. Howes invented the triple lumen venous catheter, which has been credited with helping save the lives of over 20 million critically ill patients worldwide. His catheter is the number one venous catheter in the world today and his name is well recognized in over 100 countries. He has been recognized as a humanitarian, visionary, entrepreneur, singer, songwriter, inventor and author.

He received the Harper Award for innovative research from the American College for Advancement in Medicine, served as their keynote speaker and his peers refer to him as "a walking encyclopedia on oxygen metabolism."

He is a Dr. Norman Vincent Peale Unsung Hero award winner, which recognized his awesome versatility. Additionally, even though he is humble and does not like talking about it, he is a self made multi-millionaire.

He is currently doing extensive research on cures for cancer and heart disease and development of revolutionary treatment modalities. He has written 17 books over the past 8 years on the subject of oxygen metabolism, as it relates to protection from cancer, heart disease, diabetes, malaria, HIV/AIDS, Alzheimer's disease, aging and arthritis.

He has written many scientific and medical papers and has lectured nationally and internationally. He has written over 230 medical letters to the editor on popular topics.

His research has shown that currently common antioxidant vitamins, such as vitamins A & E, (and vitamin C to a lesser extent) can be harmful and that oxygen free radicals protect us from bacterial, fungal and viral infections and they help to control cancer growth. He has developed an effective, inexpensive singlet oxygen generating system, from orthomolecular agents, for the treatment of cancer and heart disease. He is passionate about his research and hopes to have his discoveries at the patient's bedside in his lifetime. Admittedly, this is an extremely ambitious goal.

There are over 8,000 pages in his magnum opus and at the Howes World Selective Library on Oxygen Metabolism. **Over 3,000 pages of his opus are available online in a searchable format www.iwillfindthecure.org** © 2011 by R.M. Howes

The scientific method demands that we change our beliefs or theories to fit the factual data. I believe that this applies directly to the Free Radi-Crap theory. Again, I say to you, "The free radical theory has fallen and so has the mitochondrial free radical theory of aging."

Companion Papers:

Citation: R. Howes: Mythology of Antioxidant Vitamins?. *The Journal of Evidence-Based Alternative and Complimentary Medicine.* April, 2011. 16(2): 149-189.

Citation: R. Howes: Cancer Therapy: A Review with Scientific Validation for the Role of Electronically Modified Oxygen Derivatives in Oncologic Treatment Modalities. *The Internet Journal of Alternative Medicine.* 2010 Volume 8 Number 1.

Citation: R. Howes: Hydrogen Peroxide: A review of a scientifically verifiable omnipresent ubiquitous essentiality of obligate, aerobic, carbon-based life forms. *The Internet Journal of Plastic Surgery.* 2010 Volume 7 Number 1.

Howes M.D., PhD., R. (2009). Dangers of Antioxidants in Cancer Patients: A Review. *PHILICA.COM Article number 153.* Published 7th February, 2009. (20 pages)

Howes M.D., PhD., R. (2008). Aging and anti-aging claims: a review on antioxidant vitamins A, C & E. *PHILICA.COM Article number 116.* Published on 12th January, 2008. (16 pages)

Howes M.D., PhD., R. (2007). Sleep: An original "radical" proposal. *PHILICA.COM Observation number 42.* Published on 5th October, 2007. (1 page)

Howes M.D., PhD., R. (2007). Antioxidant Vitamins A, C & E; Death in Small Doses and Legal Liability? *PHILICA.COM Article number 89.* Published on 5th April, 2007. (23 pages)

Howes M.D., PhD., R. (2007). Cancer, Apoptosis and Reactive Oxygen Species: A New Paradigm. *PHILICA.COM Article number 86.* Published on 26th February, 2007. (11 pages)

Howes M.D., PhD., R. (2007). Antioxidant Vitamins A, C and E: Assessing Potential for Harm. *PHILICA.COM Article number 83.* Published on 15th February, 2007. (14 pages)

Howes M.D., PhD., R. (2007). The Consequent Downfall of the Free Radical Theory. *PHILICA.COM Article number 75.* Published on 22nd January, 2007. (9 pages)

Howes, R.M.: "The Free Radical Fantasy," The Annals of New York Academy of Sciences, 2006, Vol. 1067, pp. 22-26.

Other Books Published:

The Fire Eaters, Molding your own destiny more easily, Carnivore Press, © 1982

Uplift, The Answer Book to your plastic and cosmeticsurgery questions, Carnivore Press, © 1986

The Pundit Speaks, An Anthology of Neoclassical Poetic Philosophy, Carnivore Press, © 1990

The Pundit Speaks, Volume II, An Anthology of Neoclassical Poetic Philosophy, Free Radical Press, © 1994

The Pundit Speaks, Volume III, An Anthology of Neoclassical Poetic Philosophy, Free Radical Press, © 1996

The Fable of the Chocolate Covered Strawberry Coloring Book, Free Radical Press, © 2001

The Pundit Speaks, Volume IV, An Anthology of Neoclassical Poetic Philosophy, Free Radical Press, © 2003

The Pundit Speaks, Volume V, An Anthology of Neoclassical Poetic Philosophy, Trafford Publishing, © 2009

Death In Small Doses? Book One and Book Two. Trafford Publishing, © 2010

Antioxidant Overkill, CreateSpace and Free Radical Publishing, © 2011

Dangers of Excessive Antioxidants in Cancer Patients, CreateSpace and Free Radical Publishing, © 2011

Heart Disease and Antioxidant Failures, CreateSpace and Free Radical Publishing, © 2011

Antioxidant Failures and Dangers, CreateSpace and Free Radical Publishing, © 2011

Anti-Aging, Anti-oxidant Scams, CreateSpace and Free Radical Publishing, © 2011

Sports, Athletes, Exercise Facts & Antioxidant Myths. CreateSpace and Free Radical Publishing, © 2011

Some Material Available at:

www.philica.com

www.medi.philica.com

www.iwillfindthecure.org

DEDICATION

To the late Professor Richard H. Steele, Ph.D.
My mentor, my friend and my cerebral soul mate.
And to my other intellectual confidante,
Professor Robert C. Allen, M.D., Ph.D. FCAP
The three of us will "pow-wow" in perpetuity.

TABLE OF CONTENTS:

The only oxygen we need is one pint per breath at the rate of
only a minimum of 21,600 times per day.
Other than that....
R. M. Howes, M.D., Ph.D.
9/12/09

Professional wrestlers, used car dealers,
and politicians should all be sponsored
by antioxidant manufacturers and pushers,
since they all adhere to the same
code of veracity, whilst eschewing mendacity.
The trust they receive has been based upon and
in proportion to
decades of questionable performances, fraud,
hoaxes and fakery.
R. M. Howes, M.D., Ph.D.
10/20/11

PREFACE

Even though the sales of antioxidants have continued to increase, in response to forceful marketing campaigns, serious questions and issues have arisen concerning their efficacy and safety.

Many experts now agree that antioxidant nutrient supplementation is unlikely to yield any benefits for chronic disease prevention in healthy, well-nourished populations, except possibly in subgroups of individuals that harbor specific genetic variants (e.g. GPx (glutathione peroxidase) polymorphisms or malabsorption syndromes).

In short, **antioxidant supplements are increasingly being consider as being unnecessary, dangerous and a waste of money**.

Of particular concern is the fact that antioxidant supplements can cause significantly serious harm, especially in individuals at higher risk of disease due to lifestyle behaviors, genetic makeup, and/or pre-existing (and possibly undiagnosed) conditions, such as cancer, chronic steroid use or those with immune deficiency states.

There is now talk of legal liabilities associated with the careless pushing of the anti-oxidants upon an unsuspecting public. The level of the problem has reached that of a global public health threat. Individuals are encouraged to take injudicious, supplemental amounts of antioxidants and these are being "stacked" with those in the food chain and those used as preservatives or fortifiers of a wide range of food products.

Yet, natural foods and their contained nutrients have been used to prevent or reverse illness for centuries. In 1905, William Fletcher showed that the vitamin B1 in unpolished rice could prevent Beriberi and British sailors (limeys) used the vitamin C in citrus foods to prevent scurvy. Further back, ancient Egyptians ate liver to obtain vitamin A to prevent night blindness. (Fletcher, 1907) (Lind, 1983) (Wolf, 1978)

Vitamin C was the first vitamin (and antioxidant) to be produced and marketed on a commercial scale, in the 1930s, after it was artificially synthesized by British and Polish chemists. (Shils, et al, 2006)

Antioxidant supplements are now "claimed" to promote and maintain optimal health, boost immunity, sharpen the brain, improve sexual prowess, achieve top athletic performance and prevent a wide range of diseases and aging. Based on these assertions, everyone wants to take them. But, basically, these exuberant claims are misleading and invalid.

This is because the claimed benefits of the antioxidants are based on the nullified free radical theory (FRT) of Denham Harman. I have accumulated hundreds and hundreds of scientific studies (over 430), which have demonstrated the failure of the free radical theory to demonstrate predictability.

Antioxidants were supposed to "suck up, quench, remove, mop up, passivate, negate or neutralize" reactive oxygen species (oxygen free radicals). I now more accurately refer to ROS as electronically modified oxygen derivatives (EMODs). The whole free radical concept and the theory of oxidative stress are riddled with mistakes, errors and misinformation. Please refer to my many other books on this subject for detailed discussions.

It was erroneously proposed and assumed that EMODs were responsible for most diseases and aging. This has been proven not to be the case. Yet, the push for increased consumption of antioxidants is driven by the profit motive. Today, antioxidants are about marketing and not about science. Printed literature and the airwaves are filled with careless and dangerous advertisements pushing the over use of antioxidant supplements.

They resort to "campaigns of persuasion" to sell their dubious products.

Only since the mid 1990s have meaningful scientific studies shined the light of truth on the adverse effects of antioxidant over loading. Please refer to my book entitled, *Antioxidant Overkill*, published in 2011 and available at www.amazon.com.

Estimates are that the vitamin supplement sales market garners between $25-28 billion annually. (Supplement Business Report, 2009)

As the sales of antioxidants have risen, so have their associated risks. But, consumers continue to be kept in the dark about the harmful potential of antioxidant abuse. (Blendon et al, 2001)

The **shocking adverse effects of beta-carotene supplementation on increasing lung cancer risk in heavier smokers and drinkers** have been exposed by several scientific reviews. (Albanes, 1999) (Mayne, 1996) (Omenn, 1998)

Similarly, the ATBC trials unexpectedly revealed **statistically significant increases in lung cancer incidence (16%) and overall mortality (8%) among men ran-**

domized to receive beta-carotene supplements *versus* placebo. (ATBC group, 1994) (Albanes et al, 1996)

In the Beta-carotene and Retinol Efficacy Trial (CARET), it was unexpectedly found that after **an average of 4 years of intervention, there was a 28% increase in lung cancer risk and a 17% increase in overall mortality among participants who received the active intervention compared with the placebo.** (Omenn et al, 1996)

The sharp contrast in findings obtained from β-carotene supplementation trials and prior observational epidemiological studies of dietary intake and circulating levels of beta-carotene **led to a reconsideration of the utility and safety of this nutrient as a chemopreventive agent.**

Other antioxidants have followed in this same path, i.e., observational studies or testimonials are not supported by randomized controlled trials. (RCTs), which are the current scientific gold standard. Studies on antioxidant vitamins A, C and E, polyphenols, flavonoids, gingko, selenium, genistein, lycopene, resveratrol, EGCG, pine extract, grape seed extract, ferulic acid, quercetin, etc, have gone down the path of early exuberance, only to be followed by disappointment and evidence of harmful effects.

A very disturbing trend

Every time a new article demonstrates the ineffectiveness or harmful potential of antioxidants, their supporters claim that the authors are pawns for the pharmaceutical industry, that their studies are purely garbage or that these studies are cloaked attempts to shut down the supplement industry. They claim that regulating the supplement industry will turn its control over to Big Pharma and that costs of the supplements will necessarily sky rocket.

I would guestimate that 95% of the comments of the believers in supplements are of the above nature. It seems that they are unbelievably closed minded, even as to the validity of scientific inquiry.

It is my belief, that in the end, we must rely on scientific data. Sadly, testimonials, observational and epidemiologic studies have a history of seriously misleading us. We must open our minds to the scientific data. Our interpretations of the data may change, but the data should be reliable.

Three of the major studies were shut down nearly 2 years ahead of schedule because the supervisory physicians realized that those in the study group receiving antioxidants where being treated unethically and being exposed to unnecessary risks. To me, the actions of terminating the ATBC trial, the CARET trial and the SELECT trial, speaks volumes.

We must continue the push to inform the general public of the scientific facts. Anything less is bordering on malpractice and negligence. The data is available and denial or ignorance is no longer an option or an excuse.

Please be assured, I have no relationship to drug manufacturers in any way, shape or form. Actually, I write a weekly medical editorial for some Louisiana newspapers and I come down hard on Big Pharma.

CHAPTER ONE

Over 100 years ago

Over one hundred years ago, German neurologist Alois Alzheimer (1864-1915) described the case of his patient Auguste D, a woman who developed dementia in her 50s and died in 1906.

He documented: "Auguste D suffered from constant restlessness and anxious confusion.

"At night she was usually put in an isolation room because she could not fall asleep in the main ward; she went to other patients' beds and woke them."

His care plan included "afternoon rest, early dinners and evening bowel evacuations", as well as soothing baths and alcohol and mild sedation to aid sleep, all given in a tolerant and appropriately stimulating environment.

A century later, experts understand a little more about the disease and can spot it earlier. There is even promise of an Alzheimer's blood test. But, **there is still no cure, or way to prevent the onset of the disease.** There is still no effective treatment in sight.

We have seen many drugs fail and care has changed very little.

Alzheimer's: A looming specter

In 1906, Alois Alzheimer identified the debilitating dementia that carries his name. Unbelievably, 100 years later, scientists are currently struggling to find a cause or a cure for Alzheimer's disease.

It will claim one in 10 baby boomers, create personal nightmares for their families and drain state and federal budgeted dollars.

Medicare now pays one-third of all its healthcare funds for some 4.5 million Alzheimer's patients. Last year Medicare spent $91 billion for Alzheimer's. Within the next five years, nearly a half-million new Alzheimer's cases will be diagnosed annually, as 78 million baby boomers reach age 65.

By robbing victims of memory, Alzheimer's strips away individuality, dignity, quality of life and independence. According to Wyeth pharmaceuticals, there are 28 Alzheimer's drugs in development, with no promises of pending success.

Progress on causation and treatment is unconscionably slow considering the looming specter of this epidemic. The FDA needs to give the same priority status to Alzheimer's as it has for AIDS and cancer treatments. We need a sense of urgency to deal with this impending catastrophe.

Yet, congress remains basically quiet.

Recently, in the journal *Alzheimer's & Dementia,* a TV journalist, whose husband has Alzheimer's, stated, "Right now the majority of Alzheimer's victims and their caregivers are our parents. Their plight is our future."

At 82 years, my mother successfully underwent cardiac surgery, aided by the multi-lumened venous catheter I had invented. Hope overflowed, but shortly thereafter she developed the onset of Alzheimer's.

That was over 10 long, heart wrenching and painful years ago. We must relentlessly press hard to fund research to find answers to this scourge of mankind.

Alzheimer's disease: What to believe?

What should you believe about Alzheimer's disease gleaned from widely conflicting so-called scientific studies?

Answer: Not much!

Experimental results are all over the place and with little agreement amongst them. First, one should consider the funding source for the reported study. Money and greed are great motivators (i.e., snake oil salesmen, fakes, frauds).

Second, one needs to know if the study was done by reputable researchers. Next, it should be a randomized, controlled, double blind study.

Since my mother succumbed to Alzheimer's, I have had a keen interest in research on this devastating disease, which is increasing globally at pandemic rates.

Over the next five years, a half-million new Alzheimer's cases will be diagnosed yearly, as 78 million baby boomers reach age 65. Italian studies have found that **not one of the six clinical trials of so-called anti-Alzheimer's drugs significantly reduced the rate of progression from mild cognitive impairment (MCI) to dementia.**

Yet, they are prescribed to 25% of those diagnosed with the disease.

Heated debates have erupted over questionable benefits and enormous costs. Alzheimer's is now being linked to diabetes and blood sugar levels but this has not yielded any new advances in treatment.

Vaccines have been primarily failures and antioxidant supplements have had questionable and disappointing results. In all honesty, we still do not know the cause of Alzheimer's or of the real significance of amyloid brain deposits or of tau proteins or tangles.

Logically, cure is a long way off and palliation is a poor but necessary second choice. Also, some studies have linked the disease to low brain oxygen levels, high uric acid levels, race, inheritance, cranial blood flow, omega-3 fatty acid intake, loneliness, lack of exercise, participation in brain games, all sorts of nutrient deficiencies, education levels, head size, cholesterol levels, inactivity, alcohol intake, the Pin1 gene, short limbs, infections, fast food intake and you name it.

You get the picture! In short, we do know what causes it and do not know how to prevent or treat it. That is the truth but research can offer hope.

We have to fight to have increased funding for Alzheimer's research. We must require and demand respectful and qualified care of all Alzheimer's patients.

The word "victim" seems overused in today's media but it is truly appropriate for those suffering from the tragedy called Alzheimer's disease (AD).

Alzheimer's disease: You can't forget about it

Was that a "senior moment" or was it a sign of Alzheimer's disease (AD)? About 5.3 million (figures vary) Americans currently have AD and a new case is diagnosed every 70 seconds.

This results in annual costs of $148 billion and this is expected to sky rocket with the 70+ million baby boomer generation.

Even though it has been seen in 30 year olds, aging is a major risk factor and those surviving to age 85 have a 50% chance of having Alzheimer's.

Women, African-Americans and Hispanics are at an increased risk, as are those with diabetes and heart disease.

The medical and scientific literature is filled with conflicting reports on AD. My reviews have found the following rather curious generalities: "An increased risk of developing Alzheimer's disease is associated with short arms, loneliness, big bellies, high uric acid levels, low oxygen levels, diabetes, low cranial blood flow, the herpes cold sore virus, low physical activity levels and being overweight. (but associations are not causation)

Alzheimer's risk may be decreased by high oxygen blood levels, bilingualism, fruit and vegetable juices and increased physical activity. Several factors have been found to be of questionable value (or of no value at all) in reducing Alzheimer's risk, such as various herbal remedies, vaccines, and vitamin and antioxidant concoctions."

Several medications are currently being prescribed to treat AD, such as **Aricept, Exelon, Cognex and Razadyne** but Italian studies have found that not one of the six clinical trials of so-called anti-Alzheimer's drugs significantly reduced the rate of progression from mild cognitive impairment (MCI) to dementia.

Hot medical debates have flared up over the questionable benefits of these drugs and their enormous costs. Most of these drugs act to maintain high levels of the neurotransmitter, acetylcholine.

Even the underlying cause of AD is a hot topic for debate and unknown. One thing is for certain: AD is a severe mental disease accompanied by language disturbances, limited ability to identify people or recognize objects, behavioral problems and personality changes. In short, **it is devastating**.

We can only offer the hope of future research. We must anticipate rough times in supporting our loved ones who are victims of AD and be there for them, with love and compassion, until the very end.

Sadly, that is about the best that we can currently do.

Alzheimer's disease costs to sky-rocket

Unless research can produce a major break through, the Alzheimer's Association predicts that the combined cost for Alzheimer's disease (AD) patients over the next 40 years will exceed $20 trillion.

Current costs are about $172 billion annually and more funds are urgently needed for research, even though the government is as broke as a politician's promises.

Today, there are over 5.5 million suffering from Alzheimer's in the USA and that number is predicted to reach 13.5 million by mid-century.

The bad news is, as most experts agree, that, "Today, there are no treatments that can prevent, delay, slow or stop the progression of Alzheimer's disease." Also, sadly, there is no good evidence that any supplement, medication, diet or behavior change actually prevents Alzheimer's or other age-related cognitive decline.

Thus, even modest improvements and discoveries can have a huge impact on the development and progression of AD and its consequent costs.

Lawmakers are being encouraged to pass the National Alzheimer's Project Act to develop an overall game plan.

There is lots of talk about beta-amyloid and tau proteins and APOE genes but there has been minimal meaningful clinical application of this data.

The National Institutes of Health reviewed 250 human research studies and 25 review papers on Alzheimer's prevention and found that in all cases, the correlations were too weak to confidently point to any risk factor as a cause of Alzheimer's disease or cognitive decline but high blood pressure and diabetes appeared to show associations with cognitive decline.

I have seen disappointing results with cholesterol-lowering statin drugs, omega-3 fatty acids, gingko and antioxidants but we must keep trying to find answers for prevention and treatment.

We realize that AD can not be predicted by any specific test, or by looking into your genome, blood or spinal fluid. The good news is that there are things that can be done that will help overall, such as: brain games (cognitive training), exercise, staying socially active, staying engaged with other people and eating a healthy balanced diet. These things are not cures but they add to the patients quality of life no matter what.

I have seen some studies (not all) showing that brisk walking, treadmill or stationary bike exercise for about 40 to 60 minutes per day, 4-5 days a week seems to stall AD and improves mental agility. Unfortunately, many patients have already lost the ability to participate in these activities.

I am convinced that these activities increase brain oxygen levels, resulting in improved cognition. We are all familiar with the effects of low brain oxygen levels in airplane pilots, who can develop symptoms of confusion, delusions, poor coordination, fainting, coma or death. As I say in my lectures, "Oxygen is truly our greatest ally."

Widespread advertisements for Aricept "brag" that it is the only drug approved to treat dementia. Unfortunately, studies indicate that Alzheimer drugs do not delay dementia onset and after 6 months of treatment, they hardly alter its course.

Actually, there are three main drugs (Aricept, or donepezil; Exelon, or rivastigmine; and Reminyl, Razadyne or galantamine) which are currently approved for use in mild-to-moderate Alzheimer's disease. As I previously mentioned, not one of the six clinical trials examined by Italian researchers found that the drugs significantly reduced the rate of progression from mild cognitive impairment (MCI) to dementia.

Estimates are that upwards of one in four with MCI are given these drugs, which can cause ulcers, gastric bleeding, nausea, vomiting, diarrhea, insomnia, fatigue, fainting, muscle cramps, etc. Giving Alzheimer's drugs to people with early memory problems did not delay the onset of the disease.

Bitter debates have erupted over questionable benefits and enormous costs. Britain's National Institute for Health and Clinical Excellence said they should not be given to newly diagnosed patients with mild Alzheimer's disease.

Using predatory advertising practices, drug companies try to "shame" family members into asking our physicians to prescribe them for our affected loved ones.

We urgently need more clinical trials, using a single agreed upon definition of MCI, before we can justify use of these costly and potentially harmful drugs in pre-dementia cases. After all, we are usually making decisions to use these drugs for our loved ones, when they are most vulnerable and in their times of greatest need.

Several genes are linked with early Alzheimer's, and study might lead to better understanding of how the disease begins and how to tackle it. **Abnormalities in a gene called SORL1 increased the risk for the disease**, and this finding could help scientists develop new treatments.

People who are fully bilingual and speak both languages every day for most of their lives can delay the onset of dementia by up to four years compared with those who only know one language, according to Canadian scientists. Researchers said the extra effort involved in using more than one language appeared to **boost blood supply to the brain** and ensure nerve connections remained healthy -- two factors thought to help fight off dementia.

Alzheimer's costs to soar without effective drugs

A May 2010 report said Alzheimer's disease will rack up more than $20 trillion in treatment costs over the next 40 years in the United States, according to a report that called on Congress to increase funding for drug research. The report issued by the Alzheimer's Association found that from 2010 to 2050, the cost of caring for Americans 65 and older with Alzheimer's disease will increase more than six times to $1.08 trillion per year.

Alzheimer's disease is the sixth leading cause of death in the United States and the fifth leading cause of death for Americans 65 and older, according to the Alzheimer's Association.

Currently, $172 billion a year is spent by the government, private insurance and individuals to care for people with the disease, the most common cause of dementia.

Current drugs help manage symptoms but, so far, **no treatment can stop the progression of Alzheimer's,** which can start with vague memory loss and confusion before progressing to complete disability and death.

The Alzheimer's Association now estimates the number of Americans 65 and older with Alzheimer's will increase from **5.1 million today** to 13.5 million by mid-century.

"Alzheimer's not only poses a significant threat to millions of families, but also drives tremendous costs for government programs like Medicare and Medicaid."

The group said costs to Medicare, the federal health insurance program for the elderly, would **rise 600 percent by 2050**, from $88 billion today to $627 billion in 2050. During the same time period, Medicaid costs will rise 400 percent, from $34 billion to $178 billion.

Driving the cost increases, they said, is the fact that by 2050, 48 percent of the projected 13.5 million people with Alzheimer's will be in the severe stage of the disease, when costly, around-the-clock care is often needed.

"We know that Alzheimer's disease is not just 'a little memory loss' -- it is a national crisis that grows worse by the day," Harry Johns, president and CEO of the Alzheimer's Association, said in a statement. **"Today, there are no treatments that can prevent, delay, slow or stop the progression of Alzheimer's disease."**

"While the ultimate goal is a treatment that can completely prevent or cure Alzheimer's, we can now see that even modest improvements can have a huge impact."

They estimate that a drug that delays the onset of Alzheimer's by five years would decrease the total number of Americans age 65 and older with Alzheimer's from 5.6 million to 4 million in 2020.

And if a drug were discovered by 2015 that slowed disease progression, it could cut the number of people in the severe stage of Alzheimer's disease in half to 1.1 million by 2020, and 1.2 million in 2050, down from the projections of 6.5 million. The group is asking lawmakers to enact the National Alzheimer's Project Act, which would create a national plan to overcome Alzheimer's disease.

Doctors know **about risk factors for cognitive decline: smoking, diabetes, depression, metabolic syndrome (the constellation of conditions including high blood pressure, obesity and high cholesterol that are associated with heart disease and diabetes) and specific gene variants were all linked with increased risk of developing Alzheimer's disease.**

In addition, preventive behaviors such as eating a Mediterranean diet (high in fruits and vegetables, omega-3 fatty acids and unsaturated fats), exercising, maintaining cognitive engagement (doing puzzles, learning new things) and fostering extensive social relationships were linked to a lower risk.

The problem is that **none of these relationships were particularly robust.**

Currently, firm conclusions cannot be drawn about the association of any modifiable risk factor with cognitive decline or Alzheimer's disease.

CHAPTER TWO

Alzheimer's victims

In August of 2008, Val Brickates Kennedy wrote an article in MarketWatch on AD. The following is a excerpt of that article. **I have had personal experience with this disease and first hand knowledge of its cruelty.** (MarketWatch, V.B. Kennedy, 2008)

Alzheimer's disease, the leading cause of dementia in older people, is caused by the widespread destruction of brain cells called neurons over the span of several years.

As the destruction of neurons escalates, the ensuing brain damage slowly robs victims of the ability to learn, recall information, create and execute tasks. Judgment becomes impaired and victims become increasingly confused. At the end stages of the disease, Alzheimer's patients are generally bedridden and unable to communicate.

Because victims can become so incapacitated, Alzheimer's is often called a fatal illness. Actually, patients often die from complications associated with being bedridden. Poor communication skills often make it difficult for a patient to show being in distress, such as from a heart attack or serious infection.

Frequently, they don't even know they have AD.

Many doctors also suspect that the immune systems of Alzheimer's patients deteriorate during the course of the disease, which also can contribute to death.

Alzheimer's is the seventh leading cause of death in the U.S. According to the Alzheimer's Association, about 5.2 million American suffered from Alzheimer's in 2008. About 13% of all people aged 65 and over have the disease, with that number rocketing to about 50% at age 85.

The association predicts that by 2010, approximately 500,000 new cases of Alzheimer's will be diagnosed every year. By 2050, that number will leap to 1 million.

Many seniors with dementia actually suffer from a combination of Alzheimer's and vascular dementia, which is caused by **decreased blood flow to the brain** because of cardiovascular problems. Some may suffer only from vascular dementia. But **Alzheimer's is still the leading cause of dementia in older people, accounting up to 80% of all cases**.

While the scientific community is still searching for the exact cause of Alzheimer's, many believe that a brain protein called beta-amyloid is to blame. While younger brains are generally able to keep beta-amyloid levels in check, some older brains appear to lose that ability, allowing the protein to build up to toxic levels.

It is believed that the results of the buildup are devastating, resulting in slow but steady destruction of neurons. But, cause and effect have not been established.

In the earlier stages of Alzheimer's, patients first experience problems with remembering recent events. Sufferers also begin to have problems recalling familiar words.

As the disease progresses, patients find it difficult going about their daily activities. Mathematical skills decline, along with the ability to recall key life events. Disorientation can also occur, with patients losing track of time or where they are.

Eventually self-help skills also erode, such as eating, dressing, washing and using the bathroom. Patients also run a higher risk of hurting themselves as they become increasingly unable to gauge dangerous situations. Personality changes and/or sudden mood swings are also common, and there can be a tendency to wander from home.

In the last stage of the disease, patients lose the ability to walk, communicate coherently and recognize loved ones. Swallowing can become difficult, and muscles can grow rigid.

Not unsurprisingly, Alzheimer's patients are also susceptible to mental illness as the disease worsens. Patients might become verbally or physically aggressive, anxious or depressed. In the latter stages of the disease, hallucinations, paranoia and delusional thinking can take hold.

Several compounds are in mid-to-late stage clinical trials, and the first new drugs could hit the market in as soon as three years.

"The rate of Alzheimer's is going to explode as the baby boomers hit 65," said Dr. Sam Gandy, a leading researcher at Mount Sinai Medical Center and chairman of the Alzheimer's Association's medical board.

The current size of Alzheimer's drug market is an estimated $3 billion, with up to 12 million people suffering from the condition in the U.S., Europe and Japan. The market could possibly surpass $20 billion if the newer drugs prove to be highly effective, according to UBS analyst Roopesh Patel.

The key growth driver for Alzheimer's drugs is undoubtedly an aging population.

When Dr. Alois Alzheimer identified the disease in early 1900s, he described the illness as rare. But back then, the average American's life expectancy was 50. Now it's 78.

Because Alzheimer's patients eventually require some type of round-the-clock care, having a family member stricken with the disease can be a heavy burden, emotionally and financially. And although many patients do end up spending their final days in a nursing facility, an estimated 70% are cared for at home.

"When half of the Baby Boomers over 85 years old become demented, it's going to create a crisis," said Gandy. **"The cost of Alzheimer's will break the bank of Medicare."**

Only four drugs have been approved to treat Alzheimer's in the U.S., and they come with limitations. They're generally capable, at best, of boosting memory for up to 18 months.

After that, patients continue to decline as the disease progresses.

Basically, if you look at a time chart, all AD patients end up at the same place over a period of time, whether they received drugs or not.

Myriad (MYGN) was forced to pull the plug on its hotly-anticipated Alzheimer's drug Flurizan after a Phase III trial showed it wasn't effective. Myriad spent $60 million in the first six months of 2008 alone on the product.

In late July of 2008, shares of Wyeth and Elan were hammered on mixed Phase II news for their highly-touted antibody therapy bapineuzumab. The results showed that while the drug appeared to be quite effective on some Alzheimer's patients, **it may have triggered brain swelling in a small number of other users.** Wyeth and Elan are still moving ahead with Phase III trials.

There only four medications approved to treat AD. And none of these are superstars.

All four essentially stoke the "firing power" of the brain cells that haven't been destroyed yet by the disease. But while they can temporarily help patients think or remember things more clearly, they can't stop the disease's progression. And the drugs usually are effective for no more than 18 months.

"The current drugs out there treat symptoms of the disease," said Dr. Eric Siemers, medical director for Eli Lilly & Co.'s Alzheimer's program. "They can boost memory but they don't get to the underlying cause of the disease." **Even this is debatable.**

Autopsies of patients with Alzheimer's show their brains are riddled with piles of beta-amyloid, often referred to as plaque.

The build-up is toxic to brain cells, resulting severe brain damage over the course of several years. **Researchers estimate that Alzheimer's sufferers lose up to 6% of their brain mass every year.**

Normal "senior moments," or Alzheimer's disease?

The passing of vibrant actor Charlton Heston from late-stage Alzheimer's disease makes us all stop and think about our own mortality. In particular, it is natural to wonder about your own memory, and what is 'normal' when it comes to memory loss as a result of aging.

Occasional memory lapses, such as forgetting why you walked into a room or having difficulty recalling a person's name, become more common as we approach our 50s and 60s. It's comforting to know that this minor forgetfulness is a normal sign of aging, not a sign of dementia.

But other types of memory loss, such as forgetting appointments or becoming momentarily disoriented in a familiar place, may indicate mild cognitive impairment.

In the most serious form of memory impairment -Alzheimer's and other forms of dementia -- people often find themselves disoriented in time and place and unable to name common objects or recognize once-familiar people.

Here are examples of the types of memory problems common in normal age-related forgetfulness, mild cognitive impairment, and dementia.

Memory Condition -- Normal Age-Related Forgetfulness:

- Sometimes misplaces keys, eyeglasses, or other items.
- Momentarily forgets an acquaintance's name.
- Occasionally has to "search" for a word.
- Occasionally forgets to run an errand.
- May forget an event from the distant past.
- When driving, may momentarily forget where to turn. Quickly orients self.
- Jokes about memory loss.

Memory Condition -- Mild Cognitive Impairment:

- Frequently misplaces items.
- Frequently forgets people's names and is slow to recall them.
- Finding words becomes more difficult.
- Begins to forget important events and appointments.
- May forget more recent events or newly learned information.
- May temporarily become lost more often.
- May have trouble understanding and following a map.
- Worries about memory loss. Family and friends notice the lapses.

Memory Condition -Alzheimer's Disease and Other Forms of Dementia:

- Forgets what an item is used for or puts it in an inappropriate place.
- May not remember knowing a person.
- Begins to lose language skills. May withdraw from social interaction.
- Loses sense of time. Doesn't know what day it is.
- Short-term memory is seriously impaired. Has difficulty learning and remembering new   information.
- Becomes easily disoriented or lost in familiar places, sometimes for hours.
- May have little or no awareness of cognitive problems.

If you are concerned about memory loss in yourself or a loved one, there can be a variety of underlying causes too which can be treated, for example, temporary memory loss due to depression, or certain prescription or over the counter medications. You should discuss such concerns with your doctor.

There are a number of tests your doctor can administer right in the office which can help determine whether it is cognitive impairment or Alzheimer's disease or another form of dementia. (Johns Hopkins Health Alerts Memory Topic)

The secret to longevity
is to keep breathing oxygen.
R. M. Howes, M.D., Ph.D.
6/8/11

Antioxidants—Antioxidants are nutrients that "deactivate" reactive molecules (free radicals) and prevent (alleged) harmful chain reactions. In the body, the most prevalent forms of free radicals are the oxygen free radicals.

CHAPTER THREE

Selective summary of 105 factoids arguing against the use of supplements and antioxidants and the proposal that oxidative stress is causative of Alzheimer's disease:

Important Alzheimer's observations

- **Researchers estimate that Alzheimer's sufferers lose up to 6% of their brain mass every year.**

- **"The cost of Alzheimer's will break the bank of Medicare."** (MarketWatch, V.B. Kennedy, 2008)

- **half of all nursing home residents have Alzheimer's disease or a related disorder.** (the Scripps Institute)

- **Americans age 55 and older fear Alzheimer's disease more than any other diagnosis, even cancer.** (2006, MetLife Foundation)

- **Clearly, hypertension alone doesn't doom someone to later dementia. Far more people, nearly one in three U.S. adults, have hypertension.** But, it is a risk factor. **Hypertension is a leading cause of heart attacks, strokes and kidney failure. And, while some studies have found hypertension treatment lowered the dementia risk, others haven't.**

- **Nearly a million older Americans slide from normal memory into mild impairment each year**, researchers estimate, based on a Mayo Clinic study of

Minnesota residents. That's on top of **the half million Americans who develop full-blown Alzheimer's** or other forms of dementia.

- **Literature review shows that antioxidant therapies have enjoyed general success in preclinical studies across disparate animal models, but little benefit in human intervention studies or clinical trials.** (Kamat et al, 2008)

- **No significant change in risk of AD was found when the scientists looked at vitamin E supplements, the other antioxidants and their supplements, or a general multivitamin.** (Morris et al, 2002)

- **It is not recommended, based on current evidence in 2002, that people take high-dose vitamin E supplements or other antioxidant pills in an effort to prevent mental decline.** (Neil Buckholtz, Ph.D., head of the Dementias of Aging Branch at the NIA, 2002)

- **The failure of a potent antioxidant (vitamin E) to reduce cognitive decline substantially when used for almost a decade conveys a strong message.** (Kang et al, 2006)

- **Given that past studies on vitamin E have produced equivocal results, the investigators concluded that further studies are needed to assess the long-term balance of risks versus benefits for people with Alzheimer's disease from taking vitamin E and anti-inflammatory drugs**. (Dr. Alireza Atri, Massachusetts General Hospital (MGH), 2009)

- **Recent high-profile failures of vitamin E trials in Parkinson's disease, and nitrone therapies in stroke, have diminished enthusiasm to pursue antioxidant neuroprotectants in the clinic.** (Kamat et al, 2008)

- **there is little doubt that ingesting fruits and vegetables (which contain antioxidants) can reduce the risk of having various age-associated diseases, such as cancer, heart disease, macular degeneration and cataracts. At present there is relatively little evidence from human studies that supplements containing antioxidants lead to a reduction in either the risk of these conditions or the rate of aging**. As such, antioxidant supplements may have some health benefits for some people, but **so far there is no scientific evidence to justify the claim that they have any effect on human aging.** (Olansky, Hayflick, 2004)

- **The "amyloid hypothesis" has already produced some stunning failures in large, late-stage trials**. (Dr. Samuel Gandy, researcher at Mount Sinai School of Medicine in New York, 2009)

- Evidence from these trials indicates that **aspirin, naproxen, and celecoxib do not appear to reduce the risk for Alzheimer's. NSAIDs** have also been investigated for treatment of Alzheimer's disease. To date, rigorous **studies have failed to show a benefit**. (http://health.nytimes.com/health/guides/disease/alzheimers-disease/prevention.html). (Harvey Simon, MD, Associate Professor of Medicine, Harvard Medical School, 2008)

- **Results from the largest statin (a cholesterol lowering drug) study (LEAPe) of patients with AD showed Lipitor (R) had no significant impact on the disease.** (American Academy of Neurology meeting, 2008)

- In 2007, Dr. Kristine Yaffe of the San Francisco Veterans Affairs Medical Center and University of California at San Francisco stated, **"For the clinician, there is no convincing justification to recommend the use of antioxidant dietary supplements to maintain cognitive performance in cognitively normal adults or in those with mild cognitive impairment."** (Nov. 2007, Archives of Internal Medicine)

- **"There's no evidence that people should be on these drugs (Celebrex & Aleve anti-inflammatories) to prevent Alzheimer's disease."** (Dr. David Bennett of Chicago's Rush University Medical Center, 2008)

- Dr Alan Dangour said **claims about the benefits of oily fish in warding of dementia in older people seemed to have been oversold. "The evidence on this has always been sporadic.** What this shows is there is a link between people who eat oily fish and better cognitive function, but **if you adjust for education and mood this relationship goes." "Once age, sex and education are accounted for the research does not show any significant benefit of regularly eating oily fish."**

- *Statins.* Statins are common drugs used to lower cholesterol levels. In past years, a number of studies reported a significantly lower risk for Alzheimer's disease in patients who took statins. However, **newer studies have failed to prove that statins (cholesterol lowering drugs) can help prevent Alzheimer's disease**. (http://health.nytimes.com/health/guides/disease/alzheimers-disease/prevention.html). (Harvey Simon, MD, Associate Professor of Medicine, Harvard Medical School, 2008)

- *Hormone Therapy.* Hormone replacement therapy (HT) has been studied for years for health effects after menopause, including its effect on mental decline. **A number of studies, including a major 2003 analysis, have found no differences in mental performance or protection from Alzheimer's disease in women taking HT compared to non-users.** Based on these results, researchers from **the National Institute on Aging (NIA) recommended against prescribing combination** hormone therapy to older women for maintaining or improving cognitive function. It is even possible that women ages 65 years and older who take estrogen-only HT have a slightly increased risk of developing dementia. (http://health.nytimes.com/health/guides/disease/alzheimers-disease/prevention.html). (Harvey Simon, MD, Associate Professor of Medicine, Harvard Medical School, 2008)

- There is no evidence from randomized controlled trials that any specific diets or diet supplements prevent or treat Alzheimer's disease. (http://health. nytimes.com/health/guides/disease/alzheimers-disease/prevention.html).   (Harvey Simon, MD, Associate Professor of Medicine, Harvard Medical School, 2008)

- While some studies have described a benefit with administration of vitamin B12, or vitamin B6, there is no good evidence from randomized controlled trials that these supplements prevent Alzheimer's disease. http:// health.nytimes.com/health/guides/disease/alzheimers-disease/prevention.html. (Harvey Simon, MD, Associate Professor of Medicine, Harvard Medical School, 2008)

- High doses of B vitamins failed to slow cognitive decline in people with Alzheimer's disease. "Our results give a very clear answer that these vitamins should not be taken to treat Alzheimer's disease. They're ineffective." (Aisen et al, 2008)

- Thus far, studies have not supported the use of omega-3 in AD patients. Surprisingly, in 2009, Harvard linked fish and omega-3 fats to type 2 diabetes. Following **195,204 adults** for 14 to 18 years, researchers reported in 2009 that they had found that **the more fish or long-chain omega-3 fatty acids participants consumed, the higher their risk of developing diabetes**. (Kaushik et al, 2009)

- Meanwhile, fish oil manufacturers pinned their hopes on brain function. Maybe fish oil could make you smarter. But in 2010, researchers dashed those hopes also. A group of **867 elderly people** were randomly assigned to either **a fish-oil supplement** or placebo. After two years of supplementation, **elderly adults showed no benefit at all in tests for reaction time, spatial memory, and processing speed measurements.** (Dangour et al, 2010)

- A later 2010 JAMA report showed that **omega-3 supplements do not slow mental decline in Alzheimer's patients.** (Quinn et al, 2010)

- And at the other end of the age spectrum, babies get no benefit either from omega-3s. A JAMA report showed that **consumption of fish oil during pregnancy does not benefit babies' cognitive development**. (Makrides et al, 2010)

- In these reports, **fish oil is sounding more like snake oil**. The new findings linking higher DHA levels to cancer add yet another reason to use caution with fish oil supplements.

- **Fish oil has failed its marketing claims.** Specifically, **it is no help for heart patients, does not forestall Alzheimer's disease, does not prevent depression, and does not make babies smarter**.

- Also in 2010, the New England Journal of Medicine reported **similarly dismal results with heart patients given omega-3 fatty acids in addition to standard drug therapy**. They had **no reduction in cardiovascular events**. (Krombout et al, 2010)

- **Results from the Ginkgo biloba for the Evaluation of Memory (GEM) Study show that 240 mg of ginkgo daily has no effect on the onset of dementia or development of Alzheimer's**. The study appeared in the *Journal of the American Medical Association*. **The results were disappointing and surprising.** (DeKosky et al, 2008)

- **"We don't think it (the antioxidant, gingko biloba) has a future as a powerful anti-dementia drug."** (DeKosky et al, 2008)

- **exercise may help prevent the development of Alzheimer's disease and other forms of dementia. A 2006 study found that older adults (65 years and older) who exercised three times a week reduced their risk for Alzheimer's by about 40%.** http://health.nytimes.com/health/guides/disease/alzheimers-disease/prevention.html. (Harvey Simon, MD, Associate Professor of Medicine, Harvard Medical School, 2008)

- **Those with Alzheimer's disease had a three-fold greater risk of dying compared to those not experiencing cognitive function problems. Those with mild cognitive impairment were 50% more likely to die.** The risk of death increased as cognitive impairment became more severe. (*Archives of Neurology*, 2009)

- **There is no evidence of efficacy of Vitamin E in the prevention or treatment of people with Alzheimer's disease (AD) or Mild cognitive impairment (MCI).** (Isaac et al, 2008 CD002854)

- **There is little evidence that dietary supplements can prevent or treat AD. Multivitamins do not reduce the risk of dementia.** (Huang et al, 2006)

- **Large doses of vitamin E have little effect in slowing progression to AD among those with mild cognitive impairment.** (Isaac et al, 2008)

- **Combinations of vitamin B-12 and folic acid** in very large doses reduce homocysteine concentrations (a risk factor for cerebrovascular disease) but **fail to improve cognitive function in elderly persons with no or moderate cognitive impairment.** (Eussen et al, 2006) **nor do they slow cognitive decline in those with mild to moderate AD.** (Aisen et al, 2008)

- **Vitamin B-6, vitamin B-12, and folic acid** either alone or in various combinations **do not improve cognitive function or dementia.** (Balk et al, 2007)

- **There is inadequate evidence that fish oils or omega-3 fatty acids protect against decreases in cognitive functions and the incidence or clinical progression of dementias.** (Lim et al, 2006)

- Riboflavin, vitamin B-6, vitamin C, blueberry extract, *alpha*-lipoic acid, and the adrenal hormone dehydroepiandrosterone (DHEA) **lack evidence of efficacy in humans**. (Dwyer, Donoghue, 2010)

- *Ginkgo biloba* **has been studied extensively for its effects on memory. It lacks predictable, clinically significant benefits in persons with acquired cognitive impairments, including dementia of any degree of severity.** (Birks et al, 2007)

- **The Ginkgo Evaluation of Memory Study (GEMS), a randomized controlled trial of *G. biloba* in elderly persons aged >75 y, found no effects on all-cause dementia, on AD, or on the rate of progression to dementia in elderly persons with mild cognitive impairment.** (Dekosky et al, 2008) Also, *G. biloba* **increases the risk of bleeding when taken with aspirin.**

- **The evidence suggests that dietary supplement use is unlikely to prevent cognitive impairment or AD, nor is e4+ status an indication for their use.** Behaviors that reduce cardiovascular disease risk are more promising. (Dwyer, Donoghue, 2010)

- **vitamin E supplements should not be recommended for primary or secondary prevention of AD. Although the risks of taking high doses of vitamin C are lower than those with vitamin E, the lack of consistent efficacy data for vitamin C in preventing or treating AD should discourage its routine use for this purpose.** (Boothby et al, 2005)

- **There was no significant difference in the probability of progression from MCI to AD between the Vitamin E group and the placebo group. There is no evidence of efficacy of Vitamin E in the prevention or treatment of people with AD or MCI.** (Isaac et al, 2008, CD002854)

- **More Alzheimer's participants taking Vitamin E suffered a fall.** (Isaac et al, 2008)

Oxygen effects

- **When healthy adults older than 55 improved their fitness through aerobic exercise, there was also often an improvement in memory, attention or other mental abilities.** (Cochrane Database of Systematic Reviews, 2008)

- **This research clearly establishes that reducing the oxygen supply to neurons creates the same causes of damage as those that occur when people develop Alzheimer's disease.** (Peers et al, 2009)

- **There is a clear link between low oxygen levels in the brain and Alzheimer's disease.** (Peers et al, 2009)

- **Lowered oxygen levels, or hypoxia, seems to increase the risk of dementia.** (Peers et al, 2009)

- **A person whose blood supply (and oxygen supply) to the brain has been interrupted by a stroke is ten times more likely to develop dementia than someone who has not.** (Peers et al, 2009)

- **less oxygenated blood to the brain may mean a bigger build-up of the protein plaques that are so closely tied to Alzheimer's disease.** The Canadian team says a specific gene may be key to this process. (HealthDay News, 2006)

- **People with low blood oxygen levels caused by long-term respiratory disease are also at increased risk of developing dementia.** (PNAS, 2006)

- **lowered brain-oxygen levels, caused by reduced blood flow, increase the risk of Alzheimer's disease.** (PNAS, 2006)

- **"If we can improve blood flow to the brain, maybe we can help slow Alzheimer's progression.** This report provides the mechanics for that. Increasing blood flow for the heart also helps slow Alzheimer's disease," he said. (Song, 2006)

- **Four of five patients reported decreased fatigue (receiving hyperbaric oxygen therapy)**, while one of five patients dropped out at three weeks because of increased fatigue. **Maximum isometric voluntary contraction (MVIC) of all muscle groups except right hand grip improved significantly by up to 97%. Most improvement occurred during the four weeks after treatment.** (Steele et al, 2004)

- They also previously reported that **hyperbaric oxygen (HBO) treatment delayed the onset of weakness in the wobbler mouse.** (Steele et al, 2004)

- **An active lifestyle with moderate amounts of aerobic activity will likely improve cognitive and brain function, and reverse the neural decay frequently observed in older adults.** (Erickson, Kramer, 2009)

- Sun and colleagues defined the molecular mechanism of hypoxia leading to dementia and showed that **hypoxia leads to increased beta-secretase activity and production of beta-amyloid protein.** (Sun et al, 2006)

- **Mitochondria in AD do not exhibit striking evidence of oxidative damage, as would be expected if they produced free radicals directly.** (Cash et al, 2002)

- **There is no strong evidence of AD protection to date from using antioxidant supplements.** (*New York Times. August 9, 2008*)

- **There is no evidence from randomized controlled trials that any specific diets or diet supplements prevent or treat Alzheimer's disease.** (*New York Times. August 9, 2008*)

- **A 2006 study found that older adults (65 years and older) who exercised three times a week reduced their risk for Alzheimer's by about 40%.** (*New York Times. August 9, 2008*)

- **Neither the primary nor the secondary outcome measures could determine whether a megadose of vitamin E is efficacious in slowing disease progression in amyotrophic lateral sclerosis (ALS, Lou Gehrig's disease) as an add-on therapy to riluzol.** (Graf et al, 2005)

- **Long-term antioxidative treatment with vitamin E did not benefit patients with ALS.** (Kwiecinski et al, 2001)

- With **an array of antioxidants** with N-acetylcysteine (NAC); vitamins C and E; N-acetylmethionine (NAM); and dithiothreitol (DTT) or its isomer dithioerythritol

(DTE), **Antioxidants neither seem to harm ALS patients, nor do they seem to prolong survival**. (Vyth et al, 1996)

- **There was no such association (decreased risk of AD) with the intake of vitamins C, E, or beta-carotene, although these are abundantly present in fruit and vegetable juices; other studies have also failed to find any effect of these substances on the development of Alzheimer's**. (Dai et al, 2006, the Kame Project)

More studies showing the ineffectiveness of antioxidant in AD

- **"Today, there are no treatments that can prevent, delay, slow or stop the progression of Alzheimer's disease," said** Harry Johns, president and CEO of the Alzheimer's Association in May of 2010.

- **Currently, there is no good evidence that any supplement, medication, diet or behavior change actually prevents Alzheimer's or other age-related cognitive decline.** (LiveScience Contributor, 5-18-10)

- **The bad news is we have nothing that's been proven to prevent Alzheimer's disease,"** said Cynthia Carlsson, professor and Alzheimer's researcher at the University of Wisconsin School of Medicine and Public Health. (LiveScience Contributor, 5-18-10)

- **A panel of 15 independent scientists convened by the National Institutes of Health reviewed 250 human research studies and 25 review papers on Alzheimer's prevention and found that in all cases, the correlations were too weak to confidently point to any risk factor as a cause of Alzheimer's disease or cognitive decline.** said panel head Martha L. Daviglus, professor of preventative medicine at Northwestern University in Chicago. (LiveScience Contributor, 5-18-10)

- **Vitamin E supplements are no longer recommended for brain health, indeed, the high doses originally thought to help slow the onset of dementia with aging is now recognized to increase the risk of cerebral hemorrhage** (Ann Pharmacother, 39: 2073, 2005).

- **The available evidence is insufficient to recommend the routine use of B vitamins, vitamin E and vitamin C for the prevention of stroke.** (Sanchez-Moreno et al, 2009)

- **6 months supplementation of physiological dosages of antioxidants and B vitamins have no effect on cognitive performance in presumedly healthy and well-nourished female seniors.** (Wolters et al, 2005)

- **The study results provide no evidence for a beneficial effect of daily multi-vitamin and multimineral supplements on these domains of cognitive function in community-living people over 65 years.** (McNeill et al, 2007)

- **Intervention studies with antioxidant vitamins found no evidence for a beneficial effect of supplements.** (Stott et al, 2005) (McMahon et al, 2006) (Eussen et al, 2006) (Heart Protection Study Collaborative Group MRC/BHF Heart Protection Study, 2002)

- **Intervention studies with antioxidant vitamins and B vitamins given for 24 weeks or more in community-living older people have found no evidence for a beneficial effect of supplements.** (Durga et al, 2007)

- **Two randomized trials which used multivitamins for 24 weeks or more also found no evidence of a beneficial effect.** (Cockle et al, 2000) (Wolters et al, 2005)

- **A meta-analysis showed no significant effect of taking B vitamins or anti-oxidant vitamins on global cognitive function. There was little evidence of a beneficial effect from taking B vitamins or antioxidant supplements on global cognitive function in later life.** (Jia et al, 2008)

- **Several exogenous antioxidant compounds have been tested and found beneficial in transgenic AD mice, such as vitamins and spices.** However, **their efficacy was much more modest in human trials.** (Dumont et al, 2010)

- **Unfortunately, the randomization failed, and at baseline the placebo group was significantly better cognitively than the other groups. No benefit of either the antioxidant, deprenyl, or vitamin E was seen without adjusting for this baseline difference.** (Shoulson, 1998)

- **No motor benefit was seen for vitamin E and there was no effect of either deprenyl or vitamin E on cognitive performance in early Parkinson's disease (PD).** (Kieburtz et al, 1994)

- **A subsequent ADCS trial** (The Alzheimer's Disease Cooperative Study) **of vitamin E in MCI showed no benefit on risk of progression to AD**. (Parnetti et al, 1995)

- **there were no significant differences in rate of progression to AD between the vitamin E and placebo groups at any time point, either among all patients or among apolipoprotein E ε4 carriers.** (Jack et al, 2008)

- **it is not known whether supplementation with vitamin E significantly increases brain levels, although levels in CSF are increased.** (Vstassery et al, 1998)

- **Vitamin E reduces amyloid levels and amyloid deposition in transgenic AD mice when started before plaque deposition, but not when started after plaques appear.** (Sung et al, 2004) thus, it will not reverse AD

- **In the Honolulu-Asia Aging Study** (Masaki et al, 2000), **vitamin E and vitamin C use was determined in 3,385 Japanese American men, and 3–10 years later cognitive status was classified as AD, vascular dementia, mixed/other dementia, low test scores without dementia, or cognitively intact. There was a significant protective effect of combined vitamin E and vitamin C for non-AD dementias but not for AD. Similar results were found in the Canadian Study of Health and Aging.** (Maxwell et al, 2005)

- In the **Monongahela Valley Independent Elders Survey of 1,059 subjects**, intake of antioxidant supplements (vitamins A, C, E, *beta*-carotene, zinc, and selenium) **there were no significant differences between antioxidant users and nonusers.** (Mendelsohn et al, 1998)

- **Antioxidants studies have failed to reverse or prevent AD up to this point.** (Markesbery, 1997)

- In a prospective, community-based study of 815 non-demented subjects, vitamin E from food, but **not from supplements**, was associated with decreased incidence of AD in the highest quintile of vitamin E intake, **a protective effect seen only among subjects not carrying an apolipoprotein E *epsilon*4 allele.** (Morris et al, 2002)

- **In the Washington Heights-Inwood Columbia Aging study of 980 non-demented subjects, intake of vitamin C and carotenes, or vitamin E in supplemental or dietary (nonsupplemental) forms, was not associated with decreased incidence of AD.** (Luchsinger et al, 2003)

- In the **Age-Related Eye Disease Study**, participants were randomly assigned to receive daily antioxidants (vitamin C, vitamin E, *beta*-carotene), zinc and copper, antioxidants plus zinc and copper, or placebo, and a cognitive battery was administered to 2,166 elderly subjects after a median of 6.9 years of treatment. **There were no**

differences among the treatment groups in any of the cognitive tests. (Yaffe et al, 2004)

- **In the Women's Health Study, a double-blind, randomized, placebo-controlled trial of vitamin E in 39,876 healthy women, 6,377 women 65 years or older participated in a cognitive sub-study. There were no differences between treatment groups in global composite scores at the first or last time points or in mean cognitive change over time.** (Kang et al, 2006)

- **Several large meta-analyses suggesting that high dose antioxidant vitamin supplementation may be associated with a slight increase in all-cause mortality.** One such analysis, focused on vitamin E, combined 19 clinical trials (135,967 participants). They found that in high dose vitamin E (> 400 IU/day) trials, the pooled all cause mortality risk difference was 39 per 10000 persons, whereas in low dose (≤ 400 IU/day) trials, the risk difference was 16 per 10000. (Miller et al, 2005)

- The **Cochrane Hepato-Biliary Group** attempted to analyze all randomized trials in adults involving *beta*-carotene, vitamin A, vitamin C, vitamin E, and selenium. When all qualified randomized trials were included (68 trials, 232,606 participants), there was no significant effect on mortality. However, **in "low-bias" trials (180,938 participants), antioxidant supplementation was associated with a slight (~5%) but statistically significant increase in mortality. Specifically, there were slight but statistically significant increases in all-cause mortality with *beta*-carotene (~7% increase), vitamin A (~16% increase), and vitamin E (~4% increase).** (Bjelakovic et al, 2007, JAMA) (Bjelakovic et al, 2008:CD007176)

- **The ADCS trial** (The Alzheimer's Disease Cooperative Study) **found no significant effect in 536 subjects randomized to placebo or 3 doses of the antioxidant, idebenone. There was a benefit in cognition when all 3 idebenone groups were combined, but this effect was deemed too small to be clinically significant.** (Thal et al, 2003)

- In a small 6-month pilot trial, 34 subjects with AD were randomized to placebo or two doses of the antioxidant, **curcumin. There was no cognitive decline in the placebo group, and no improvement was observed with curcumin.** (Baum et al, 2008)

- **The more recent CONNECTION trial, based in the US, Europe, and South America, showed no benefit for latrepirdine in any parameter for AD.** (ClinicalTrials.gov. A safety and efficacy study of oral Dimebon in patients with mild-to-moderate Alzheimer's disease (CONNECTION) [Accessed March 10, 2010];2009 July 14; http://clinicaltrials.gov/ct2/show/NCT00675623) (Alzheimer Research Forum.

Dimebon disappoints in Phase 3 trial. [Accessed March 10, 2010];2010 March 4; http://www.alzforum.org/new/detail.asp?id=2387)

- Antioxidant/mitochondrial-based therapies have presented a mixed picture. **Many have not proved significantly effective in treatment of AD or MCI (mild cognitive impairment).** (Dumont et al, 2010)

- **Many scientists firmly believe exercise is more likely to help than existing pharmaceuticals or supplements, which have failed to show preventive effects in clinical trials.** (January 2010, Archives of Neurology)

- **After six months, the aerobic exercisers showed significant gains in mental agility, while the non-aerobic group showed continuing decline in tests of thinking speed, fluency with words and ability to multi-task.** (January 2010, Archives of Neurology) **Please read my 2011 book, *Sports, Athletes, Exercise Facts and Antioxidant Myths*.** It will explain the significance of exercise and increased EMODs.

- **"We know some level of exercise is critical, we just don't know how much is needed,"** said Laura Baker, a research scientist at the Puget Sound VA, assistant professor at UW. (January 2010, Archives of Neurology)

- The Seattle study is one of the first human **randomized clinical trials showing that exercise is a source of brain protection.** (January 2010, Archives of Neurology)

> EMODs are not as harmful as you might've imagined,
> not as destructive as you might've thought
> and not the "inner enemy" you might've feared.
> In fact, your life depends on them.
> R. M. Howes, M.D., Ph.D.
> 5/28/10

(EMODs, electronically modified oxygen derivatives, formerly called reactive oxygen species, ROS)

CHAPTER FOUR

Consensus statements on the fall of the free radical theory

The reason antioxiants do not prevent AD is because this premise is based on the outdated and nullified free radical theory. The following is a listing of pertinent comments by respected investigators, whereby they express their discontent with the free radical theory.

Basically, many researchers are perplexed by the continued attempts to make good data conform to the flawed free radical theory.

Some authors argue that the hypothesis that antioxidants could prevent chronic diseases has now been disproved and that the idea was misguided from the beginning. (Hail et al, 2008)

The hype about antioxidants creates a false sense of security. There is no such thing as a super-food. (Jeffrey Blumberg, 2005)

The scientific understanding of radicals has not yet led to any therapeutic application. (Wingler et al, 2009)

For many years, scavenging already formed radicals with antioxidants was considered to be the most promising therapeutic approach, but clinical trials based on this principle have yielded mostly negative results. (Wingler et al, 2009)

The current lack of sufficient data does not permit the systematic recommendation of anti-oxidants. (Bonnefoy et al. 2002)

The results of the large, randomized controlled studies, has been disappointing and arguably provides the strongest evidence against the oxidative modification hypothesis of atherosclerosis. (Stocker, Keaney, 2004)

Supplementation with antioxidant vitamins does not lower serum lipid and lipoproteins or blood pressure. (Hodis et al, 2002)

Collectively, for the most part, clinical trials have failed to demonstrate a beneficial effect of antioxidant supplements on CVD morbidity and mortality. With regard to the meta-analysis, the lack of efficacy was demonstrated consistently for different doses of various antioxidants in diverse population groups. (Kris-Etherton et al, 2004)

The relevance of the antioxidant hypothesis for the treatment of patients with atherosclerosis has not been definitively proven. Results of randomized trials with 'antioxidant' vitamins have been disappointing. (Tardif, 2006)

The obtained results suggest that supplementation of antioxidants cannot be recommended for the normal population. (Siekmeier et al, 2006)

Overall results of clinical studies investigating antioxidant effects have been disappointing given the consistent and promising findings from experimental investigations, clinical observations, and epidemiological data. (Parvicini, Touyz, 2008)

Much of the U.S. public has been misled by manufacturers and have an unhealthy faith in the benefits of nutritional supplements (Blendon et al, 2001)

Ironically, clinical trials of antioxidant supplements have shown that the oxidative theory lacks predictability but antioxidants continue to be widely used, even by physicians (Muntwyler et al, 2002)

There is **no convincing evidence that taking supplements of vitamin C prevents any disease. No one should take beta carotene supplements.** (Vitamin supplements. The Medical Letter on Drugs and Therapeutics, 1998)

Findings add to the growing body of evidence that certain supplemental antioxidant regimes have limited benefit in patients with cardiovascular disease. (Freedman, 2001)

The absence of efficacy and safety data from randomized trials precludes the establishment of population-wide recommendations regarding vitamin E supplementation. (Tribble et al, 1999)

In 2003, **the U.S. Preventive Services Task Force (USPSTF) concluded there is insufficient scientific evidence to recommend vitamin supplements as a**

way to prevent cancer or heart disease. (U.S. Preventive Services Task Force, New Topic, 2003)

In 2004, after reviewing their results, **the American Heart Association Council on Nutrition, Physical Activity, and Metabolism concluded that antioxidants have little or no proven value for preventing or treating cardiovascular disease**.

In 2007, Cochrane Collaboration team concluded that commonly taken antioxidant supplements may do more harm than good. (Bjelakovic et al, Feb. 2007)

With respect to antioxidants and other phytochemicals, the key question is whether supplementation has been proven to do more good than harm. So far, the answer is no, which is why the FDA will not permit any of these substances to be labeled or marketed with claims that they can prevent disease. (Barrett, Quackwatch report, 2003)

Intervention studies have failed to show a consistent beneficial effect of high doses of antioxidant supplementation against chronic diseases, including cardiovascular disease. (Barrett, Quackwatch report, 2003)

The initial promising reports on beneficial effects with antioxidant therapies against atherosclerosis, derived from observational studies, were followed by generally negative results reported from large randomized controlled trials. (Riccioni et al, 2007)

Clinical trials with classic vitamin antioxidants have generally failed to demonstrate any benefit in cardiovascular outcomes. (Sachidanandam et al, 2005)

Despite the wealth of data supporting a role of ROS in hypertension and other cardiovascular diseases, treatment with commonly employed antioxidants have failed, and in some cases have proven harmful, prompting a reconsideration of the concept of oxidative stress. (Harrison et al, 2007)

Even if antioxidant supplementation is receiving growing attention and is increasingly adopted in Western countries, supporting evidence is still scarce and equivocal. (Fusco et al, 2007)

Given the lack of efficacy of antioxidants in clinical trials to date, antioxidant vitamin combinations above the recommended dietary allowances should not be recommended for prevention or treatment of cardiovascular disease. (Kuller, 2001)

The existing scientific database does not justify routine use of antioxidant supplements for the prevention and treatment of CVD. (Kris-Etherton et al, 2004)

There is enough evidence from large, well-designed studies to discourage the use of vitamin E in Parkinson's disease, cataract, and Alzheimer's disease. (Pham and Plakogiannis, 2005)

It has now been proven that the "biological rationale rendered by the oxidative modification hypothesis" is wrong. (Steinberg et al, 1989)

The overwhelming majority of large, randomized and prospective trials of antioxidant supplements in CVD have yielded disappointing results. (Dagenais et al, 2000) (ATBC Study, 1994) (GISSI-Prevenzione Investigators;1999) (Yusuf et al. 2000 HOPE) (Omenn et al, 1996) (Hennekens et al, 1996) (Wilson et al, 1973)

A number of prospective, randomized, placebo-controlled, 3- to 6-year clinical trials (HOPE, GISSI, ATBC, Hennekens study, Omenn's study, Brown's study, MRC/BHF, Vivekananthan's meta-study, Miller's meta-study) have been published, testing the effect of vitamin E and other antioxidant vitamins or their combinations on clinical manifestations of cardiovascular disease and cancer. (Yusuf et al. 2000 HOPE) (GISSI-Prevenzione Investigators;1999) (Virtamo et al, 1998) (Heinonen et al, 1994 ATBC Study) (Hennekens et al, 1996) (Omenn et al, 1996) (Brown et al, 2001) (MRC/BHF, 2002) (Vivekananthan et al, 2003) (Miller et al, 2005). **These trials have surprisingly yet consistently shown that commonly used antioxidant vitamin regimens (vitamins E, C, beta carotene, or a combination thereof) do not significantly reduce overall cardiovascular events or cancer.**

By extending HOPE and adding to the growing list of neutral prospective vitamin E trials (HOPE, GISSI-IV, ATBC, HPS, HATS), this report effectively closes the door on the prospect of a major protective effect of long-term exposure to vitamin E, taken in moderately high dosage, against complications of atherosclerosis and overall cancer incidence. (Brown et al, 2001)

The public health viewpoint would have to be that there's really nothing to support widespread use of these vitamins. (Dr. Ian Graham quote, a professor of cardiology, 2005)

Antioxidants -- compounds in foods and supplements that prevent cell damage -- may actually increase the chances of getting diabetes, at least

in the early stages, antioxidants may contribute to early development of insulin resistance. (Tiganis quote, 2009)

Although some levels of antioxidant vitamins and minerals in the diet are required for good health, there is considerable doubt as to whether these antioxidant supplements are beneficial or harmful, and if they are actually beneficial, which antioxidant(s) are needed and in what amounts. (Stanner et al, 2004)

Some but not all studies have reported a direct association between uric acid (an antioxidant) concentrations and atherosclerosis, hypertension, and cardiovascular mortality. (Rao et al, 1991)

A 2009 review of experiments in mice concluded that almost all manipulations of antioxidant systems had no effect on aging. (Pérez et al, 2009)

Antioxidant vitamin supplementation has no detectable effect on the aging process, so the effects of fruit and vegetables may be unrelated to their antioxidant contents. (Thomas quote, 2004)

Antioxidant supplements do not appear to increase life expectancy in humans. (Green, 2008)

Antioxidant supplements have no clear effect on the risk of chronic diseases such as cancer and heart disease. (Stanner, 2004)

Nutrition expert, Marian L. Neuhouser, said, **"Consumers spend money on dietary supplements with the thought that they are going to improve their health, but there's no evidence for this."**

In 2006, Dr. David Gems said in Science Daily. **"But there is no clear evidence that dietary antioxidants can slow or prevent aging." "Oxidative damage is clearly not a universal, major driver of the aging process." "The free radical theory of aging has filled a knowledge vacuum for over 50 years now, but it just doesn't stand up to the evidence."**

Hekimi believes that the findings of Van Raamsdonk (i.e., removing SODs from C. elegans increases their lifespan) throws a wrench in the entire free radical theory of aging. Bart Braeckman of Ghent University also does not think that the free radical theory is the only answer. Braeckman states, "The final conclusion was similar in all these papers: **there is a problem with the free radical theory.**"

References for this section on the consensus of the FRT can be found in my book entitled, *Heart Disease and Antioxidant Failures, 2011.*

CHAPTER FIVE

Harmful effects of antioxidants summary

In summary, some antioxidant study reports have selectively shown the following:

Antioxidants have increased mortality by as high as 17% and 19%.

Antioxidants have increased lung cancer by 18% and 28%, esophageal cancer deaths by 14% and 22.1%, breast cancer by 19%, hemorrhagic stroke deaths by 50%, ischemic heart disease by 11%, and cardiovascular disease by 18%.

Increase risk of prostate cancer by 17%.

Antioxidants have increased prostate cancer deaths, elevated the risk of squamous cell carcinoma, doubled the risk of adenoma recurrence, increased the rate of second primary cancers, and increased recurrence of head and neck tumors.

Antioxidants increased the incidence of melanoma in women by 4 fold. (Hercberg et al, 2007, VITAL)

Patients taking an antioxidant were 1.65 times more likely to suffer a return of their original cancer.

Three major studies were stopped early due to unexpected harmful outcomes and adverse effects for study participants: ATBC, CARET and SELECT. (Heinonen et al, 1994, ATBC) (Omenn et al, 1996, CARET) (Lippman et al, 2009, SELECT) respectively.

Antioxidants have increased ischemic heart disease, deaths from fatal coronary heart disease, increased risk of nonfatal and fatal myocardial infarction, decreased platelet function, increased intima-to-media thickness, negated statin effects, increased risk of hospitalization for heart failure and hypertension, altered liver function tests, increased blood pressure, and increased blood loss after cardiac surgery.

Antioxidants have increased hemorrhagic stroke deaths as much as 22% to 50%, increased risk of subarachnoid hemorrhage 50% and increased risk of intracerebral hemorrhage 62% and increased risk of fatal subarachnoid hemorrhage 181%.

Antioxidants have increased wheezing, productive coughs, and risk of asthma.

In diabetics, antioxidants have increased pre-diabetic changes in glucose metabolism, increased severity of diabetic retinopathy, and increased blood pressure.

Antioxidant have increased preterm deliveries, premature rupture of membranes and low birth weight, increased gestational hypertension, increased risk of hospitalization, altered liver function tests, increased risk for severe preeclampsia, and fetal loss or perinatal death in women at risk for preeclampsia.

Antioxidants have increased risk of tuberculosis by 72% and pneumonia by 14%, indicating an altered immune system.

Antioxidants have adversely affected muscle performance and hampered endurance capacity.

Antioxidants increased risk of cataracts by 38% and by 56% in hormone replacement users, and increased risk of age-related macular degeneration (AMD).

Antioxidants increased the risk of hip fractures, damaged sperm DNA, increased epistaxis (nose bleed) and mother to child transfer of HIV.

Other than that....

Now, you can make up your own mind.

Cancer concern and antioxidants

Also, we must keep in mind the fact that antioxidants protect cancer cells in vitro.

Human cancer cell types (27 human & 9 murine) shielded by antioxidants

If you are worried about cancer, just take a look at the human cell types that are protected by antioxidants from cell death in lab experiments.

Unbelievably, there are twenty seven (27) types of human cancer cell types and nine (9) murine cancer cell types that can be killed by EMODs and in which the killing can be blocked by antioxidants, thereby providing antioxidant protection and shielding of the cancer cells. Published data has shown that antioxidants blocked the killing of the following human and murine (rodent) cancer cell types by EMODs:

- **human breast cancer** (J. Nutr. 134, 2004) (Gundimeda et al, 1996) (Peralta et al, 2006) (Aykin-Burns et al, 2009) (Xiao et al, Mol Cancer Ther. 2006)
- **human prostate carcinoma** (Xiao et al, 2006) (Wu et al, 2005) (Singh et al, 2005) (Cho et al, 2005) (Milanesa et al, 2000)
- **human non-small cell lung cancer** (Ling et al, 2003) (Wu et al, 2006)
- **human colon adenocarcinoma** (Wenzel et al, 2005)
- **human colon cancer** (Wenzel et al, 2004) (Aykin-Burns et al, 2009)
- **human colorectal carcinoma** (Chen et al, 2004) (Gali-Muhtasib et al, 2008)
- **human ovarian cancer cells** (Pak et al, 2011)
- **human melanoma** (Marcin et al, 2005) (Okroj et al, 2006) (Nishikawa et al, 2004) (Grimm et al, 2011)
- **human metastatic melanoma** (Kirshner et al, 2008)
- **human head and neck cancer** (Mattson et al, 2009) (Simons et al, 2007)
- **human lymphoma** (J. Nutr. 134, 2004) (Mansat-De Mas et al, 1999)
- **human leukemia** (Hileman et al, 2004) (McKallip et al, 2006) (Hou et al, 2005) (Feng et al, 2007) (Yedjou et al, 2008) (Hiraoka et al, 1998)
- **human hepatoma** (Wu et al, 2004) (Wu, Ng, Lin, 2004)
- **human hepatocellular liver carcinoma** (Shimoda et al, 2003)
- **human pancreatic cancer** (Maehara et al, 2004)
- **human multiple myeloma** (Grad et al, 2001) (Ahmad et al, 1997) (Gupta et al, 2000) (Nakazato et al, 2005) (Isham et al, 2007)
- **Burkitt's lymphoma** (Ahmad et al, 1997) (Gupta et al, 2000) (Nakazato et al, 2005) (Ahmad et al, 1997)
- **human chronic lymphocytic leukemia** (Kay, 2006) (Chandra et al, 2003) (Shanafelt et al, 2005) (Mow et al, 2002) (Biswas S, et al, 2010)
- **human acute myeloid leukemia** (Kay, 2006) (Chandra et al, 2003) (Shanafelt et al, 2005) (Mow et al, 2002)
- **human promyelocytic leukemia** (Hou et al, 2005)
- **human erythromyeloid leukemia** (Wagner et al, 2000)
- **human epithelial cancer cells** (breast and colon) (Aykin-Burns et al, 2009)
- **human endometrial cancer** (Llobet et al, 2008)
- **human bladder cancer cells** (Miyajima et al, 1999)
- **human invasive bladder cancer** (Miyajima et al, 1999 - human bladder cancer KU-1 cell line)
- **human glioblastoma cells** (Lee et al, 2004)
- **human osteosarcoma** (Ahmad et al, 2005)

- **murine pheochromocytoma** (Jang, Surh, 2001)
- **murine retinoblastoma** (Salganik et al, 2000)
- **murine thymoma** (Tome et al, 2001)
- **murine lymphoma- six cell types** (Nathan et al, vol 153, 1981)
- **murine leukemia** (Wagner et al, 1996)
- **murine fibrosarcoma** (Teicher et al, 1994)
- **murine neuroblastoma** (Prasad et al, PNAS. 1979)
- **murine mammary cancer** (Bracke et al, 1999)
- **murine brain cancer** (Zeisel (2), 2004)

Part of this list was compiled in 2009 and has been updated for this book. (Howes, Philica. Feb 7, 2009). **It is evident to many investigators that the in vitro apoptogenic agents function as prooxidants.** (Hail et al, 2008). Note: References for this list are available in my book, *Dangers of Excessive Antioxidants In Cancer Patients, 2011*.

Organizations not recommending antioxidant vitamins

Contrary to the common impression, major health organizations do not recommend the antioxidant vitamins A, C and E.

THE FOLLOWING LIST PROVIDES THE MAJOR MEDICAL AND SCIENTIFIC ORGANIZATIONS WHICH DO NOT RECOMMEND THE USE OF ANTIOXIDANT VITAMINS

The following either do not recommend antioxidant vitamins or have found inconclusive evidence of their benefit:

- **The U.S. Food and Drug Administration (FDA)**
- **The American Heart Association (AHA)**
- **The American Cancer Society (ACS)**
- **The National Cancer Institute (NCI)**
- **Institute of Medicine of the National Academies**
- **The American College of Cardiology**
- **The American College of Chest Physicians (ACCP)**
- **The American Diabetes Association**
- **The American Academy of Family Physicians**
- **Scientific Statement From the American Heart Association and the American Diabetes Association**
- **The American College of Cardiology/American Heart Association Task Force on Practice Guidelines**

- **United States Preventive Services Task Force (USPSTF)**
- **The American Cancer Society Guidelines on Nutrition and Physical Activity for Cancer Prevention**
- **The Nutrition Committee of the American Heart Association Council on Nutrition, Physical Activity, and Metabolism**
- **The AHA Scientific Position of the American Heart Association**
- **The Canadian Task Force on Preventive Health Care (CTFPHC)**
- **Food and Nutrition Board, Institute of Medicine**
- **The Food and Nutrition Board of the National Academy of Sciences**
- **National Academy of Sciences**
- **The 2006 AHA Diet and Lifestyle Recommendations**
- **The Medical Letter**
- **The Oregon Health and Science University**
- **Food Standards Agency/ the British Nutrition Foundation (BNF)**
- **Quackwatch**
- **American College of Cardiology Foundation Task Force on Clinical Expert Consensus Documents**
- **National Institutes of Health State-of-the-Science Conference**
- **The American Heart Association Atherosclerosis, Hypertension, and Obesity in Youth Committee, Council of Cardiovascular Disease in the Young, With the Council on Cardiovascular Nursing**
- **The Physicians Health Study**
- **The 2008 VITAmins and Lifestyle (VITAL) study**
- **The Physicians' Health Study II Randomized Controlled Trial**
- **The Swedish Council of Technology Assessment**
- **National Heart Foundation of Australia's Nutrition and Metabolism Advisory Committee**

Although their conclusions are not iron clad, many prestigious scientific organizations have concluded that, "taking antioxidant vitamins - such as vitamins A, C and E - serves no purpose, and in some cases could likely be harmful."

Such a list is rather astounding because broadcast media presents a never-ending cycle of advertisements pushing the wonders of antioxidants and antioxidant vitamins. One would assume that such advertisements would have the backing of major medical and scientific organizations, but that is not the case.

The above 32 conclusions or recommendations are apparently some of the best kept secrets in America, since antioxidants are being fortified or added to a wide spectrum of commercial products including foods, cosmetics, dermatologics, pet products, beverages, energy drinks, energy bars, fruits drinks, fruit juices, chewing gum, shampoos, etc. **Genetic engineers are hurriedly creating "super foods," which will be "antioxidant-rich."** (Howes R.M. 2009, Am J Cosm Surg)

CHAPTER SIX

What is on the AD horizon?

Here's a listing of some of the most talked-about drugs in development that "**might**" be able to slow down the progression of Alzheimer's.

Eli Lilly (LLY) has been working on two Alzheimer's treatments that stimulate the immune system to ward off plaque.

Currently in Phase III clinical testing, LY450139 is aimed at inhibiting an enzyme called gamma-secretase, which plays a role in the production of amyloid-beta.

Lilly is also developing an antibody-based product code-named LY2062430. On July 30, 2008, the drugmaker announced it plans to begin Phase III testing for the therapy in 2009.

Lilly added that the product, as opposed to some other antibody therapies, did not appear to trigger any treatment-related brain-swelling, bleeding or similar negative side effects.

"The Phase III drug (LY450139) slows down the body's ability to make amyloid-beta," explained Siemers. "The antibody helps get amyloid-beta out of the brain."

Wyeth and Elan

Madison, N.J.-based Wyeth and Irish drugmaker Elan have teamed up on two Alzheimer's drug candidates, an antibody treatment called bapineuzumab and a vaccine called ACC-001.

According to Menelas Pangalos, who heads Wyeth's Alzheimer's program, the antibody binds to a-beta plaque deposits and removes them from the brain.

"We're hoping it stops disease progression," said Pangalos. "We're actually trying to hit the disease process itself."

Pangalos said that if all goes well, bapineuzumab could be on the market in three to five years. The drug began Phase III trials in December 2008.

ACC-001 is intended to stimulate a patient's immune system to manufacture antibodies that recognize a-beta in their system. The product is in Phase II testing.

Both drugs, however, have been haunted by safety concerns.

On July 29, Wyeth and Elan unveiled relatively favorable Phase II results for bapineuzumab. **But the study also showed the compound was ineffective on a subgroup of patients who have a genetic mutation called ApoE4**, which has been associated with an inherited form of Alzheimer's.

Even more worrisome, **a handful of bapineuzumab users, particularly those who had the ApoE4 mutation, developed brain swelling**.

The ACC-001 program has also had trouble. **It was put on hold earlier this year after a patient developed a potentially dangerous skin reaction**. Wyeth received the green light from regulators to resume clinical testing in May.

Baxter International

Deerfield, Ill.-based Baxter International (BAX) has been testing its hematology drug **GammaGard** as a treatment for Alzheimer's.

Originally used to treat children with severe immune deficiencies, GammaGard is really a mélange of antibodies derived from human blood. The product is known generically as Immune Globulin Intravenous, or IGIV.

IGIV researchers think the therapy can battle Alzheimer's by stimulating the body to generate antibodies that discourage plaque build-up.

"It's like a gentle vacuuming," said Dr. Norman Relkin, a leading Alzheimer's researcher at Weill Cornell Medical Center in New York City. He added that because the product has already been on the market for decades, its safety-profile has been well-established.

GammaGard is about to begin Phase III clinical trials for Alzheimer's. According to Baxter, the company could be ready to file for regulatory approval for that indication between 2011 and 2012.

One potential downside of the product, however, is that because it is garnered from donated blood, IGIV is often in short supply.

Medivation (MDVN), like Baxter, is also trying to teach an old drug new tricks.

Originally approved about 25 years ago in Russia as an antihistamine, San Francisco-based Medivation has been testing Dimebon for not just for Alzheimer's but the equally devastating Huntington's disease as well.

According to Medivation Chief Executive Officer Dr. David Hung, **Dimebon works by tinkering with a cellular component called mitochondria, which plays a role in cellular death.** The drug is currently in Phase III testing for Alzheimer's.

"We've shown in pre-clinical trials that Dimebon inhibits neuron death," said Hung, adding that Alzheimer's patients can lose up to 6% of their brain mass each year as brain cells die.

A recent study published in the prestigious British medical journal Lancet also noted that Dimelbon users appeared to steadily improve over the course of 12 months, rather than just level off, as users of current medications tend to do.

Epix and Glaxo

Lexington, Mass.-based Epix Pharmaceuticals (EPIX) has teamed up with U.K. pharmaceutical giant GlaxoSmithKline (GSK) on a drug code-named PRX-03140.

Currently in Phase II testing, Epix researchers said they've been primarily testing the product as a "brain booster," to help improve cognitive function. But they add that the drug, at least in animal studies, also appears to be able to slow progression of the disease.

The company has particularly heartened by Phase IIa results for the product, released at the beginning of the year.

"We saw significant improvement in cognition in just two weeks," former Epix Chief Executive Officer Michael Kauffman, told MarketWatch in late June. He noted that **drugs currently on the market can take up to six months to have an effect.**

Epix said the drug works in part by stimulating neurons that researchers believe become dormant in the brains of Alzheimer's patients.

"The fact we're able to get an effect that quickly indicates you're taking the neurons that were asleep and waking them up, and also making the existing neurons work harder," said Kauffman.

Prana Biotechnology

Australia-based Prana Biotechnology Ltd. is also diligently working on a beta-amyloid inhibitor, called PBT2.

According to Prana's co-founder, Harvard University geneticist Rudolph Tanzi, PBT2 is **based on the theory that the metals copper and zinc play a key part in the toxicity of beta-amyloid**. PBT2 neutralizes toxicity of beta-amyloid by blocking the interaction with these metals.

"The product disrupts the aggregation of a-beta (beta-amyloid)," said Tanzi. "It works in the 'nip it in the bud' stage, before the build-up."

Prana released positive Phase IIa data on PBT2 in February, 2011. Val Brickates Kennedy is a reporter for MarketWatch in Boston.

Experimental AD drug shows some promise

For the first time, as of July 2008, an experimental drug shows promise for halting the progression of Alzheimer's disease by taking a new approach: breaking up the protein tangles that clog victims' brains.

The encouraging results from the drug called **Rember**, reported at a medical conference in Chicago, electrified a field battered by recent setbacks. The drug was developed by Singapore-based TauRx Therapeutics.

Even if bigger, more rigorous studies show it works, Rember is still several years away from being available, and experts warned against overexuberance. But they were excited.

"These are the first very positive results I've seen" for stopping mental decline, said Marcelle Morrison-Bogorad, director of Alzheimer's research at the National Institute on Aging. "It's just fantastic."

The federal agency funded early research into the tangles, which are made of a protein called tau and develop inside nerve cells.

For decades, scientists have focused on a different protein — beta-amyloid, which forms sticky clumps outside of the cells — but have yet to get a workable treatment.

The drug is in the second of three stages of development, and scientists are paying special attention to potential treatments because of the enormity of the illness, which afflicts more than 26 million people worldwide and is mushrooming as the population ages.

The four Alzheimer's drugs currently available just ease symptoms of the mind-robbing disease.

TauRx's chief is Claude Wischik, a biologist at the University of Aberdeen in Scotland who long has done key research on tau tangles and studies suggesting that Rember can dissolve them.

He is an "esteemed biologist," and the research "comes with his credibility attached to it," said Dr. Sam Gandy of Mount Sinai School of Medicine in New York. He heads the scientific advisory panel of the Alzheimer's Association.

In the study, 321 patients were given one of three doses of Rember or dummy capsules three times a day. **The capsules containing the highest dose had a flaw in formulation that kept them from working, and the lowest dose was too weak to keep the disease from worsening,** Wischik said.

However, the middle dose helped, as measured by a widely used score of mental performance.

"The people on placebo lost an average of 7 percent of their brain function over six months whereas those on treatment didn't decline at all," he said.

After about a year, the placebo group had continued to decline but those on the mid-level dose of Rember had not. At 19 months, the treated group still had not declined as Alzheimer's patients have been known to do.

Two types of brain scans were available on about a third of participants, and they show the drug was active in brain areas most affected by tau tangles, Wischik said.

"This is suggestive data," not proof, Wischik warned.

The main chemical in Rember is available now in a different formulation in a prescription drug sometimes used since the 1930s for chronic bladder infections — **methylene blue**. However, it predates the federal Food and Drug Administration and was never fully studied for safety and effectiveness, and not in the form used in the Alzheimer's study, Wischik and other doctors cautioned.

I have been studying methylene blue for decades because it is a good source of singlet oxygen, when exposed to photoexcitation. Please see the section on methylene blue and the treatment of AD and Parkinson's disease.

At the International Conference on Alzheimer's Disease, other researchers reported encouraging results from a test of a different experimental drug that also targets tau tangles. That drug, by British Columbia-based Allon Therapeutics Inc., was tested in people with an Alzheimer's precursor, mild cognitive impairment.

The tau-drug results are in stark contrast to the flop of Flurizan, which was aimed at blocking enzymes that form the beta-amyloid clumps. Myriad Genetics announced in June 2008 that it would abandon development of Flurizan after the failure, the biggest clinical trial of any Alzheimer's drug to date. Full results were presented at the conference.

Also due out are full results of a closely watched test of bapineuzumab, an experimental drug that aims to enlist the immune system to clear out the sticky brain clumps.

Its developers — New Jersey-based Wyeth and the Irish company Elan Corp. PLC — previously announced that the 240-patient study missed its main goal of improving patients' mental performance at 18 months.

But the company found a silver lining — the drug appeared to help the roughly 60 percent of people in the study who did not have a gene that scientists think makes Alzheimer's disease more severe.

Scientists were eager for information on side effects and possible magnitude of benefit for the drug, which the companies have already said will move on to late-stage testing in more than 4,000 patients.

Vaccine triggers immune response, prevents AD

A vaccine created by University of Rochester Medical Center scientists **prevents the development of Alzheimer's disease-like pathology in mice without causing inflammation or significant side effects.**

Vaccinated mice generated an immune response to the protein known as amyloid-beta peptide, which accumulates in what are called "amyloid plaques" in brains of people with Alzheimer's. The vaccinated mice demonstrated normal learning skills and functioning memory in spite of being genetically designed to develop an aggressive form of the disease.

The Rochester scientists reported the findings in an article in the May 2008 issue of *Molecular Therapy*, the journal of The American Society of Gene Therapy.

"Our study demonstrates that we can create a potent but safe version of a vaccine that utilizes the strategy of immune response shaping to prevent Alzheimer's-related pathologies and memory deficits," said William Bowers, associate professor of neurology and of microbiology and immunology at the Medical Center and lead author of the article. "The vaccinated mice not only performed better, we found no evidence of signature amyloid plaque in their brains."

Alzheimer's is a progressive neurodegenerative disease associated with dementia and a decline in performance of normal activities. Hallmarks of the disease include the accumulation of amyloid plaques in the brains of patients and **the loss of normal functioning tau, a protein that stabilizes the transport networks in neurons**. Abnormal tau function eventually leads to another classic hallmark of Alzheimer's, neurofibrillary tangle in nerve cells. After several decades of exposure to these insults, neurons ultimately succumb and die, leading to progressively damaged learning and memory centers in the brain.

The mice that received the vaccines were genetically engineered to express large amounts of amyloid beta protein. They also harbored a mutation that causes the tau-related tangle pathology. Prior to the start of the vaccine study, the mice were trained to navigate a maze using spatial clues. They were then tested periodically during the 10-month study on the amount of time and distance traveled to an escape pod and the number of errors made along the way.

"What we found exciting was that by targeting one pathology of Alzheimer's - amyloid beta - we were able to also prevent the transition of tau from its normal form to a form found in the disease state," Bowers said.

The goal of the vaccine is to prompt the immune system to recognize amyloid beta protein and remove it. To create the vaccine, Bowers and the research group use a herpes virus that is stripped of the viral genes that can cause disease or harm. They then load the virus container with the genetic code for amyloid beta and interleukin-4, a protein that stimulates immune responses involving type 2 T helper cells, which are lymphocytes that play an important role in the immune system.

The research group tested several versions of a vaccine. Mice were given three injections of empty virus alone, a vaccine carrying only the amyloid beta genetic code, or a vaccine encoding both amyloid beta and interlueikin-4, which was found to be the most effective.

"We have learned a great deal from this ongoing project," Bowers said. "Importantly, it has demonstrated the combined strengths of the gene delivery platform and the immune shaping concept for the creation of customized vaccines for Alzheimer's disease, as well as a number of other diseases. We are currently working on strategies we believe can make the vaccine even safer."

Bowers expects the vaccine eventually to be tested in people, but due to the number of studies required to satisfy regulatory requirements, it could be three or more years before human trials testing this type of Alzheimer's vaccine occur.

'Pre-dementia' is rising, especially in men

In July of 2008, it was reported that a milder type of mental decline that often precedes Alzheimer's disease is alarmingly more common than has been believed, and in men more than women, doctors reported Monday. **Nearly a million older Americans slide from normal memory into mild impairment each year**, researchers estimate, based on a Mayo Clinic study of Minnesota residents.

That's on top of **the half million Americans who develop full-blown Alzheimer's** or other forms of dementia — a problem sure to grow as baby boomers age (those born between 1946 to 1964). "We're seeing that there's a much larger burgeoning problem out there" of people at risk of developing dementia, said Dr. Ronald Petersen, the Mayo scientist who led the study.

Dr. Ralph Nixon, a New York University psychiatrist and scientific adviser to the Alzheimer's Association, was blunt. "We're facing a crisis," he said. **There are no treatments now to prevent this mental slide or reverse it once it starts.**

But that may be changing. Researchers reported early, somewhat encouraging results from an experimental nose spray that seemed to improve certain memory measures in a study of mildly impaired people.

The drug, for now just called AL-108, needs testing in a longer, larger study. It is being developed by Allon Therapeutics Inc., based in Vancouver, B.C.

Doctors said it shows the potential for new types of medicines that target the protein tangles that kill nerve cells, instead of targeting the sticky brain deposits that have gotten most of the attention up to now. The studies were reported at the International Conference on Alzheimer's Disease in Chicago.

Petersen is the scientist who defined **mild cognitive impairment, or MCI**, as a transition phase between healthy aging and dementia. It is more than "senior moments" like forgetting where you parked the car, but not as severe as having dementia, where you forget what a car is for. People with it have impaired memory but not other problems like confusion, inattention or trouble putting thoughts into words.

The Alzheimer's Association says **more than 5 million Americans have Alzheimer's**, but no estimate for this "pre-dementia" has been available until now.

Petersen's federally funded study involved roughly **1,600 people, ages 70 through 89,** living in Olmstead County, which surrounds the Mayo Clinic in Rochester, Minn. All tested normal when they were enrolled in the study, but more than 5 percent had developed mild impairment when evaluated a year later.

Men were nearly twice as likely as women to develop it. That's a surprise, because some studies have found more women with Alzheimer's than men. But there may be a simple explanation:

Even though more men may be impaired, women outlive them and therefore have more time to develop full-blown dementia.

"This is a very large and important issue for our country and for the world," said Duke University psychologist Brenda Plassman. A smaller study she published earlier this year backs up the Mayo study's findings.

The mild impairment rate is two to three times larger than many researchers had expected, Petersen said.

"It's the iceberg under the tip," agreed Dr. R. Scott Turner, incoming director of the memory disorders program at Georgetown University Medical Center. **A prime goal is finding drugs to treat the mild impairment before Alzheimer's develops.**

The AL-108 study tried to do that. Scientists gave **144 people** with mild impairment either a low or high dose of the drug or a dummy drug for 12 weeks. The study missed its main goal — a composite of various memory scores — and **the low dose showed no effect.** But those on the higher dose improved on some memory tasks after one month and benefits lasted a month after they stopped treatment, said the study's leader, Dr. Donald Schmechel of Duke University.

The study was sponsored by the drug maker. Please keep this in mind.

In another study presented at the conference and published on the Internet by the British medical journal The Lancet, researchers reported that **dementia rates in developing countries may be considerably higher than official estimates and closer to rates in wealthy countries.**

Scientists used a more liberal definition of dementia more suitable to poorer, less educated populations, where respect for family often means relatives don't regard dementia as a burden so much and may be less likely to report problems.

The study involved nearly **15,000 people** in 11 sites from China, India, Cuba, Mexico and other nations. **Dementia rates ranged from nearly 6 percent in rural China to nearly 12 percent in the Dominican Republic**, said co-author Martin Prince of King's College in London.

The World Health Organization and the Alzheimer's Association were among the study's sponsors.

Alzheimer's Disease: Bad News and Good News

The overall consensus is sobering: **Currently, there is no good evidence that any supplement, medication, diet or behavior change actually prevents Alzheimer's or other age-related cognitive decline.** (LiveScience Contributor, 5-18-10)

Such a grim verdict on a much-dreaded disease might seem like cause for despair. It's not, say researchers. **"The bad news is we have nothing that's been proven to prevent Alzheimer's disease,"** said Cynthia Carlsson, a professor and Alzheimer's researcher at the University of Wisconsin School of Medicine and Public Health, who was not on the panel that reviewed the research. **"But the good news is we're really at a tremendous point in understanding more about the disease causes."**

Ongoing research has pinpointed several biological markers, or indicators that someone is at risk for Alzheimer's (just as blood pressure is a biomarker for risk for cardiovascular disease). These include proteins called **beta-amyloid and tau**, found in the spinal fluid during the early stages of the disease. In full-blown Alzheimer's, these proteins form plaques and tangles in the brain which seem to interfere with the functioning of neurons. Exactly what causes the proteins to form isn't known, but variations on a gene called **APOE seem to increase the risk.**

But when it comes to behavioral risk factors, the evidence isn't as strong.

A panel of 15 independent scientists convened by the National Institutes of Health reviewed 250 human research studies and 25 review papers on Alzheimer's prevention and found that in all cases, the correlations were too weak to confidently point to any risk factor as a cause of Alzheimer's disease or cognitive decline. In most cases, the studies were too small and the associations too limited to draw firm conclusions, said panel head Martha L. Daviglus, a professor of preventative medicine at Northwestern University in Chicago.

While the NIH-convened panel found no strong evidence for Alzheimer's prevention, **the scientists did say some factors showed very limited evidence of protection against Alzheimer's, including omega-3 fatty acids and a diet low in saturated fat and high in vegetables. But, this has not been proved.**

A few studies also showed that increased cognitive engagement and physical activity might keep older people sharp and possibly keep their brains clear of dementia, while **high blood pressure and diabetes showed associations with cognitive decline. None of this evidence met the panel's criteria for high-quality evidence.**

Doctors can't yet predict who will develop Alzheimer's just by peering into the individual's genome or spinal fluid. But biomarkers like the APOE gene variation and measurements of beta-amyloid and tau proteins can predict a person's risk for getting the disease, just as high blood pressure predicts risk for cardiovascular disease.

And while the plaques and tangles on the brain can't be seen, improved brain imaging can track blood flow in the brain, giving insights into which parts of the brain are experiencing decline. Detailed neuropsychological tests that measure memory and judgment are another common research tool.

Diet, exercise, staying socially active, staying engaged with people, those things are going to improve your quality of life no matter what.

The disorder is marked by memory loss, confusion and the inability to function independently.

Abnormal Heart Rhythm Linked to Alzheimer's

In April of 2010, it was reported that people with atrial fibrillation, a form of abnormal heart rhythm, are more likely than others to develop dementia, including Alzheimer's disease.

The presence of atrial fibrillation also predicted higher death rates in dementia patients, especially among younger patients in the group studied, meaning under the age of 70.

"This leaves us with the finding that atrial fibrillation, independent of everything else, is a risk factor [for dementia]," said Dr. Gary Kennedy, director of geriatric psychiatry at Montefiore Medical Center in New York City. "This is adding one more brick in the road toward understanding that cardiovascular disease is a major risk factor for dementia."

"Alzheimer's disease, in particular, is one where we don't quite understand the risk factors and what causes it, so studies [like this] that try to investigate the causative effect will help us understand that and ultimately design therapies and approaches to prevent or minimize disease," added Dr. Jared Bunch, lead author of a study appearing in the April edition of the *HeartRhythm Journal* and a cardiologist/ electrophysiologist with Intermountain Medical Center in Murray, Utah.

This study, however, was not specifically set up to establish a direct cause-and-effect relationship. The authors looked at **37,025 patients without atrial fibrillation or dementia**, aged 60 to 90, over a five-year period.

Individuals who developed atrial fibrillation had a higher risk of all types of dementia, even when other risk factors were taken into account. Alzheimer's disease is by far the most common form of dementia.

More surprising was that **those in the younger group -- under age 70 -- who had atrial fibrillation had the highest risk of developing dementia, even though dementia is normally associated with aging**. People in this group were also at a 38 percent higher risk of dying.

Among the 764 patients who developed both conditions, **diagnosis of atrial fibrillation usually happened first, followed by a diagnosis of dementia.**

The authors hypothesized that both atrial fibrillation and dementia may arise from the same risk factors, such as hypertension. Another possibility is that atrial fibrillation increases inflammation, and **dementia has been shown to be higher in people with signs of systemic inflammation.**

"From a public health perspective, the best thing we can do to decrease the coming epidemic of Alzheimer's disease is to do a much better, more aggressive job of helping people with heart disease," Kennedy said. "**That means diet and exercise**, of course -- everyone knows that. A heart-healthy diet and lifestyle are really the best means we have available to prevent dementia."

About 2.2 million Americans have atrial fibrillation, while an estimated 5.5 million suffer from AD.

Aerobic exercise can protect brain, improve mental agility

A January 2010 study reported there is no proven way to prevent Alzheimer's disease, but a new Seattle-area study provides some of the strongest evidence yet **that regular exercise can protect the brain -- and even improve cognitive performance -- in older adults showing signs of mental decline.**

I believe this is support for my theory whereby I contend that EMODs are essential for normal brain function and that exercise increases the supply of EMODs during times of EMOD insufficiency.

Researchers at the University of Washington School of Medicine and Veterans Affairs Puget Sound Health Care System tested the effects of aerobic training in a clinical trial with **33 women and men** diagnosed with **mild cognitive impairment (MCI)**, often a prelude to Alzheimer's disease.

Twenty-three of the volunteers, selected randomly, began an intense program of aerobic exercise, **spending 45 to 60 minutes on a treadmill or stationary bike four days a week.** The remaining 10, the study's control group, spent the same amount of time performing non-aerobic stretching and balance exercises.

After six months, the aerobic exercisers showed significant gains in mental agility, while the non-aerobic group showed continuing decline in tests of thinking speed, fluency with words and ability to multi-task. (January 2010, Archives of Neurology)

Please read my 2011 book, *Sports, Athletes, Exercise Facts and Antioxidant Myths.* It will explain the significance of exercise and increased EMODs.

While it remains unknown whether fitness training can prevent Alzheimer's, **many scientists firmly believe exercise is more likely to help than existing pharmaceuticals or supplements, which have failed to show preventive effects in clinical trials.** (January 2010, Archives of Neurology)

"We know some level of exercise is critical, we just don't know how much is needed," said Laura Baker, a research scientist at the Puget Sound VA, assistant professor at UW, and lead author of the study published in **January 2010, Archives of Neurology.**

The Seattle study, funded by the Alzheimer's Association and the Department of Veterans Affairs, is one of the first human **randomized clinical trials showing that exercise is a source of brain protection**, said Dr. Jeffrey Kaye, director of the Layton Aging and Alzheimer's Disease Center at Oregon Health & Science University, who was not involved in the study.

"The bottom line is, movement and activity does really seem to be good for your brain," Kaye said. The challenge now, he said, "is to understand, at a scientific level, what elements of activity really do enhance brain function, and what level, what dose of activity is needed."

I believe that all of the good effects of exercise are due to increased EMOD production.

Scientists don't fully understand how Alzheimer's disease wipes out memory, scrambles the ability to think and erodes personality. Nerve cells die and the brain shrivels as the disease advances.

The damage seems to begin with the clustering of protein fragments, called **amyloid plaques**, among brain cells. Larger, tangled strands of another protein soon appear inside brain cells. Generally, the more plaques and tangles, the more severe the symptoms of dementia.

Because lifestyle factors seem to lower the risk, some researchers suspect that physical fitness, overall health and mental stimulation provide a buffer, or reserve, that allows the brain to withstand more damage and still function normally. Strong social connections also seem to help, perhaps by ameliorating stress.

It's clear that uncontrolled high blood pressure and diabetes contribute to the loss of brain cells. **High blood pressure destroys small blood vessels that bring oxygen and nutrients to brain cells. Diabetes, in which the body loses control of energy metabolism, worsens blood pressure and artery damage**.

Aerobic exercise probably protects the brain in several ways, Baker said. It builds heart and artery resilience, which **boosts blood flow to the brain. I believe this increases oxygen in the brain, which also increases EMOD levels.**

Exercise keeps energy metabolism stable, preventing and even reversing diabetes. Exercise also relieves stress, preventing damaging chain-reactions unleashed by the build-up of stress hormones.

Dr. Michael Mega, a neurologist and neuroscientist with the Providence Brain Institute in Portland, said the Seattle study fits with the emerging view that heart health and brain health go hand in hand.

I believe it should be said that oxygen and EMOD levels and brain health go hand in hand.

"All of the things that cause your heart to stop working well -- sedentary lifestyle, high cholesterol, diabetes, smoking -- are also the risk factors that come right underneath advanced age as factors increasing risk for Alzheimer's disease," Mega said.

Mega found one result jarring in the new study: exercise didn't improve performance on memory tests.

In a previous study, a moderate exercise program -- brisk walking -- improved memory after one year in Dutch women and men with mild cognitive impairment. Kaye said memory gains may take longer than six months to emerge or require a different type or intensity of exercise than used in the Seattle study.

For reasons that remain unclear, **aerobic training helped women's mental agility substantially more than it helped men's.** "It might be that this was the perfect dose of exercise for women but not men," said Baker, the study author.

But people who aren't exercising regularly shouldn't wait for more scientific data to get going, Baker said. "Don't worry about the intensity. **You can start by walking 20 minutes a day,"** she said. "Just get moving. You don't need to join a gym or hire a personal trainer."

Aerobic exercise may shield aging brain

Keeping the heart fit with aerobic exercise may also boost older adults' brainpower, a research review suggests.

In an analysis of pooled data from previous clinical trials, researchers in the Netherlands found that **when healthy adults older than 55 improved their fitness through aerobic exercise, there was also often an improvement in memory, attention or other mental abilities.** (Cochrane Database of Systematic Reviews, 2008)

The findings appear in the Cochrane Library, a publication of the Cochrane Collaboration, an international organization that evaluates medical research.

Aerobic exercise is any activity, such as brisk walking, that gets the heart rate up and improves endurance, over time. This type of exercise has proven benefits for the heart.

At the same time, research has linked regular exercise to better cognitive function in older adults -- but it has not been clear whether this is related specifically to aerobic exercise and gains in cardiovascular fitness.

To investigate, Dr. Maaike Angevaren and colleagues at the University of Applied Sciences in Utrecht reviewed **11 clinical trials** conducted in the U.S., France and Sweden that involved a total of **670 adults older than 55.**

Some studies tested the effects of aerobic exercise against no exercise only; others also included comparison activities, like flexibility or strength training, or social activities. In eight of these studies, the researchers found, participants who engaged in aerobic exercise showed an average improvement in their fitness levels. That improvement coincided with gains in certain measures of mental acuity.

Still, **it's not clear that the improved physical fitness bestowed the benefit, according to Angevaren and her colleagues. When the researchers excluded non-exercisers from the analysis, there was no consistent evidence that aerobic exercise was more beneficial than other forms of exercise.**

"It needs to be established whether the same effects can be achieved with any type of physical exercise," Angevaren said in a statement. However, she also pointed to reasons why aerobic exercise, or improved cardiovascular fitness in particular, would benefit the brain.

"Improvements in cognition as a result of improvements in cardiovascular fitness are being explained by **improvements in cerebral blood flow, leading to increased brain metabolism** which, in turn, stimulates the production of neurotransmitters and formation of new synapses," Angevaren explained.

It is due to OXYGEN, folks! EMODs.

Neurotransmitters are chemicals that carry messages between nerve cells, and synapses are the connections through which this communication takes place.

Improved cardiovascular fitness may also protect the brain by lowering the risks of heart disease and stroke, Angevaren said. **Cardiovascular disease is known to contribute to problems with mental function.** SOURCE: Cochrane Database of Systematic Reviews, online April 16, 2008.

CHAPTER SEVEN

Alzheimer's linked to high blood pressure

An article in early 2010 announced, "If the cardiologist's warnings don't scare you, consider this: Controlling blood pressure just might be the best protection yet known against dementia."

In a flurry of new research, scientists scanned people's brains to **show hypertension fuels a kind of scarring linked to later development of Alzheimer's disease** and other dementias. Those scars can start building up in middle age, decades before memory problems will appear.

The evidence is strong enough that the National Institutes of Health soon will begin enrolling thousands of hypertension sufferers in a major study to see if aggressive treatment — pushing blood pressure lower than currently recommended — better protects not just their hearts but their brains,

"If you look ... for things that we can prevent that lead to cognitive decline in the elderly, **hypertension is at the top of the list**," Dr. Walter Koroshetz, deputy director of NIH's National Institute of Neurological Disorders and Stroke, told The Associated Press.

Age is the biggest risk factor for Alzheimer's disease and other forms of dementia that affect about one in eight people 65 or older.

Scientists have long noticed that some of the same triggers for heart disease — **high blood pressure, obesity, diabetes — seem to increase the risk of dementia**, too. But for years, they thought that link was with "vascular dementia," memory problems usually linked to small strokes, and not the scarier classic Alzheimer's disease.

Now those lines are blurring as specialists realize that many if not most patients have a mix of the two dementias. Somehow, factors like hypertension — blood pressure readings of 140 over 90 or higher — that weaken arteries also seem to spur Alzheimer's disease-like processes.

One suspect: **Scarring known as white matter lesions.** White matter acts as the brain's telephone network, a system of axons, or nerve fibers, that allow brain cells to communicate with each other. Even slightly elevated blood pressure can damage the tiny blood vessels that nourish white matter, interrupting those signals.

Among the strongest new studies:

_MRI scans showed women 65 and older with high blood pressure had significantly more white matter lesions in their brains eight years later. The study included 1,403 women who were enrolled in a memory subset of the landmark Women's Health Initiative that tracked postmenopausal health. **The worse their blood pressure, the higher volume of white matter damage,** says the study published in the Journal of Clinical Hypertension.

"This is a silent disease in the brain," says lead researcher Dr. Lewis Kuller of the University of Pittsburgh. "It's evolving over time and it leads to very bad outcomes."

_The journal Stroke just published similar evidence from a Johns Hopkins University-led study that tracked **983 people for more than 15 years, starting in middle age. The longer people spent with uncontrolled high blood pressure, the more white matter damage they accumulated.** The researchers could see a change with each 20-point jump in too-high systolic pressure, the top number in a blood-pressure reading.

Clearly, hypertension alone doesn't doom someone to later dementia. Far more people, nearly one in three U.S. adults, have hypertension.

And there are plenty of other reasons to lower blood pressure: **Hypertension is a leading cause of heart attacks, strokes and kidney failure.**

But **while some studies have found hypertension treatment lowered the dementia risk, others haven't.**

Enter the **NIH's SPRINT study**, which is to begin enrolling 7,500 hypertension patients age 55 and older around the country. The test: Whether aggressive treatment to lower systolic blood pressure below 120 — what's considered normal — will prove healthier than today's guidelines that urge getting it below 140, or 130 for diabetics.

With dementia rising fast as the population grays, **even a small effect from better blood pressure control could have a big public health impact**, says Dr. William Thies of the Alzheimer's Association.

Other dementia-preventing efforts, such as targeting the sticky amyloid plaques in Alzheimer's patients brains, haven't panned out so far — while hypertension control has little downside, notes Pittsburgh's Kuller.

Uric acid levels tied to impaired thinking in the elderly

Uric acid is one of the most prominent antioxidants in the human body.

Even mildly elevated levels of uric acid in the elderly are associated with slower thinking and memory problems, according to a report by researchers at Yale and Johns Hopkins Schools of Medicine in Neuropsychology.

The researchers found that **elderly individuals with uric acid levels at the high end of the normal range had the lowest scores on tests measuring mental processing speed, verbal memory and working memory**. The study included among 96 persons between the ages of 60 and 92.

"These findings suggest that **high normal concentrations of serum uric acid should be added to the growing list of cardiovascular and metabolic biomarkers of mild cognitive impairment among elderly adults**," said Godfrey Pearlson, M.D., psychiatry professor at Yale and co-author of the study.

Uric acid is produced from digested food and the breakdown of the body's cells. Most uric acid is filtered out by the kidneys and passes out of the body in urine. The level of uric acid in the blood increases if too much is being produced or if the kidneys are not able to remove it from the blood normally.

The researchers said the mechanism linking uric acid levels and cognitive functioning is unknown. **I believe uric acid helps create an EMOD insufficiency state.**

Elevated uric acid commonly accompanies hypertension, increased concentration of lipids in the bloodstream, obesity, renal disease, insulin resistance, and the metabolic syndrome. The investigators found that the relationship of uric acid to cognition survived correction for most of these factors.

One question raised in the study was how the findings **could be reconciled with evidence that uric acid is an antioxidant that might protect against the development of Alzheimer's and Parkinson's disease.**

These investigators would call this another paradox.

"One possibility," said Pearlson, "is that despite being an antioxidant, uric acid can acquire pro-oxidant properties that damage the vascular endothelium in certain conditions and might even play a key role in the development of accelerated atherosclerosis." (Schretlen et al, 2007)

I believe that I have predicted the association of the increasing antioxidant, uric acid, with age and the onset of EMOD insufficiency diseases, such as atherosclerosis, diabetes, obesity, dementia and hypertension. I would suspect there is also an increased risk for cancer and arthritis and cataracts.

Investigators said that "It is odd that uric acid is linked with cognitive decline, since it has antioxidant properties that are thought to be protective in other situations."

The link between uric acid and dementia is likely due to an EMOD insufficiency as I have predicted in my books.

HIV patients face increased risk of diabetes and dementia

In January of 2005, Edwin J. Bernard (Source: Aidsmap) published in the Journal of AIDS a report that **HIV patients who develop diabetes as a result are more prone to developing HIV-associated dementia** also. Researchers state that higher fasting glucose levels are responsible for the increased risk of dementia and it is thus imperative that optimal blood sugar control is achieved in AIDS patients who have diabetes. **Research results from another study found that diabetes produced a trebled risk of dementia in people without HIV.** Unrelated studies report that 15% of HIV patients develop dementia and up to 30% develop some signs of neurological impairment. Other studies have found that the prevalence of diabetes was 2.11 times higher in HIV patients not taking HAART and 5.36 times higher in those taking HAART compared to healthy men. More research needs to be done to determine the mechanism by which HIV patients are more prone to dementia and diabetes.

Dementia, Type 2 diabetes, vascular disease increased in black Americans

America's black population has the highest incidence of Alzheimer's of any other American group. This is probably due to the fact that **black Americans also have a greater incidence of type 2 diabetes and vascular diseases such**

as high blood pressure and high cholesterol. Blacks face a 60% higher risk of type 2 diabetes than whites and 15% greater incidence of hypertension. The Alzheimer's Association claims that hypertension or high cholesterol double the risk of Alzheimer's disease. Studies show that black American's face a 14-100% greater risk of dementia and 44% of direct relatives of black Alzheimer's sufferers also face a risk of dementia. The other handicap that black dementia sufferers face is a general mistrust of doctors, lack of health care and economic reasons. This leads to later diagnosis and hence a poorer outcome. **I believe that this is related to decreased EMOD levels and represents a part of what I call an EMOD insufficiency syndrome.**

Much of Alzheimer's research has focused on so-called amyloid plaques, a buildup of proteins inside the brain between cells that appears to contribute to dementia. But Geschwind and his colleagues looked at tangles, another part of the puzzle. **These tangles of protein, called tau, are associated with cognitive decline in Alzheimer's and similar "tauopathy" diseases.**

Alzheimer's disease appears to have multiple causes, and scientists are slow at unraveling them.

The following was taken from: http://health.nytimes.com/health/guides/disease/alzheimers-disease/prevention.html

The emerging role of infection in Alzheimer's disease

A number of chronic diseases are in fact caused by one or more infectious agents. For example, stomach ulcers are caused by **Helicobacter pylori**, chronic lung disease in newborns and chronic asthma in adults are both caused by **Mycoplasmas and Chlamydia** pneumonia, while some other pathogens have been associated with atherosclerosis. The realization that pathogens can produce slowly progressive chronic diseases has opened new lines of research into Alzheimer's disease.

In a special issue of the *Journal of Alzheimer's Disease* published May 2008, guest editors Judith Miklossy, from The University of British Columbia, and Ralph N. Martins, from Edith Cowan University and Hollywood Private Hospital, Perth, Western Australia, and a group of experts explore this exciting topic.

Alzheimer's disease (AD), the most frequent cause of dementia, is a form of amyloidosis. It has been known for a century that dementia, brain atrophy and amyloidosis can be caused by chronic bacterial infections, namely by Treponema pallidum in the atrophic form of general paresis in syphilis. Bacteria and viruses are powerful stimulators of inflammation. It was **suggested by**

Alois Alzheimer and his colleagues a century ago that microorganisms may be contributors in the generation of senile plaques in AD.

The fact that pathogens may suppress, subvert or evade host defenses and establish chronic or latent infection has received little attention in the past. **During infection, active oxygen and nitrogen species generated by inflammatory cells may allegedly cause DNA damage, induce apoptosis, and modulate enzyme activities and gene expression**. Depending upon the biology of the pathogen and the host defense mechanisms the organism can persist in the infected tissues and cause chronic inflammation and amyloid deposition. The outcome of infection is as much determined by the genetic predisposition of the patient as by the virulence and biology of the infecting agent. Environmental factors and nutrition are critical determinants of disease expression as well.

In this special issue a series of reviews draws attention to both historic and recent observations related to this emerging field of AD research. **The first review shows the importance of chronic inflammation in AD, followed by three articles presenting evidence on the involvement of spirochetes, Chlamydia pneumoniae and Herpes simplex virus type 1 in AD**. These are followed by a review of amyloid proteins, which occur in many cellular forms in Eukaryotes and Prokaryotes.

According to Miklossy and Martins, "The historic and new observations reviewed in this special issue clearly show that high priority should be given for further research in this field as it may have major implications for public health, treatment, and prevention as adequate anti-bacterial and anti-viral drugs are available. **Treatment of a bacterial infection and associated viral infection may result in regression** and, if started early, prevention of disease. The impact on reducing healthcare costs would be substantial."

CHAPTER EIGHT

Nonsteroidal Anti-Inflammatory Drugs (NSAIDs) as Prevention

Several trials have investigated the use of anti-inflammatory drugs (including aspirin) in preventing Alzheimer's disease. The trials were based on the premise that because inflammation may be involved in the process of Alzheimer's disease, anti-inflammatory drugs may help to prevent it.

Evidence from these trials indicates that **aspirin, naproxen, and celecoxib do not appear to reduce the risk for Alzheimer's.** Also, some non-steroid anti-inflammatory drugs (NSAIDs) and Cox-2 inhibitors have been associated with cardiovascular risks.

NSAIDs have also been investigated for treatment of Alzheimer's disease. To date, rigorous **studies have failed to show a benefit**.

Heart-Protective Medications and Behaviors

The same lifestyle and medical choices that reduce risk factors for heart disease and diabetes may help lower the risk for Alzheimer's disease.

Blood Pressure Drugs. Because high blood pressure is associated with increased risk of Alzheimer's, researchers have been studying whether blood pressure medication can reduce this risk. Good blood pressure control **may** help to prevent the onset of Alzheimer's.

Statins. Statins are common drugs used to lower cholesterol levels. In past years, a number of studies reported a significantly lower risk for Alzheimer's disease in patients who took statins. However, **newer studies have failed to prove that statins can help prevent Alzheimer's disease**.

Lipitor(R) has no significant impact on AD

Results from the largest statin study (LEAPe) of patients with AD showed Lipitor (R) had no significant impact on the disease. (American Academy of Neurology meeting, 2008)

In April of 2008, a study in patients with mild-to-moderate Alzheimer's disease (AD), the addition of Lipitor (atorvastatin calcium tablets) 80 mg to Aricept® (donepezil HCl) 10 mg showed **no significant differences in cognition or global function** (key measures of Alzheimer's progression) compared to placebo plus Aricept 10 mg. Furthermore, **no statistically significant differences were seen on various cognitive, behavioral and functional secondary endpoints.** However, **the Lipitor arm was not associated with greater cognitive decline than the placebo arm in this trial.** The results were presented today at the annual **American Academy of Neurology** meeting in Chicago.

The **18-month study, called Lipitor's Effect on Alzheimer's Dementia (LEADe), included 640 patients** and is the largest statin study in Alzheimer's disease.

While rates of decline in cognition and global function were similar for both the Lipitor and placebo groups, there were some interesting findings from the trial:

In a sub set of 64 patients for whom MRI scans were available, **patients in the Lipitor arm had significantly less decline in hippocampal volume in the brain** compared to the placebo arm. While the clinical significance of this result is not yet fully understood, less decline in hippocampal volume may be beneficial since declines have been associated with the progression of Alzheimer's disease. This finding requires further investigation and analysis.

In a sub-analysis completed after the trial, **men in the Lipitor arm had a significantly slower rate of decline in cognition** compared to men in the placebo arm. **There was no difference in the rate of decline in cognition in women in the Lipitor arm** compared to women in the placebo arm. However, **no definitive conclusions can be drawn from this post-hoc analysis.**

"The results of our investigation of Lipitor on the symptoms of Alzheimer's disease have been long awaited," said Professor Howard Feldman, chair of the LEADe Steering Committee and professor and head of the division of neurology, University of British Columbia Hospital in Canada. "While **the LEADe study on Lipitor did not demonstrate significant benefits on the symptoms of mild to moderate Alzheimer's disease**, there are some noteworthy findings that require further analysis and should inform further research to determine the potential for statin use in this population."

Lipitor 80 mg was shown to be well tolerated and the incidence of liver and muscle adverse events in patients was low.

Aricept was selected as the background therapy since it is proven effective for treating the symptoms of Alzheimer's and is the most widely used cholinesterase inhibitor. The effect of Aricept on Alzheimer's was not investigated in this study.

"Over the past 15 years, Pfizer has been committed to researching the potential benefit of Lipitor in patients at various levels of cardiovascular risk as well as in non cardiovascular diseases such as Alzheimer's disease," said Dr. Rochelle Chaiken, vice president of the cardiovascular/metabolic team in Pfizer global medical. "While we are not planning additional studies with Lipitor in patients with Alzheimer's disease at this time, LEADe provides the medical community with important data.

Alzheimer's disease is a progressive degenerative brain disorder that gradually destroys a person's memory and ability to learn, reason, make judgments, communicate, and carry out daily activities. As the disease progresses, patient may experience changes in personality and behavior, such as anxiety, suspiciousness or agitation, as well as delusions or hallucinations.

Pfizer claims **Lipitor is the most prescribed cholesterol-lowering therapy in the world, with nearly 144 million patient-years of experience. Lipitor is supported by an extensive clinical trial program involving more than 400 ongoing and completed trials with more than 80,000 patients.** Lipitor is not for everyone. It is not for those with liver problems. And it is not for women who are nursing, pregnant or may become pregnant. Patients taking Lipitor should tell their doctors if they feel any new muscle pain or weakness. This could be a sign of rare but serious muscle side effects.

The manufacturer claims **ARICEPT is the number-one prescribed AD medication worldwide, with more than 3 billion patient days of ARICEPT therapy sold. Nearly 2.3 million people in the United States alone have begun ARICEPT therapy.**

ARICEPT is well tolerated but may not be for everyone. **People at risk for stomach ulcers or who take certain other medicines should tell their doctors because serious stomach problems, such as bleeding, may get worse. Some people who take ARICEPT may experience fainting. Some people may have nausea, vomiting, diarrhea, bruising, or not sleep well. Some people may**

have muscle cramps or loss of appetite or may feel tired. In studies, these were usually mild and temporary.

Male and Female Hormone Replacement Therapies

Hormone Therapy. Hormone replacement therapy (HT) has been studied for years for health effects after menopause, including its effect on mental decline. **A number of studies, including a major 2003 analysis, have found no differences in mental performance or protection from Alzheimer's disease in women taking HT compared to non-users.** Based on these results, researchers from **the National Institute on Aging (NIA) recommended against prescribing combination hormone therapy to older women for maintaining or improving cognitive function. It is even possible that women ages 65 years and older who take estrogen-only HT have a slightly increased risk of developing dementia.**

I believe this is due to the antioxidant properties of estrogens.

In contrast, Some testosterone converts to estrogen, which may be why older men appear to have a lower risk for Alzheimer's disease than older women. **Animal studies have suggested that testosterone may help reduce levels of beta amyloid.** There is also some evidence that low testosterone levels may be a particular risk factor in men with the ApoE4 gene. Some experts believe that giving testosterone to elderly men, and combinations of testosterone and estrogen to older women, may prove to be protective. However, **the evidence is far from conclusive and does not come from high quality studies.** Side effects of testosterone in women include increased body hair, acne, fluid retention, anxiety, and depression. Long-term benefits or serious adverse effects are unknown.

DHEA. Dehydroepiandrosterone (DHEA) is a male-like hormone in the body that declines with age. Some studies claim that it may help reduce mental decline in older women, **but not in older men. Evidence is far from conclusive**, however. While its effect on cancer-cell growth is unknown, **some evidence indicates that high levels may increase cancer risk. In any case,** DHEA is not regulated, and brands vary widely in their content.

Failed antioxidant studies in Alzheimer's disease

New York Times. August 9, 2008. **Antioxidant Supplements.** Much research on Alzheimer's disease has indicated that oxidation (release of damaging unstable particles) may play an important role in the disease process. Some reports, including a large 2002 population study, have suggested that vitamin E intake, from food or supplements, may protect against mental decline. Other studies suggest that vitamin E protects only those who carried the ApoE4 gene. Most of the evidence finding any benefits from other antioxidants comes from using a combination of antioxidant vitamins, such as vitamins C and E, but not from using them separately. However, **there is no strong evidence of AD protection to date from using antioxidant supplements.** (*New York Times. August 9, 2008*)

Physical Exercise. Studies indicate that exercise may help prevent the development of Alzheimer's disease and other forms of dementia. **A 2006 study found that older adults (65 years and older) who exercised three times a week reduced their risk for Alzheimer's by about 40%.** (*New York Times. August 9, 2008*)

Exercise in the study included walking, hiking, aerobics, calisthenics, swimming, water aerobics, weight training, and stretching.

CHAPTER NINE

Mental Exercise. Cognitive training that includes exercises to stimulate memory, reasoning, and mental processing speed may help improve both mental ability and enable patients to handle daily living tasks -- such as performing housework, managing money, and preparing meals. Other studies indicate that participating in intellectually engaging activity (such as doing crossword puzzles or learning a new language) may help reduce the risk of Alzheimer's disease

Because Alzheimer's disease rates vary among different populations, investigators are researching how diet can help in prevention. Caloric intake itself may play a role in brain health. However, **there is no evidence from randomized controlled trials that any specific diets or diet supplements prevent or treat Alzheimer's disease.** (*New York Times. August 9, 2008*)

Fighting memory loss through brain games, exercise and rest

The following was from a column, *growingolder@seattletimes.com*.

Brain-game claims are spreading like spring weeds across the media, promising to help us reduce memory loss and even prevent Alzheimer's disease as we grow older.

The reasoning: By exercising our minds through difficult new thinking tasks such as crossword puzzles and memory games, and by learning to use e-mail or speak French, we can keep our minds flexible and healthy.

Playing games to preserve our brains is a seductive idea, fueled by our fear of Alzheimer's. A survey in 2006 by MetLife Foundation showed **Americans age 55 and older fear Alzheimer's disease more than any other diagnosis, even**

cancer. I understand. Since my mom died of Alzheimer's, and my name- and word-finding skills are plummeting, I want to know whether these claims are valid.

Some memory tasks stick with us better than others. You're much more likely to recognize that you've met someone before, for example, than you are to remember her name. But your failure to remember her name and many other things begins early in life. The average 45-year-old has a 35 percent loss in remembering a name compared with when he was 25. **By age 65, there's a 62 percent deficit (compared to age 25) and by age 75, a 74 percent deficit.**

Whew! So far, I feel normal.

It's called **"Age-Associated Memory Impairment,"** a normal decline of memory as we age that's not associated with developing Alzheimer's disease. That's according to Thomas H. Crook, former chair of the National Institute of Mental Health and American Psychological Association Task Forces on the Diagnoses and Treatment of Age-Associated Memory Impairment. Crook wrote the excellent new book, "The Memory Advantage: Improve Your Memory, Mood and Confidence Throughout Life" (*SelectBooks, Inc; $21.95*).

There are other causes of memory loss in older people: some medications, stress, depression, heart disease, not drinking enough water, not eating nutritiously and certain medical problems. Diabetes, for example, is associated with memory loss among people with type 2 diabetes over age 65. "It's almost as if diabetes speeds up the normal process of brain aging," writes Crook.

At the University of Washington's VA Memory Wellness Program in Seattle, research is under way to explore the relationship between insulin, blood sugar and memory loss in older adults. One out of three Americans over age 60 has poor blood-sugar regulation — a factor related to memory loss, says lead investigator Suzanne Craft. Perhaps improving insulin activity will have a positive effect on memory, giving researchers new treatments in the future.

But what about now? Does playing games help?

The jury's still out, but here's some of what we know:

The most important way to keep your memory strong, experts agree, is to keep your brain healthy. That includes, "Think, Think, Think," says a great little flier published by the American Geriatrics Society (AGS) Foundation for Health in Aging (available at www.healthinaging.org/public_education/cognitive_vitality.pdf). Pushing your brain to try new games, recipes, languages, driving routes, technology and other new skills won't hurt you, and it's likely to help

— because using your brain in new ways stimulates new neuron pathways or brain cells.

"A lot of studies are now using brain stimulation," says Jane Tornatore, a consultant with the Alzheimer's Association in Seattle and a therapist in private practice specializing in memory problems and mid-life transitions, "and some show memory improvement. While they may not actually prevent a dementing illness, they give families hope — something to do that may be helpful."

Unfortunately, there's no miracle. "But from all of my reading and experience," says Tornatore, **"exercise is the best thing we can do to keep our minds healthy."** Echoes the AGS flyer: **"Exercise increases blood flow to the brain, which helps keep the brain healthy and working well. Exercise may even help new brain cells grow."**

Another critical factor is diet. "Results **from two recent studies suggest that people who exercise regularly or eat healthy diets are less likely to develop Alzheimer's disease**," reports Craft, with even better results for those who do both. As an added benefit, "a healthy diet and regular exercise can improve your mood and help control your weight and blood pressure," all factors in keeping your brain working better.

Getting enough sleep and reducing stress are also important. "Older adults don't need less sleep than younger adults," says the AGS. Sleeping less than seven or eight hours can make it harder to concentrate and remember. And, over time, stress can make it hard to get a good night's rest. So finding ways to reduce your stress through exercise, prayer and meditation may help you sleep, plus improve your memory. *growingolder@seattletimes.com or www.seattletimes.com/growingolder/.*

Loneliness could boost Alzheimer's risk

In 2007, HealthDay News reported that **being lonely may increase the risk of developing Alzheimer's disease later in life**, new research suggests.

Researchers at the Rush University Medical Center in Chicago assessed loneliness and dementia in **823 people**, averaging almost 81 years of age, for up to four years. At the start of the study, the participants' overall average loneliness score was 2.3 on a scale from 1 (lowest) to 5.

Seventy-six people developed Alzheimer's disease during the course of the study, which is published in the February 2007 issue of the journal Archives of General Psychiatry. According to the researchers, each point of increase on the loneliness score was associated with about a 51 percent increased risk of developing Alzheimer's. This would mean that **a person with a high loneliness score (3.2) would be about 2.1 times more likely to develop Alzheimer's than someone with a low score (1.4), they said.**

Autopsies performed on 90 people who died during the study revealed that loneliness in life was not related to any of the characteristic brain changes -- such as nerve plaques and tangles -- that are associated with Alzheimer's disease. So, **the actual mechanism linking loneliness and Alzheimer's is unclear**, the researchers said. It's unlikely that Alzheimer's actually causes the loneliness, they said.

"In human beings, loneliness has been associated with impaired social skills. Thus, neural systems underlying social behavior might be less elaborated in lonely persons and, as a result, be less able to compensate for other neural systems compromised by age-related neuropathy," the study authors wrote.

Alzheimer's is unique. **It costs taxpayers three times as much to treat an Alzheimer's patient as any other patient under Medicare.**

If both parents have Alzheimer's, your risk soars

If both your parents have Alzheimer's disease, you probably are more much likely than other people to get it, researchers said.

Their study focused on 111 families in which both parents were diagnosed with Alzheimer's disease, the most common form of dementia among the elderly, and assessed the risk for developing it among the offspring.

The parents had 297 children who lived into adulthood. Of the 98 men and women who were at least 70 years old, 41 of them -- about 42 percent -- developed Alzheimer's disease, researchers at the University of Washington in Seattle found.

"That's greater than you would expect in the general population in that age group," Dr. Thomas Bird, one of the researchers, said in a telephone interview.

In the general population, risk for the disease begins to rise at about age 65, with the number of people developing the disease doubling every five years beyond that, experts say.

But about two-thirds of the adult offspring in the study still had not reached age 70. Counting all 297 of these adult offspring regardless of age, 23 percent already had been diagnosed with Alzheimer's disease, with the disease diagnosed on average at age 66, the researchers found.

Bird said that compares to the roughly one in 10 chance that the average person will develop the disease.

"I think it confirms that there's a strong genetic component in the disease and that's not a surprise," said Bird, whose study was published in the **Archives of Neurology**.

Scientists do not yet fully understand the causes of Alzheimer's disease, although genetics plays an important role. There is no cure.

Bird said there is only one gene, known as ApoE, that is generally agreed among researchers as a risk factor for the disease but there likely are many more.

The ApoE gene is involved in making a substance in the body that helps carry cholesterol in the bloodstream and the gene seems to influence the age of onset of Alzheimer's.

The researchers have been doing the study for about two decades and intend to continue for at least another decade.

"The numbers will be interesting to follow as they get older and older," Bird said.

Bird said the study is not examining the Alzheimer's risk for people who have one but not two parents who develop the disease.

In order to confirm that both parents actually had Alzheimer's, the researchers reviewed the medical records and in many cases the brain autopsies of those who had died, and tried to meet in person to assess those who were still living.

In people with Alzheimer's disease, healthy brain tissue degenerates, causing an inexorable decline in memory and mental abilities. **The average length of time from diagnosis to death is about eight years.**

People live 4.5 years after dementia strikes

Michael Kahn reported that **people with dementia survive an average four-and-a-half years after diagnosis**, researchers said on Friday in a study they hope might help care-givers plan for patients with Alzheimer's and other, similar illnesses.

Researchers know dementia raises the risk of dying early but the study is the first to estimate how long people are likely to survive with the condition, said Carol Brayne, a researcher at the Institute of Public Health at the University of Cambridge.

"This gives people a rough idea of how long they are looking at," said Brayne, who led the study published in the British Medical Journal. "This can add more to the information that physicians and families have."

An estimated 24 million people worldwide have the mental confusion marked by memory loss and problems with orientation that signals Alzheimer's disease and other forms of dementia.

The researchers, who said the number of people with dementia was expected to rise to 81 million globally by 2040, studied 13,000 people aged 65 or older who were assessed for the condition at regular intervals between 1991 to 2005.

During this time, 438 people developed dementia, of whom 81 percent died. **Age, gender and disability were the main factors determining how long a person survived,** the researchers said.

Women lived for 4.6 years compared to 4.1 years for men. There was nearly seven years difference in survival between the youngest and oldest, with people aged 65 to 69 living 10.7 years and those over 90 living 3.8 years, the researchers found.

"The type of care and the environment where a person is living is also important," Brayne said in a telephone interview.

The study also found that the most frail patients died on average three years sooner than people who are more robust, even with age factored in.

The findings might help policy makers, families and health professionals better plan and care for people with dementia to determine things such as how long a person might be in an institution, the researchers said.

"Some of these results may seem self-evident but they answer questions asked by those caring for and advising people with dementia," the researchers wrote.

"We hope the estimates will be valuable to patients, clinicians, carers, service providers and policy makers."

Most older adults have brain disease

Megan Rauscher reported that **results of a brain autopsy study indicate that most older adults have significant brain pathology (disease), regardless of the presence or absence of outward signs of dementia.**

As part of the long-term Rush Memory and Aging Project, researchers evaluated the spectrum of abnormalities found in the brains of 141 older adults, with and without clinically evident dementia.

At the time of death, only 20 persons (14.2 percent) were free of brain disease, Dr. Julie A. Schneider, from Rush University Medical Center, Chicago, and colleagues found.

Most older persons with dementia (i.e., memory and other cognitive impairments) had more than one type of pathology in their brain causing the impairment, Schneider told Reuters Health.

"This most commonly was Alzheimer's disease pathology and cerebral infarcts (strokes), followed by Alzheimer's disease and Lewy body disease, a disease related to Parkinson's disease," she said.

Older persons without dementia also frequently had brain disease, most commonly Alzheimer's-like disease, but also multiple other abnormalities, Schneider noted. Having more than one disease in the brain significantly increased the likelihood that symptoms of dementia will be present.

"Older persons can often handle one pathology in their brain, but the burden of more than one pathology may tip them over the threshold of clinical dementia," Schneider said.

Therefore, prevention of not only Alzheimer's disease but these other pathologies, particularly stroke and those things that may increase the risk of stroke, like high blood pressure, high cholesterol, cigarette smoking, obesity, "are likely to significantly decrease the prevalence of dementia," Schneider added.

The findings are published in the journal **Neurology,** December 11, 2007.

Based on this study, write two neurologists in an accompanying editorial, "we may wish to maximize medical management of vascular risk factors in the growing elderly population, regardless of whether cognition is still normal or there are signs of overt dementia."

CHAPTER TEN

Dietary factors and AD

Because Alzheimer's disease rates vary among different populations, investigators are researching how diet can help in prevention. Caloric intake itself may play a role in brain health. However, **there is no evidence from randomized controlled trials that any specific diets or diet supplements prevent or treat Alzheimer's disease**.

Fats and Oils. **Some studies suggest an association between fat and Alzheimer's disease, including a lower prevalence of Alzheimer's disease in countries where fat intake is low.**

In general, the recommended dietary goal is to limit total fat intake to 25 - 35% of total daily calories. But not all fats are alike. Unhealthy fats include saturated fats (contained in animal products such as meat) and trans-fatty acids (contained in fast foods and commercially baked products). The American Heart Association recommends limiting saturated fat intake to less than 7% of total daily calories and trans-fatty acid intake to less than 1% of total daily calories.

Omega-3 fish oil. **Omega-3 fatty acids are excellent sources of unsaturated fats.** Docosahexaenoic acid (DHA) is a type of omega-3 fatty acid found in fish oil. In 2007, the U.S. National Institutes of Health launched a large-scale clinical trial to evaluate whether DHA supplements can slow the progression of cognitive and functional decline in people with mild-to-moderate Alzheimer's disease.

Thus far, studies have not supported the use of omega-3 in AD patients. Surprisingly, in 2009, Harvard linked fish and omega-3 fats to type 2 diabetes. Following **195,204 adults** for 14 to 18 years, researchers reported in 2009 that they had found that **the more fish or long-chain omega-3 fatty acids participants consumed, the higher their risk of developing diabetes**. (Kaushik et al, 2009)

Meanwhile, fish oil manufacturers pinned their hopes on brain function. Maybe fish oil could make you smarter. But in 2010, researchers dashed those hopes also. A group of **867 elderly people** were randomly assigned to either **a fish-oil supplement** or placebo. After two years of supplementation, **elderly adults showed no benefit at all in tests for reaction time, spatial memory, and processing speed measurements.** (Dangour et al, 2010)

A later 2010 JAMA report showed that **omega-3 supplements do not slow mental decline in Alzheimer's patients.** (Quinn et al, 2010)

And at the other end of the age spectrum, babies get no benefit either from omega-3s. A JAMA report showed that **consumption of fish oil during pregnancy does not benefit babies' cognitive development.** (Makrides et al, 2010)

In these reports, **fish oil is sounding more like snake oil.** The new findings linking higher DHA levels to cancer add yet another reason to use caution with fish oil supplements.

Fish oil has failed its marketing claims. Specifically, **it is no help for heart patients, does not forestall Alzheimer's disease, does not prevent depression, and does not make babies smarter.**

A 2011 study in rats shows that fish oils can block chemotherapy drugs. So, be cautious with their use. Prof Emile Voest University Medical Centre Utrecht said, "**Using drugs to block the production of the fatty acids prevented this form of resistance which "significantly enhances the chemotherapy."**

Also in 2010, the New England Journal of Medicine reported **similarly dismal results with heart patients given omega-3 fatty acids in addition to standard drug therapy.** They had **no reduction in cardiovascular events.** (Krombout et al, 2010)

Oily fish dementia boosts queried

A UK study has cast doubt on claims that eating oily fish can protect against dementia in old age. Data from a trial of more than 800 older people initially showed that those who eat plenty of oily fish seem to have better cognitive function. But factors such as education and mood explained most of the link.

Researchers need to clarify what, if any, benefits fish oil has on the ageing brain, they wrote in the Journal of Nutrition, Health and Ageing. In recent years, there has been increasing interest in diet as a way of preventing dementia. Much focus has been on omega 3 fatty acids found in oily fish, such as salmon and mackerel. And there are biological reasons, backed by tests in the laboratory, why in theory, these fatty acids would be neuroprotective.

The latest study found a significant association between eating a couple of portions of fish a week and better scores on tests of cognitive function. But **when the researchers, from the London School of Hygiene and Tropical Medicine, took into account education and psychological health the association almost disappeared.**

Experts advise eating a couple of portions of fish a week, with at least one being an oily fish, because there are proven benefits on the heart.

Study leader Dr Alan Dangour said **claims about the benefits of oily fish in warding of dementia in older people seemed to have been oversold.** "The evidence on this has always been sporadic. **"What this shows is there is a link between people who eat oily fish and better cognitive function, but if you adjust for education and mood this relationship goes, so it's not at all clear that healthy older people get any benefit from eating fish oil."**

The evidence collected by Dr Dangour was for a study due to report later comparing fish oil supplements with placebo. He added that this randomised, controlled study should provide clarification.

Neil Hunt, chief executive of the Alzheimer's Society, said: "One of the best ways to reduce your risk of dementia is by eating a Mediterranean diet rich in fruit, vegetables, grains, fish and poultry. "However, we still do not know which components of this sort of diet help the most. "Unfortunately this study does not add to our understanding.

"Once age, sex and education are accounted for, the research does not show any significant benefit of regularly eating oily fish."

Rebecca Wood, of the Alzheimer's Research Trust, said: "Research into the effects of oily fish and other foodstuffs attracts much interest because it may offer a relatively inexpensive way to fight dementia, a devastatingly costly condition.

"Many scientists believe there is a link between diet and reducing dementia risk. More research is desperately needed to understand the effects of diet, including omega-3 fatty acids, on the brain."

Fruits and Vegetables. **A 2006 study of over 3,000 elderly adults found that consumption of vegetables (especially green leafy vegetables) helped reduce the rate of cognitive decline, but fruit intake had no effect.** http://health.nytimes.com/health/guides/disease/alzheimers-disease/prevention.html

Alcohol. Some **studies have suggested that moderate intake of alcohol (one or two drinks a day) may protect the aging brain**, possibly by releasing acetylcholine, the chemical in the brain that is deficient in Alzheimer's disease. **Not all studies have been positive.** In any case, heavy alcohol consumption offers no protection and is dangerous.

Alzheimer's starts earlier for heavy drinkers, smokers

Heavy drinkers and heavy smokers develop Alzheimer's disease years earlier than people with Alzheimer's who do not drink or smoke heavily, according to research presented at the American Academy of Neurology 60th Anniversary Annual Meeting in Chicago, April 12-19, 2008.

"These results are significant because it's possible that if we can reduce or eliminate heavy smoking and drinking, we could substantially delay the onset of Alzheimer's disease for people and reduce the number of people who have Alzheimer's at any point in time," said study author Ranjan Duara, MD, of the Wien Center for Alzheimer's Disease at Mount Sinai Medical Center in Miami Beach, FL, and Fellow of the American Academy of Neurology.

"It has been projected that a delay in the onset of the disease by five years would lead to a nearly 50-percent reduction in the total number of Alzheimer's cases," said Duara. "In this study, we found that the combination of heavy drinking and heavy smoking reduced the age of onset of Alzheimer's disease by six to seven years, **making these two factors among the most important preventable risk factors for Alzheimer's disease."**

The study looked at **938 people** age 60 and older who were diagnosed with possible or probable Alzheimer's disease. The researchers gathered information from family members on drinking and smoking history and determined whether the participants had **the epsilon 4 gene variant of the APOE gene, which increases the risk of Alzheimer's disease.** People with the **epsilon 4 variant** also develop Alzheimer's at an earlier age than those who do not have the gene variant.

Seven percent of the study participants had a history of heavy drinking, which was defined as more than two drinks per day. Twenty percent had a history of heavy smoking, which was defined as smoking one pack of cigarettes or more per day. And 27 percent had the APOE epsilon 4 variant.

Researchers found that people who were **heavy drinkers developed Alzheimer's 4.8 years earlier** than those who were not heavy drinkers. **Heavy smokers developed the disease 2.3 years soone**r than people who were not heavy smokers.

People with APOE epsilon 4 developed the disease three years sooner than those without the gene variant.

Adding the risk factors together led to earlier onset of the disease. People who had all three risk factors developed the disease 8.5 years earlier than those with none of the risk factors. The **17 people in the study** with all three risk factors developed Alzheimer's at an average age of 68.5 years; the **374 people with none** of the three risk factors developed the disease at an average age of 77 years.

This research adds to the weight of evidence on drinking and smoking habits and the risk of developing dementia. **Smoking, drinking heavily and having high cholesterol can all lead to an increased risk of developing this devastating condition** and the risk is further increased for individuals with **a particular genetic variant**. Not only is dementia devastating for the individual and their family, it also places a huge burden on society. If we can reduce the number of people living with dementia we can increase the quality of life and independence of older people in our communities.

Cholesterol

High cholesterol levels in your 40s may raise the chance of developing Alzheimer's disease decades later, according to a study underscoring the importance of health factors in middle age on risk for the brain ailment.

The study involving **9,752 people** in northern California found that **those with high cholesterol levels between ages 40 and 45 were about 50 percent more likely than those with low cholesterol levels to later develop Alzheimer's disease.**

The findings were presented on 4/16/08 at a meeting of the American Academy of Neurology in Chicago.

"Alzheimer's disease does not happen overnight," Dr. Alina Solomon of the University of Kuopio in Finland, who helped lead the study, said in a telephone interview.

"Alzheimer's disease has a very long preclinical phase -- a silent phase -- when you don't see any signs of the disease, but the disease is there. The pathological changes in the brain can sometimes develop over decades."

Alzheimer's disease is the most common form of dementia among older people, and researchers have been working to understand its causes and risk factors.

The findings come just weeks after another study showed that **having a big belly in middle age may greatly increase one's risk of later developing Alzheimer's disease or another form of dementia.**

Rachel Whitmer of the Kaiser Permanente Division of Research in Oakland, California who led that study also was involved in the new one on cholesterol levels.

"Cholesterol is just one piece of the puzzle. There are other risk factors like hypertension and obesity. The more risk factors you have, the higher the risk gets," Solomon said.

Solomon said previous research had looked at the issue of high cholesterol levels in middle age as a risk factor for later development of dementia, but did not focus specifically on Alzheimer's disease.

The people in the new study underwent detailed health evaluations between 1964 and 1973 when they were ages 40 to 45, including blood cholesterol measurements. The researchers then looked at the cholesterol measurements of the 504 people in the study who developed Alzheimer's disease decades later.

High levels of cholesterol -- a waxy, fat-like substance that occurs naturally in the body -- in the blood can raise one's risk of heart disease. Physical inactivity, obesity and a fatty diet can contribute to high cholesterol.

"The association between cholesterol and cardiovascular disease is well known. What we know now is that minding heart health may protect your brain as well," Solomon said.

Exercise and eating more fruits and vegetables can lower cholesterol, and there are cholesterol-lowering drugs as well.

Folate and Vitamin B12. **While some studies have described a benefit with administration of vitamin B12, or vitamin B6, there is no good evidence from randomized controlled trials that these supplements prevent Alzheimer's disease.** http://health.nytimes.com/health/guides/disease/alzheimers-disease/prevention.html

Homocysteine, vitamin B12 impact risk of Alzheimer's

High levels of homocysteine and low levels of vitamin B12 may increase the risk of Alzheimer's disease. Babak Hooshmand, MD, and his colleagues at the Karolinska

Institute, Sweden, measured blood levels of homocysteine and "holotranscobalamin," the

active form of vitamin B12, in the blood of **271 people** ages 65 to 71 years. Elevated levels of homocysteine, which can usually be controlled with supplemental folic acid and vitamin B12, are a risk factor for heart disease, stroke, and Alzheimer's. None of the subjects had any signs of dementia at the beginning of the study. Seven years later, 17 of

the subjects had been diagnosed with Alzheimer's disease. **People with high levels of homocysteine and relatively low levels of vitamin B12 were more likely to develop Alzheimer's disease.** (Hooshmand et al, 2010)

Eating less cuts AD symptoms in mice

In 2006 it was proposed that eating fewer calories may help prevent the symptoms of Alzheimer's disease, researchers reported. A study in mice suggests a lower-calorie diet can help trigger the production of a protein that protects the brain from the disease, said researchers at the Mount Sinai School of Medicine in New York City.

In the study, the mice in one group were permitted to eat as they wished, while the other group of mice was fed only 70 percent of that amount. When the animals were killed six months later, researchers discovered the brains of the calorie-restricted mice held significantly higher levels of **an anti-aging protein, SIRT1**, the researchers reported in the July issue of the Journal of Biological Chemistry.

That protein has been shown to curtail and reverse the production of plaque in the brain, a typical symptom of Alzheimer's disease. Researchers have found the protein can also enhance the function of a patient's metabolism, kidneys and liver. "The real message is that, **in an animal model of Alzheimer's disease, caloric restriction led to the elevation of molecules that are associated with longevity and good health**," said Dr. Giulio Pasinetti, a professor of psychiatry and neuroscience who led the study. "This may be the reason why caloric restriction may work to prevent Alzheimer's disease."

According to the National Institute of Aging, **about 4.5 million Americans** are living with Alzheimer's disease, the most common cause of elderly dementia.

Its first symptom is often a mild forgetfulness that escalates into an inability to care for oneself and, eventually, death. **There is no cure**, and treatments merely delay the progression of the disease for a short time.

The Mount Sinai study bolsters other research that has found a relationship between what and how much people eat and risk for the disease in general. "The same things that we know are good for your body -- particularly your vascular system -- are all part of maintaining healthy brain function," said Dr. Bill Thies, a staff pharmacologist at the Alzheimer's Association.

Pasinetti said his team had already replicated their experiment in monkeys and recorded similar results. They hope to begin a human version of the study by the end of the year. Subjects would likely be near 70 years of age and submit to a more modest calorie reduction of perhaps 10 or 15 percent.

Antioxidant Supplements. **Some reports, including a large 2002 population study, have suggested that vitamin E intake, from food or supplements, may protect against mental decline. Other studies suggest that vitamin E protects only those who carried the ApoE4 gene.** However, **there is no strong evidence of protection to date from using antioxidant supplements.**

In 2007, Dr. Kristine Yaffe of the San Francisco Veterans Affairs Medical Center and University of California at San Francisco stated, **"For the clinician, there is no convincing justification to recommend the use of antioxidant dietary supplements to maintain cognitive performance in cognitively normal adults or in those with mild cognitive impairment."** (Nov. 2007, Archives of Internal Medicine)

Scyllo-inositol delays Alzheimer's

Certain variants of a simple sugar ameliorate Alzheimer's-like disease in mice, according to a new study by Canadian researchers. Although the new studies are still in the early stages, the findings could lead to new therapies that prevent or delay the onset of Alzheimer's disease. The new studies show that some types of a sugar called **cyclohexanehexol**—also known as inositol—**prevented the accumulation of amyloid β deposits**, a hallmark of Alzheimer's disease. Scyllo-inositol treatment also improved cognitive abilities in the mice and allowed them to live a normal lifetime. The study appeared in advance online publication of the journal **Nature Medicine on June 11, 2006**.

HHMI international research scholar and senior author Peter St George-Hyslop cautioned that the chemicals tested in these studies are not the type of inositol sold commercially as a nutritional supplement. That type—**myo-inositol—has been shown previously to be ineffective at breaking up amyloid aggregates**, he said.

In the brain of a person with Alzheimer's disease, small proteins called amyloid β aggregate into plaques, and a protein called tau clumps into neurofibrillary tangles.

The brain becomes inflamed and neurons atrophy and die. It's not completely clear what kind of amyloid β peptide (monomers, oligomeric aggregates, or fibrillar aggregates) is responsible for the onset of disease, said St George-Hyslop of the University of Toronto. "Because we were able to show that scyllo-inositol specifically dispersed the high-molecular-weight oligomeric aggregates, this study confirms that the initiating event is the accumulation of oligomeric aggregates of amyloid β peptide," he said.

Previous work by JoAnne McLaurin, also of the University of Toronto and lead author of the Nature Medicine paper, showed that several types of inositol could stop amyloid proteins from aggregating in test tubes. To see if these compounds could do the same in vivo, St George-Hyslop, McLaurin, and colleagues tested them in transgenic mice with human genes that predispose them to an Alzheimer's-like disease.

When the researchers treated these mice with scyllo-inositol, all of the animals' disease symptoms improved. Cognitive function was improved, amyloid plaques disappeared, inflammation declined, and the mice lived longer. The scientists found that scyllo-inositol conferred these benefits not only if the mice were treated when they were very young and disease-free, but also if they were treated after the onset of disease.

As a model system, these mice "are pretty good, but they're not a perfect replica of the disease," St George-Hyslop said. The mice do not develop tau tangles, he explained, but they are prone to amyloid plaques, brain inflammation, cognitive disturbance, and early death, just like humans with Alzheimer's disease.

The researchers found that scyllo-inositol worked better than the epi-inositol version. Scyllo-inositol produced more dramatic benefits overall, while epi-inositol worked only transiently and only when given before disease symptoms appeared. Scyllo-inositol "is an exciting experimental therapy, but until it has actually been tested in humans, it should not be considered the cure for Alzheimer's disease," St George-Hyslop said. "There are many things that are very promising when done in animal models that turn out to either not work in humans or to have unexpected toxicity."

A public Canadian company called Transition Therapeutics has regulatory approval for clinical trials of scyllo-inositol in humans with Alzheimer's disease. Phase one trials began about a week ago. St George-Hyslop has a small financial interest in the company.

St George-Hyslop and his colleagues are optimistic that scyllo-inositol will be less toxic to humans than some previous drug candidates for Alzheimer's disease. A vaccine designed to destroy amyloid β, for example, was first tested successfully in the same type of mice used in the scyllo-inositol studies, but the vaccine turned out to be toxic in some humans. It caused an autoimmune reaction in about 10 percent of patients who were immunized, St George-Hyslop said.

Autoimmune responses shouldn't be a problem with scyllo-inositol. "This compound works by a different mechanism and doesn't involve immunizing a patient with his own protein, which was probably the origin of the allergic reaction to the vaccine," the researcher said.

Another complication with previous attempts to treat Alzheimer's disease has been that some compounds—such as beta secretase inhibitors—cannot enter the brain easily, St George-Hyslop explained. Scyllo-inositol, on the other hand, readily passes through the blood-brain barrier where it is made available to the central nervous system. Even if scyllo-inositol does prove safe and effective in humans, patients will likely still need drugs designed to attack other aspects of Alzheimer's pathology, such as tau neurofibrillary tangles, St George-Hyslop said.

"Alzheimer's disease is probably going to be treated by a cocktail of drugs," he predicted. "Some of them might be this compound, or one like it, that blocks the toxicity and aggregation of amyloid."

CHAPTER ELEVEN

Physical exercise

Physical Exercise. Studies indicate that **exercise may help prevent the development of Alzheimer's disease and other forms of dementia. A 2006 study found that older adults (65 years and older) who exercised three times a week reduced their risk for Alzheimer's by about 40%.**

Very few Americans physically active

Nearly everyone understands that regular physical activity can reduce the risk of overweight, diabetes, cardiovascular diseases, and cancer. But a team of American researchers has found that very few people actually engage in any type of daily vigorous

activity. **In a study of almost 80,000 Americans, the researchers reported that only 5 percent of people exercised vigorously** (not including people whose jobs involved physical activity). The most common types of exercise were using cardiovascular equipment and running. One-fourth of the subjects described food and drink preparation as their physical activities, although the researchers classified these activities as sedentary. (Tudor-Locke, 2010)

Aerobic activity may reverse mental decline

Summing up, Kramer and Erickson point out that "many questions remain unanswered" regarding the effects of exercise on the brain. However, "we can safely argue that **an active lifestyle with moderate amounts of aerobic activity will likely improve cognitive and brain function, and reverse the neural decay frequently observed in older adults**," they conclude. Regular aerobic exercise can not only stave off the decline in brain function that often comes with age, it can also help turn back the clock on brain aging, two experts in the field report, based on a critical review of published studies.

In people with or those without signs of dementia or Alzheimer's disease, regular moderate physical activity, enough to make a person breathless, has been shown to boost not only the speed and sharpness of thought but also the actual volume of brain tissue and the way in which the brain functions, Kramer and Erickson note. (Erickson, Kramer, 2009)

Exercise not proven as dementia treatment

In July of 2008, investigators released a statement saying physical activity is a good thing for nearly everybody and clearly boosts alertness and a sense of well-being. So can we use it as a treatment for elderly patients with dementia? That's a good question, **but existing research doesn't provide an answer, according to a new Cochrane Library review**.

"Physical activity may be beneficial for persons with dementia. But due to the small number of studies we have not been able to demonstrate this," said review lead author Dorothy Forbes, an associate professor with the faculty of health sciences at the University of Western Ontario, in Canada.

On the other hand, **there is no evidence that physical activity is harmful either**, she said.

Estimates indicate that dementia known in the past as **senility affects about 14 percent of Americans ages 71 and older**. More than one-third of Americans over 90 likely suffer from the condition, which causes forgetfulness, confusion and muddled thinking. A variety of medical conditions causes dementia, including Alzheimer's disease and stroke.

Physicians are unlikely to prescribe physical activity as a treatment for dementia patients because there is little evidence to support its value, Forbes said. Nevertheless, exercise is not impossible for many dementia patients, who might be able to walk, swim and exercise in groups with assistance, she said.

Researchers have shown that exercise can improve cognition and mental health in older adults, and some studies suggest that it could delay dementia from three to six years or reduce the risk that patients will develop cognitive problems, Forbes said.

"It is less clear if physical activity manages or improves other symptoms among persons with a diagnosis of dementia," she said.

In the new review, Forbes and colleagues sought to shed some light on that issue.

The review appears in The Cochrane Library, a publication of The Cochrane Collaboration, an international organization that evaluates medical research. Systematic reviews draw evidence-based conclusions about medical practice after considering both the content and quality of existing medical trials on a topic.

While evidence from animal research indicates that physical activity could be a useful treatment for dementia, **the review authors only found four studies that examined the effects of exercise in humans**.

Two of the studies were not included in the analysis because the reviewers could not get details from the original study authors.

Both of the remaining studies were small and only included Alzheimer disease patients. One looked at just 11 patients; the other examined 134, but many of those did not complete their exercise regimens.

Still, the researchers in the latter study found that **those who did exercise seemed to do better at handling the tasks of daily living.**

None of the studies looked at the effects on caregivers or on overall health-care costs.

Why have there been so few high-quality studies? Research into dementia is in its early stages, and largely has focused on diagnosis, assessment of severity and drug treatments, Forbes said.

To make things more challenging, funding is limited and it can be difficult to study people who might not be able to give consent or comply easily with the requirements of a study.

Dr. William Thies, vice president of medical and scientific relations for the Alzheimer's Association, agreed that the studies reviewed are not conclusive. "It's true that the studies had a trend toward benefits, but that's not enough to say that physical exercise ought to be a necessary element of everyone's dementia care."

Still, the review findings do not change the fact that exercise remains crucial to long-term health, he said. "The person who has built physical activity into their lifestyle is going to be in better health, more functional and probably happier over the long run," he said.

More fit Alzheimer's had less brain atrophy

Patients in the early stages of Alzheimer's disease who performed better on a treadmill test had less atrophy in the areas of the brain that control memory, according to a study released July 27, 2008. Magnetic resonance imaging (MRI) showed less shrinkage in the hippocampus region of patients' brains in the Alzheimer's patients with higher fitness scores. In Alzheimer's the hippocampus is one of the first parts of the brain to suffer damage.

Exercise and physical fitness have been shown to slow age-related brain cell death in healthy older adults.

The new study was released at the International Conference on Alzheimer's Disease in Chicago. Researchers at the University of Kansas Medical Center in Kansas City, Kan., studied the connection between cardiorespiratory fitness and regional brain volume in more than **100 people** over 60. About half were healthy older adults and half were in the early stages of Alzheimer's.

In a statement, lead researcher Robyn A. Honea said the study suggests "that maintaining cardiorespiratory fitness may positively modify Alzheimer's-related brain atrophy."

But **it isn't clear whether exercise helped avoid brain damage or if brain-damaged people had less ability to exercise**.

The study was funded by the National Institute on Aging and National Institute on Neurological Disorders and Stroke.

Physical fitness may slow Alzheimer brain atrophy

Getting a lot of exercise (and its associated increase of oxygen intake) may help slow brain shrinkage in people with early Alzheimer's disease, a preliminary study suggests. Analysis found that **participants who were more physically fit had less brain shrinkage than less-fit participants**. However, they didn't do significantly better on tests for mental performance.

That was a surprise, but maybe the study had too few patients to make an effect show up in the statistical analysis, said Dr. Jeffrey Burns, one of the study's authors. He also stressed that the work is only a starting point for exploring whether exercise and physical fitness can slow the progression of Alzheimer's. The study can't prove an effect because the participants were evaluated only once rather than repeatedly over time, he said.

While brains shrink with normal aging, the rate is doubled in people with Alzheimer's, he said. Burns, who directs the Alzheimer and Memory Program at the University of Kansas School of Medicine in Kansas City, reports the work with colleagues in July 15, 2008 issue of the journal Neurology.

The study included **57 people** with early Alzheimer's. Their physical fitness was assessed by measuring their peak oxygen demand while on a treadmill, and brain shrinkage was estimated by MRI scans. Dr. Sam Gandy, who chairs the medical and scientific advisory council of the Alzheimer's Association, said the result fits in with previous indications that things people do to protect heart health can also pay off for the brain. **I believe that this indicates that oxygen deficiency can be related to brain atrophy. The greater the oxygen consumption, the better was the effect on Alzheimer's.**

Inactivity link to mental decline

Being a slob puts you at risk of mental health problems, experts have warned.

A lack of physical activity leads to depression and dementia, evidence presented at the British Nutrition Foundation conference shows.

It comes as new research from the University of Bristol found that **being active cuts the risk of Alzheimer's disease by around a third.**

Currently only 35% of men and 24% of women reach the recommended weekly amount of physical activity.

Professor Nanette Mutrie, an expert in exercise and sport psychology at the University of Strathclyde, told the conference that mental health was not a trivial issue. "It's only recently that people have begun to see the link between physical activity and mental health.

"It's important for increasing people's self esteem, general mood, coping with stress and even sleeping better.

"And we now have very strong evidence that physical activity can prevent depression."

She said **inactive people had twice the risk of becoming depressed and there was also very good evidence that exercise is a useful treatment for depression.**

Dementia risk

Researchers at the University of Bristol carried out an analysis of 17 trials looking at the effects of physical activity on dementia and Alzheimer's disease.

They found that **in both men and women physical activity was associated with a 30-40% drop in the risk of Alzheimer's.**

It is unclear why there is such a great effect but it could be associated with benefits to the vascular system as well as release of chemicals in the brain.

I believe that it is due to increased EMOD production.

Professor Mutrie added:"It could be a simple case of use it or lose it.

"It is estimated that over 700,000 people in the UK currently suffer from dementia and more research is needed to determine how this condition can be prevented."

Professor Judy Buttriss, director general at the BNF, said with people living longer the implications of such studies were "enormous".

"There has already, justifiably, been a lot of emphasis on good nutrition but we must also find ways of helping people to be more physically active to ensure that they maintain health and quality of life in later years."

Department of Health figures show the majority of adults do not do the recommended 30 minutes of moderate activity at least five times a week.

Children are also leading increasingly inactive lives.

Around 30% of boys and almost 40% of girls fail to reach the recommended hour of moderate intensity activity per day.

Professor Chris Riddoch, expert in sport and exercise science at the University of Bath, said: **"We have half a Century of evidence showing active people have lower levels of disease.**

"We also have a very good handle on how much exercise people should take."

But he added efforts to get people to be more active had not been very successful to date.

Mental Exercise. Cognitive training that includes exercises to stimulate memory, reasoning, and mental processing speed may help improve both mental ability and enable patients to handle daily living tasks -- such as performing housework, managing money, and preparing meals. Other studies indicate that participating in intellectually engaging activity (such as doing crossword puzzles or learning a new language) may help reduce the risk of Alzheimer's disease. (Harvey Simon, MD, Associate Professor of Medicine, Harvard Medical School, 2008)

Four things that keep a mind sharp

New research reveals a host of factors that may contribute to a sharper mind late in life, including **exercise, education, non-smoking behavior and social activity**.

The study tested the cognitive ability of **2,500** people aged 70 to 79 over eight years. More than half of the subjects showed normal age-related decline in mind function and 16 percent had a considerable decline during the course of the study. But 30 percent of participants did not show a change in their cognitive skills, and some even improved on the tests.

The researchers then looked to see what could account for this difference.

EXERCISE: **They found that people who exercised moderately to vigorously at least once a week were 30 percent more likely to maintain a sharp mind than those who did not work-out as often.**

EDUCATION: **People with at least a high school education were almost three times more likely to keep up their cognitive ability than those without this education.** And those who had a ninth grade literacy level were nearly five times more likely to maintain the ability (a specific word recognition test was administered during the study to assess the subject's literacy level.)

NOT SMOKING: There was also a connection between smoking and brain function in old age. **Non-smokers were almost twice as likely to stay quick-minded as those who smoked.**

SOCIALIZING: Finally, some **social activity may also be good for the mind.** The results showed that subjects who volunteered, worked or lived with someone else were 24 percent more likely to keep up their cognitive function.

"Some of these factors such as exercise and smoking are behaviors that people can change," said Alexandra Fiocco, a study author and research at the University of California, San Francisco. "Discovering factors associated with cognitive maintenance may be very useful in prevention strategies that guard against or slow the onset of dementia."

The results were published in a **June, 2009 issue of Neurology**. The research was funded by the National Institutes of Health.

The study supports past research that has pointed to exercise as a way to protect your brain and prevent the development of cognitive disorders. Exercise stresses your body, and causes it to release certain growth factors that can strength neurons and keep them healthy.

Surprisingly, increased amyloid may delay thinking deficit

A surprising study came out on June 15, 2009. **Dimebon, Medivation Inc's promising experimental Alzheimer's drug, significantly raised levels of a toxic protein in the brains of mice, yet has been shown to delay thinking problems in human dementia patients**, U.S. researchers said.

"This is an unexpected result," said Dr. Samuel Gandy, a researcher at Mount Sinai School of Medicine in New York, whose findings were presented at an Alzheimer's meeting in Vienna. The study raises new questions about how the drug works and new worries about drugs meant to remove telltale clumps of a protein called beta amyloid from the brain as a way to reverse Alzheimer's disease.

Researchers are not sure whether amyloid is a cause or a symptom of Alzheimer's but, either way, getting rid of it had appeared to be a good thing. "We think we want amyloid levels to go down," Gandy said in a telephone interview. "Here is this compound that is looking very promising clinically that is making amyloid levels go up."

Dimebon, first sold in Russia as an antihistamine, is being developed jointly with Pfizer Inc, maker of the Alzheimer's drug Aricept. Researchers see Dimebon as the best hope for a new treatment for the incurable, mind-robbing disease that affects 26 million people globally. Now in late-stage testing, Dimebon seems to delay thinking problems in people but it is not clear how.

"We wanted to know what Dimebon was doing to amyloid," Gandy said. His team tested mice genetically engineered to have a human form of Alzheimer's. The drug increased amyloid outside nerve cells.

"It certainly means this medicine is not acting by an acute amyloid-lowering effect, which is what we were looking for in the lab," Gandy said.

Separately, Israeli researchers reported promising results from a study in mice that takes aim at a less-studied brain protein called tau, which is strongly associated with dementia in Alzheimer's disease. Hanna Rosenmann of Hadassah University Hospital in Jerusalem and colleagues found that **injecting mice with tau-fighting antibodies reduced the number of tangles in the brain by 40 percent and produced tau antibodies in the blood**. "That looks to me like a viable therapeutic avenue," said Dr. Gary Kennedy of Montefiore Medical Center in New York.

The "amyloid hypothesis" has already produced some stunning failures in large, late-stage trials. They include a drug by Canadian biotech Bellus Health, formerly known as Neurochem Inc, and one last year with Flurizan, dealing a blow to its backers Myriad Genetics and Lundbeck. "You have to wonder if maybe we have been thinking about this wrong," Gandy said.

And he wonders about **bapineuzumab, a highly watched drug for Alzheimer's being developed by Wyeth and Irish drugmaker Elan Corp and Johnson & Johnson. Last year, the drug failed to meet its primary goal in a mid-stage trial and caused brain swelling at higher doses.**

I believe that this again points out the simple fact that we are basically in the dark when it comes to understanding the cause or the treatment of Alzheimer's disease.

Alzheimer's hastens death

Also, in 2009, it was found that older adults with mild cognitive impairment or Alzheimer's disease have a shorter life span than other older adults, but **the risk of death is no greater for whites or blacks,** a new study says. The study, conducted by researchers **at Rush University Medical Center in Chicago, contradicts earlier information indicating blacks with Alzheimer's live longer than whites with the disease.**

Researchers examined **1,715 older adults** with an average age of 80 from four adjacent neighborhoods in Chicago. About 52 percent of participants were black. Each participant had a clinical evaluation that included medical history, a neurological examination and a series of thinking, learning and memory tests to determine cognitive function.

About 17.3 percent were found to have Alzheimer's disease, 34.8 percent had mild cognitive impairment, 1.2 percent had other forms of dementia and 46.8 percent had no cognitive impairment. During up to **10 years of follow-up**, 37 percent of the participants died, including 25.8 percent of those without cognitive impairment, 40.4 percent of those with mild cognitive impairment, 59.1 percent of those with Alzheimer's disease and 60 percent of those with other forms of dementia.

Those with Alzheimer's disease had a three-fold greater risk of dying compared to those not experiencing cognitive function problems. Those with mild cognitive impairment were 50 percent more likely to die. The risk of death increased as cognitive impairment became more severe. The study appeared in the June, 2009 issue of *Archives of Neurology*.

Alzheimer's disease reduces life expectancy and has emerged as a leading cause of death in the United States, according to the study. Two previous national surveys found that life expectancy among black Alzheimer's patients might be longer than for whites. But the current study, which was based on uniform clinical exams and not medical records of varying degrees of completeness, found **race had no bearing on life expectancy.**

I believe that **AD** is directly related to oxygen levels, especially at the organelle level, especially **EMODs** levels. **AD** is one of the coexistent diseases associated with **EMOD** insufficiency.

Tracking Alzheimer's-linked protein in live brains

The following was excerpted from an article by Lauran Neergaard, AP Medical Writer on Aug 28, 2008.

Scientists for the first time have peered into people's brains to directly measure the ebb and flow of a substance notorious for its role in Alzheimer's disease. The delicate research was performed not with Alzheimer's patients but with people suffering severe brain injuries — because **a brain injury increases the risk of developing dementia later in life.**

A team of scientists from Missouri and Italy got a surprise. **Too much of that Alzheimer's-related protein, called beta-amyloid, is thought to be harmful**. So the team had expected beta-amyloid levels to spike right after the injury and then drop as patients recovered.

Instead, beta-amyloid levels increased as patients improved and dropped if they got worse, lead researcher Dr. David Brody, a neurologist at Washington University in St. Louis, reported Friday in the journal Science. What's going on?

Beta-amyloid seems to be a marker of increased brain activity as patients improved.

If so, what started as a study of Alzheimer's risk might have implications for how the brain-injured are tracked in intensive-care units — although that will take much more research to prove. "Our study is just the beginning," Brody said. **"Amyloid-beta measurements in the brain may turn out to be a good indicator of how well the cells are communicating with each other."**

Beta-amyloid is best known as the sticky goo that makes up the hallmark plaques inside the brains of Alzheimer's victims. But it doesn't start out as gunk. Soluble forms are found in the fluid that bathes the brain, although scientists don't understand its purpose, or just what happens to trigger formation of those bad plaques.

Nor do they understand how brain trauma so often leads to later Alzheimer's. One possibility is that extra beta-amyloid speeds whatever dementia-forming process might be lurking among brain cells. Another theory is that the injury decreases a person's "cognitive reserve," so that symptoms merely become apparent sooner.

These patients were undergoing brain surgery anyway. What if surgeons could insert an extra tiny tube at the same time that would allow hour-to-hour sampling of brain fluid, to measure beta-amyloid? It's a technique called **intracerebral microdialysis**, and colleagues at Washington University already had performed it in mice — linking increased synaptic activity, or communication between brain cells, to increased beta-amyloid.

Brody teamed with Dr. Sandra Magnoni of the Ospedale Maggiore Policlinico, a major trauma center in Milan that has experience with the technique. They asked the families of patients suffering brain injuries from car crashes, falls or hemorrhages from burst blood vessels if they'd agree to the experiment. **Eighteen said yes**.

Roughly 24 hours after the initial injury, the catheter was placed in patients' brains, where it stayed for three to seven days. ICU doctors and nurses otherwise provided routine care, tracking patients' neurologic changes with a standard tool called the **Glasgow Coma Score.**

Brody tracked the beta-amyloid levels and found they mirrored that coma score, with a direct relationship to each patient's neurological status. That means the findings agreed with the previous research on mice. That's important, as so much Alzheimer's research must be performed in animals, said Dr. Ramona Hicks, a specialist in traumatic brain injury at the National Institutes of Health, which helped fund the work.

Brody cautions that beta-amyloid might have spiked in everyone right at the time of injury, something his study started too late to measure. Also, **it only measured total beta-amyloid levels, not a strung-together form that's thought to be toxic to cells**.

While the work raises more questions than it answers, it brings researchers a valuable new tool for studying both Alzheimer's risk and just what happens during brain-injury recovery. "It sort of sets a platform for future studies," said NIH's Hicks.

CHAPTER TWELVE

Vitamin E and C supplements and risk of dementia (Laurin, Foley, 2002)

A controlled trial of vitamin E supplementation among patients with AD found delayed time to institutionalization, but no specific effect on cognitive function. In contrast to the previous analysis from the Honolulu-Asia Aging Study (HAAS), based on prevalent cases, we did not find a significant association of vitamin E or vitamin C supplement use and incident dementia. Our results are based on incident cases and a longer period between the 1988 report of supplement use and assessment of dementia. Our data suggest that **supplemental intake of both vitamins E and C does not alter the risk for dementia**. (Laurin, Foley, 2002)

Brain mitochondrial dysfunction in aging, neurodegeneration, and Parkinson's disease

Brain senescence and neurodegeneration occur with a mitochondrial dysfunction characterized by impaired electron transfer and by oxidative damage. Brain mitochondria of old animals show **decreased rates of electron transfer in complexes I and IV,** decreased membrane potential, **increased content of the oxidation products** of phospholipids and proteins and increased size and fragility. This impairment, with complex I inactivation and oxidative damage, is named "complex I syndrome" and is recognized as characteristic of mammalian brain aging and of neurodegenerative diseases. Mitochondrial dysfunction is more marked in brain areas as rat hippocampus and frontal cortex, in human cortex in Parkinson's disease and dementia with Lewy bodies, and in substantia nigra in Parkinson's disease. The molecular mechanisms involved in complex I inactivation include the synergistic inactivations produced by ONOO- mediated reactions, by reactions with free radical intermediates of lipid peroxidation and by amine-aldehyde adduction reactions. **The accumulation of oxidation products prompts the idea of antioxidant therapies. High**

doses of vitamin E produce a significant protection of complex I activity and mitochondrial function in rats and mice, and with improvement of neurological functions and increased median life span in mice.

Mitochondria-targeted antioxidants, as the Skulachev cations covalently attached to vitamin E, ubiquinone and PBN and the SS tetrapeptides, are negatively charged and accumulate in mitochondria where they exert their antioxidant effects. Activation of the cellular mechanisms that regulate mitochondrial biogenesis is another potential therapeutic strategy, since the process generates organelles devoid of oxidation products and with full enzymatic activity and capacity for ATP production. (Navarro, Boveris, 2010)

Here is my question: Since EMODs are believed to be produced at complex I, how does decreasing electron flow at this site increase oxidative products?

Coffee may reverse Alzheimer's

A report in July of 2009 found that coffee drinkers may have another reason to pour that extra cup. When aged mice bred to develop symptoms of Alzheimer's disease were given caffeine – the equivalent of five cups of coffee a day – their memory impairment was reversed, according to University of South Florida researchers at the Florida Alzheimer's Disease Research Center.

Back-to-back studies published online July 6, 2009 in the *Journal of Alzheimer's Disease*, show caffeine significantly decreased abnormal levels of the protein linked to Alzheimer's disease, both in the brains and in the blood of mice exhibiting symptoms of the disease. Both studies build upon previous research by the Florida ADRC group showing that caffeine in early adulthood prevented the onset of memory problems in mice bred to develop Alzheimer's symptoms in old age.

I would predict that caffeine has prooxidant properties (as reported by Barry Halliwell) or to the prooxidant character of caffeine, which is responsible for its anti-Alzheimer's effect.

"The new findings provide evidence that caffeine could be a viable 'treatment' for established Alzheimer's disease, and not simply a protective strategy," said lead author Gary Arendash, PhD, a USF neuroscientist with the Florida ADRC. "That's important because caffeine is a safe drug for most people, it easily enters the brain, and it appears to directly affect the disease process."

Based on these promising findings in mice, researchers at the Florida ADRC and Byrd Alzheimer's Center at USF hope to begin human trials to evaluate whether caffeine can benefit people with mild cognitive impairment or early Alzheimer's disease, said Huntington Potter, PhD, director of the Florida ADRC and an investigator for the caffeine studies. The research group has already determined that **caffeine administered to elderly non-demented humans quickly affects their blood levels of beta-amyloid, just as it did in the Alzheimer's mice.**

"These are some of the most promising Alzheimer's mouse experiments ever done showing that **caffeine rapidly reduces beta amyloid protein in the blood, an effect that is mirrored in the brain**, and **this reduction is linked to cognitive benefit**," Potter said. "Our goal is to obtain the funding needed to translate the therapeutic discoveries in mice into well-designed clinical trials."

Arendash and his colleagues became interested in caffeine's potential for treating Alzheimer's several years ago, after **a Portuguese study reported that people with Alzheimer's had consumed less caffeine over the last 20 years than people without the neurodegenerative disease.**

Since then, **several uncontrolled clinical studies have reported moderate caffeine consumption may protect against memory decline during normal aging.** The highly controlled studies using Alzheimer's mice allowed researchers to isolate the effects of caffeine on memory from other lifestyle factors such as diet and exercise, Arendash said.

The Florida ADRC study included **55 mice** genetically altered to develop memory problems mimicking Alzheimer's disease as they aged. After behavioral tests confirmed the mice were exhibiting signs of memory impairment at age 18 to 19 months – about age 70 in human years – the researchers gave half the mice caffeine in their drinking water. The other half got plain water. **The Alzheimer's mice received the equivalent of five 8-oz. cups of regular coffee a day. That's the same amount of caffeine – 500 milligrams -- as contained in two cups of specialty coffees like Starbucks, or 14 cups of tea, or 20 soft drinks.**

At the end of the two-month study, the caffeinated mice performed much better on tests measuring their memory and thinking skills. In fact, **their memories were identical to normal aged mice without dementia.** The Alzheimer's mice drinking plain water continued to do poorly on the tests.

In addition, **the brains of the caffeinated mice showed nearly a 50-percent reduction in levels of beta amyloid**, a substance forming the sticky clumps of plaques that are a hallmark of Alzheimer's disease. Other experiments by the same investigators indicate that caffeine appears to restore memory by reducing both enzymes needed to produce beta amyloid. The researchers also suggest that caffeine suppresses inflammatory changes in the brain that lead to an overabundance of beta amyloid.

Since caffeine improved the memory of mice with pre-existing Alzheimer's, the researchers were curious to know if it might further boost the memory of non-demented (normal) mice administered caffeine from young adulthood through old age. It did not. Control mice given regular drinking water throughout their lives performed as well on behavioral tests in old age as normal mice who received long-term caffeine treatment, Arendash said. "This suggests that caffeine will not increase memory performance above normal levels. Rather, it appears to benefit those destined to develop Alzheimer's disease."

The researchers do not know if an amount lower than the 500 mg. daily caffeine intake received by the Alzheimer's mice would be effective, Arendash said. **For most individuals, however, this moderate level of caffeine intake poses no adverse health effects,** according to both the National Research Council and the National Academy of Sciences. Nonetheless, Arendash said, individuals with high blood pressure or those who are pregnant should limit their daily caffeine intake.

If larger, more rigorous clinical studies confirm that caffeine staves off Alzheimer's in humans, as it does in mice, this benefit would be substantial, Arendash said. **Alzheimer's disease attacks nearly half of Americans age 85 and older, and Alzheimer's and other dementias triple healthcare costs for those age 65 and older,** according to the Alzheimer's Association.

In addition to the Florida ADRC, Byrd Alzheimer's Center and Eric Pfeiffer Suncoast Alzheimer's and Gerontology Center at USF, researchers from the Bay Pines VA Healthcare System; Saitama Medical University, Saitama, Japan; and Washington University School of Medicine, St. Louis, collaborated on the research. The studies were supported by grants to investigators in the Florida ADRC, a statewide project sponsored by the National Institute on Aging and housed at the University of South Florida's Byrd Alzheimer's Center. (Arendash et al, 2009) (Cao et al, 2009)

In vitro prooxidant effect of caffeine

Caffeine is a methylxanthine compound that acts as a stimulant in humans. It is the most widely consumed behaviourally active substance in the western world and it affects calcium influx and release in living cells. Caffeine is present in various substances such as tea, coffee and some medications. This article is focused on the impact of caffeine on oxidation. Caffeine promoted the peroxidation of linoleic acid emulsions used by 32.5, 48.9, and 54.3%, respectively, at 15, 30 and 45 µg/mL concentrations. Standard antioxidants such as α-tocopherol and trolox, a water-soluble analogue of tocopherol, inhibited 76.2 and 93.2% peroxidation of linoleic acid emulsion at 45 µg/mL concentration. Also, PC_{50} value (caffeine concentration that produced a 50% increase in linoleic acid peroxidation) of caffeine was found to be 185 μM. (Gulcln, 2008). **This is the prooxidant action of caffeine as I had predicted.**

Antioxidant and prooxidant properties of caffeine, theobromine and xanthine

Caffeine, along with its catabolic products theobromine and xanthine, is a key component of tea and coffee. These compounds are structurally similar to uric acid, a known antioxidant which is present in blood at relatively high concentrations, but also shows prooxidant activity. In view of the structural similarity between uric acid and caffeine and its metabolites, we studied the antioxidant and prooxidant properties of these compounds. MATERIAL/METHODS: Antioxidant activity was determined by measuring the quenching effect of the compounds on oxidative DNA degradation by a hydroxyl radical generating system. Prooxidant activity was studied by measuring the ability of the compounds to oxidatively degrade DNA in the presence of copper ions. RESULTS: Caffeine, theobromine and xanthine have a quenching effect on the production of hydroxyl radicals, as well as on oxidative DNA breakage by hydroxyl radicals. **Consistent with previous observations that many known antioxidants of plant origin are also capable of prooxidant action, the purine alkaloids also show oxidative DNA breakage in the presence of transition metal ions.** CONCLUSIONS: **The alkaloid caffeine and its catabolic products theobromine and xanthine exhibit both antioxidant and prooxidant properties.** The results lead to the observation that caffeine and its metabolites may also contribute to the overall antioxidant and chemopreventive properties of caffeine-bearing beverages, such as tea. (Sonish et al, 2003)

Caffeine increases oxidative stress in athletes

Caffeine is a commonly used ergogenic aid in endurance sports. However, its role is not well known on oxidative stress during exercise: pro-oxidative or antioxidant substance? In a randomized double-blind study involving 20 active males, we examined plasma lactate, oxidative stress markers (malondialdehyde), antioxidative systems (vitamins A, E, C), and ergospirometric response before and after steady 30 min steady-state tests 75% V_{O2max} (placebo and caffeine).

They concluded that **5 mg/kg of caffeine ingestion could increase the oxidative stress** whereas its consumption may not have a clear metabolic advantage in certain aerobic activities. (Science and Sports, 2008)

Clearing plaque with vaccine does not restore lost learning and memory

A promising vaccine being tested for Alzheimer's disease does what it is designed to do - **clear beta-amyloid plaques from the brain - but it does not seem to help restore lost learning and memory abilities**, according to a University of California, Irvine study.

The findings suggest that treating the predominant pathology of Alzheimer's disease - beta-amyloid plaques - by itself may have only limited clinical benefit if started after there is significant plaque growth. However, a combination of vaccination with therapies that also target related neuron damage and cognitive decline may provide the best treatment opportunity for people with this neurodegenerative disease. Study results appeared in the April 2, 2008 issue of the *Journal of Neuroscience*.

"We've found that reducing plaques is only part of the puzzle to treat Alzheimer disease," said study leader, UC Irvine neurobiologist Elizabeth Head. "Vaccines such as this one are a good first step for effective Alzheimer's treatment, but complimentary treatments must be developed to address the complexity of the disease."

Head and colleagues studied for a two-year period in aging canines the effect of a vaccine that is currently under clinical development for treating patients with Alzheimer's disease. **The vaccine contains the beta-amyloid 1-42 protein and stimulates the immune system to produce antibodies against this same protein that is in the brain plaques**. Dogs are used for such studies because beta-amyloid plaques grow naturally in their brains and they exhibit cognitive declines similar to those seen in humans.

After the aged dogs with beta-amyloid-plaque growth were immunized (which is similar to starting a treatment in patients with Alzheimer's disease), the researchers found, in comparison with non-treated aged dogs, little difference in the results of behavioral tests that measure cognitive loss. Later, **brain autopsies showed that although plaques had been cleared from multiple brain regions - including the entorhinal cortex, a region of the brain involved with learning and memory and primarily affected by Alzheimer's - damaged neurons remained.**

Head said this discovery helps explain why there was little difference in the behavioral test results between immunized and nonimmunized dogs. In addition, she added, it implies that after clearing beta-amyloid plaques from the brain, the next step is to repair these neurons. This approach will be critical for treating and reversing the effects of the Alzheimer's disease.

Currently, Head and her colleagues are developing approaches to repair these damaged neurons and hope to test them clinically.

CHAPTER THIRTEEN

Vitamin supplements, cognitive decline and confusing data

Surprisingly, **among those who had taken supplements for about 10 y, the delayed recall scores on the East Boston Memory Test were higher for the women who took only vitamin C than for those who took vitamins E and C or vitamin E alone.** No information on any dose-response relation is offered, so the implications for recommended doses are unclear.

Inflammation and oxidation are an important part of current investigations into the causes, treatment, and prevention of cognitive impairment and dementia. Elevations in C-reactive protein and corticosteroids may be reduced by supplementation with vitamins E and C. **Other work suggests that very high amounts of vitamin E alone may actually increase oxidation and that the combination of vitamins E and C may reduce the oxidative properties of high-dose alpha-tocopherol.** Most work has focused on supplementation with vitamin E, for which the primary variant is alpha-tocopherol, but dietary vitamin E is primarily gamma-tocopherol.

Some authors have suggested that gamma-tocopherol may have stronger antioxidant properties than does alpha-tocopherol. Alpha-Tocopherol supplementation may actually reduce gamma-tocopherol concentrations. Gamma-Tocopherol may inhibit cyclooxygenase activity and may be a more effective antioxidant and anti-inflammatory agent than is alpha-tocopherol.

What are the implications of these findings for further study, for lifestyle modifications, or for treatment of elderly patients?

Because the Nurse's Health Study is an observational cohort study, **residual confounding cannot be ruled out.** Nurses who take supplements, particularly specific single supplements such as a combination of vitamins E and C, are inevitably different in a myriad of often-unmeasured ways from women who are not nurses and who do not take supplements. Even extensive adjustments and sophisticated statistical modeling cannot completely account for this. The modest benefits reported in this study could be a result of residual confounding by lifestyle and socio-demographic differences. **The inconsistency in these results with regard to duration of use and the types of cognitive function that are affected indicate that this study does not provide definitive evidence that vitamin E or C supplementation is a preventivie treatment for cognitive decline.** Taken alone, **these results do not strongly support a recommendation for supplementation.**

The lack of information about any dose-response relation is also limiting. If high doses of alpha-tocopherol actually do deplete gamma-tocopherol, vitamin E supplementation (which is mainly alpha-tocopherol) may not prevent cognitive decline. **High doses of vitamin E are also associated with some adverse effects, such as bleeding, that should be taken into account in any risk-benefit analysis.** (Haan, 2003)

Vitamin C and E for Alzheimer's disease not recommended

CONCLUSIONS: In the absence of prospective, randomized, controlled clinical trials documenting benefits that outweigh recently documented morbidity and mortality risks, **vitamin E supplements should not be recommended for primary or secondary prevention of AD. Although the risks of taking high doses of vitamin C are lower than those with vitamin E, the lack of consistent efficacy data for vitamin C in preventing or treating AD should discourage its routine use for this purpose.** (Boothby et al, 2005) (Vitamin C and Vitamin E for Alzheimer's Disease. Lisa A Boothby, Paul L Doering. The annals of pharmacotherapy. Published Online, 14 October 2005, www.theannals.com., DOI 10.1345/aph.1E495).

Vitamin E fails in Alzheimer's disease and mild cognitive impairment 2008 (Isaac et al, 2008, CD002854)

Vitamin E is a dietary compound that functions as an antioxidant scavenging toxic free radicals. Evidence that free radicals may contribute to the pathological processes of cognitive impairment including Alzheimer's disease (AD) has led to interest in the use of Vitamin E in the treatment of Alzheimer's disease and Mild Cognitivie Impairment (MCI). OBJECTIVES: To assess the efficacy of Vitamin E in the treatment of Alzheimer's disease and prevention of progression of Mild Cognitive Impairment to Alzheimer's disease. SEARCH STRATEGY: **The Cochrane Dementia and Cognitive Improvement's Specialized Register** was searched on 8 January 2007 using the following terms: "Vitamin E", vitamin-E, alpha-tocopherol. The **CDCIG Registers** contains records from major health care databases and ongoing trial databases and is updated regularly. SELECTION CRITERIA: All unconfounded, double blind, randomized trials in which treatment with Vitamin E at any dose was compared with placebo for patients with Alzheimer's disease or Mild Cognitive Impairment. DATA COLLECTION AND ANALYSIS: Two reviewers independently applied the selection criteria and assessed study quality and extracted and analysed the data. For each outcome measure data were sought on every patient randomized. Where such data were not available an analysis of patients who completed treatment was conducted. MAIN RESULTS: Only 2 studies met the inclusion criteria. The primary outcome used in the AD study was survival time to the first of 4 endpoints: death, institutionalisation, loss of 2 out of 3 basic activities of daily living and severe dementia (defined as a global Clinical Dementia Rating of 3). The investigators reported the total numbers in each group who reached the primary endpoint within two years for participants completing the study ("completers"). There appeared to be some benefit from Vitamin E with fewer participants reaching endpoint - 58% (45/77) of completers compared with 74% (58/78) - a Peto odds ratio of 0.49, 95% confidence interval 0.25 to 0.96. However, more participants taking Vitamin E suffered a fall (12/77 compared with 4/78; odds ratio 3.07, 95% CI 1.09 to 8.62). It was not possible to interpret the reported results for specific endpoints or for secondary outcomes of cognition, dependence, behavioral disturbance and activities of daily living. The primary outcome used in the MCI study which had 769 participants (257 in the Vitamin E group and 259 in the placebo group; a third Donepezil group of 253 was not included in this review) was the time to progression from MCI to possible or probable AD. A total of 214 of the 769 participants had progression to dementia, with 212 being classified as having possible or probable AD. **There was no significant difference in the probability of progression from MCI to AD between the Vitamin E group and the placebo group.** There was no significant difference between the placebo group and the Vitamin E group in adverse events. Five subjects died in each group and 72 discontinued treatment in the Vitamin E group and 66 in the placebo group. AUTHORS' CONCLUSIONS: **There is no evidence of efficacy of Vitamin E in the prevention or treatment of people with AD or MCI.** More research is needed to identify the role of Vitamin E, if any, in the management of cognitive impairment. (Isaac et al, 2008, CD002854)

Altered plasma antioxidant status in subjects with AD and vascular dementia

Oxygen--free radicals and lipid hydroperoxides may have an aetiological role in the development of lesions in the central nervous system in patients with Alzheimer's disease and in those with vascular dementia. This study aimed to make a cross-sectional comparison of blood markers of oxidative stress in two groups of patients with these disorders and a control group. Design: Cross-sectional comparative study. Setting: Established memory clinics in Cardiff organized by a University Department of Geriatric Medicine within an acute care NHS Trust. Methods: Following a dietary assessment, postprandial venous blood samples were obtained from the following: 25 subjects with probable Alzheimer's disease (AD) (mean age 74.3; 10 F, 15 M); 17 subjects with probable vascular dementia (VD) (mean age 75.5; 5 F, 12 M); and 41 controls (mean age 73.4; 24 F, 17 M) for measurement of circulating lipid peroxides (LP), total antioxidant capacity (TAC), vitamin C (VitC), vitamin E (VitE) and beta-carotene (BC). Results: Plasma levels of VitC were significantly lower in subjects with vascular dementia compared with controls (VD, 6.5 (4.8, 8.2); controls, 10.0 (8.38, 11.6); VD vs controls, $p=0.015$), but **no significant difference was seen between controls and patients with Alzheimer's disease** (AD, mean 8.3 (6.2, 10.4)). VitE levels were significantly lower in subjects with AD compared with controls (31.1 (28.2, 34.0) vs 36.0 (32.8, 39.2), $p=0.035$). **BC levels were similar in subjects with AD and controls, but significantly elevated in those with VD** (AD, 0.28 (0.2, 0.34); VD, 0.40, (0.27, 0.53); controls, 0.28 (0.22, 0.34); VD vs controls, $p=0.046$). **There were no significant differences in LP or TAC between the three groups. Conclusions:** Subjects with dementia attributed to Alzheimer's disease or to vascular disease have a degree of disturbance in antioxidant balance which may predispose to increased oxidative stress. This may be a potential therapeutic area for antioxidant supplementation. (Sinclair et al, 1999)

I conclude from Sinclair et al that there were no significant vitamin C or beta carotene differences in AD patients but there was lower vitamin E levels in AD patients.

Drink Fruit or Vegetable Juices and Avoid Alzheimer's?

Fruit and vegetable juices and Alzheimer's disease: The Kame project.

(Dai et al, 2006, the Kame Project) (#1,836)

Summary: A glass of fruit or vegetable juice 3 or more times weekly may fend off Alzheimer's disease, due to their polyphenol content, rather than vitamin antioxidants. **Introduction:** Oxidative damage is regarded today as one of the keys to the development of Alzheimer's. That's why many people take antioxidants in the hopes of delaying its onset. One of the targets of oxidative damage is the beta-amyloid peptide, and **hydrogen peroxide has been suggested as a possible mediator.** This has led to the use of polyphenols, which are described as being the most abundant dietary antioxidants, with stronger neuroprotection against hydrogen peroxide than antioxidant vitamins.

Polyphenols are usually found in the skin and peel of fruits and vegetables; when the produce is mechanically squeezed, the polyphenols pass into the juices. A study done in Japanese Americans, reported in the *American Journal of Medicine*, has explored the role of drinking juices in the development of Alzheimer's disease over a 9-year period.

What was done: The *Kame* project is part of a larger study of dementia in Japanese people living in Japan and the USA. The *Kame* cohort consists of participants aged 65 and older living in Washington State, USA. There were **1,836 subjects** who were free of dementia at enrollment in 1992-1994. At baseline the Cognitive Abilites Screening Instrument (CASI) was used to assess cognitive function; this was repeated every two years for a total of 4 times. A much broader neuropsychological exam was given to anyone scoring less than 87 out of 100 points on the CASI. Food-frequency questionnaires were completed by 87% of the participants at baseline; the questions used were appropriate for Asian populations. The usual dietary intake of nutrients, including calories, vitamins C and E, and beta-carotene were calculated for each person. Other baseline information included smoking, alcohol use, birthplace, education level, physical activity, usual eating preference (Asian or Western), and use of antioxidant vitamin supplements. The sense of smell was ascertained, and the apolipoprotein E (ApoE) gene status was determined. The participants were classified three times according to their intake of tea, wine, and juices (fruit and vegetable). Each classification used three categories, or 'tertiles': "less than once a week", "once or twice a week", and "at least 3 times a week". These tertiles were used to analyze the risks, or Hazards Ratios, of subjects in each category of developing Alzheimer's disease.

What was found: The average age at enrollment was 72; just over half of the subjects were women. One in five of them possessed an ApoE4 gene, which means they were at increased risk of developing Alzheimer's. Over the follow-up period (average duration 6.3 years) 81 cases of Alzheimer's disease were diagnosed; 63 of these had provided food frequency data at baseline, and were included in the analysis. Tea drinking, the most popular beverage in these studies, was not associated with Alzheimer's disease risk. Only a few participants drank wine, and although there may have been a trend towards a 'protective' effect of wine on the development of Alzheimer's, this was not statistically significant and so should be ignored. There was no association found for intake of vitamins E, C, or beta-carotene. After adjusting for factors that might bias the results, such as smoking, education, physical activity, and fat intake, it was found that those reporting drinking fruit or vegetable juice once or twice a week were 16% less likely to develop signs of Alzheimer's; this result was not statistically significant. But **those who drank juices three or more times a week were 76% less likely to develop the disease, a statistically significant finding.** The 'protective' effect of drinking juices was somewhat greater in those participants who were inactive, had a history of smoking, and who carried an ApoE4 gene.

What these results mean: This study shows that **Japanese Americans who drank fruit or vegetable juice 3 or more times a week were 76% less likely to develop the symptoms and signs of Alzheimer's in the next 6 years,**

compared with those who drank juices less than once a week. Importantly, there was no such association (decreased risk of AD) with the intake of vitamins C, E, or beta-carotene, although these are abundantly present in fruit and vegetable juices; other studies have also failed to find any effect of these substances on the development of Alzheimer's.

This suggests that some other constituents were responsible for the benefit shown by the juices. The obvious candidates are polyphenols, such as quercetin, which are able to cross the blood-brain barrier and get to the brain, and which have a neuroprotective effect against hydrogen peroxide. (The major polyphenol in tea, catechin, is ineffective against hydrogen peroxide, which may explain why teas had no protective effect in this study.) The researchers say their results require confirmation in more studies, especially ones designed to detect which polyphenol is most effective, and which fruits and vegetables confer the greatest protection. In the meantime, while waiting for results, we suggest you include fruit and vegetable juices in your nutrition plan. They taste good, and carry numerous other health benefits, as well. (Dai et al, 2006, the Kame Project)

Dai's guess is that the responsible agents are polyphenols but there is no proof for this. It is merely wishful thinking to interject yet another antioxidant as the hero and protector.

Some support for vitamin E in 2002 in reducing AD risk

A July 2002 article found a new population-based study of antioxidants, appearing in the "Journal of the American Medical Association" ("JAMA"), suggesting that a diet rich in foods containing vitamin E **may help protect some people against Alzheimer's disease** (AD). The study was also noteworthy for its finding **that vitamin E in the form of supplements was not associated with a reduction in the risk of AD.**

The "JAMA" study was conducted by Martha Clare Morris, Sc.D., of the Rush Institute for Healthy Aging at Rush-Presbyterian-St. Luke's Medical Center, Chicago, IL, Denis A. Evans, M.D., and colleagues. **A related study by Morris and colleagues, "in press" in the July 2002 Archives of Neurology, a "JAMA" publication, also associates vitamin E with protection against more general cognitive decline.** Both studies were supported by the National Institute on Aging (NIA) at the National Institutes of Health.

The June 26, 2002 issue of "JAMA" included similar findings from scientists in The Netherlands, who also reported a link between high dietary intake of vitamins C and E and protection against AD in certain people. In addition, the journal contains an editorial on the epidemiological study of dietary intake of antioxidants and the risk of AD by Daniel J. Foley, M.S., of the NIA's Laboratory of Epidemiology, Demography, and Biometry, and Lon White, M.D., Pacific Health Research Institute, Honolulu.

"This and a number of important population studies have pointed to vitamin E as **possibly** protective against oxidative damage or other mechanisms associated with cognitive decline and dementia," says Neil Buckholtz, Ph.D., head of the Dementias of Aging Branch at the NIA. "The only way this association can really be tested is through clinical studies and trials now underway. These will help us determine whether vitamin E in food or in supplements -- or taken together -- can prevent or slow down the development of mild cognitive impairment or AD."

It is not recommended, based on current evidence in 2002, that people take high-dose vitamin E supplements or other antioxidant pills in an effort to prevent mental decline, Buckholtz says. While population-based studies and animal research have suggested that antioxidants may be neuroprotective, clinical trials to test that notion are currently in progress.

Little is known about safety, effectiveness, and dosages of various antioxidant supplements that are proposed for neuroprotective purposes, Buckholtz emphasizes. **In excessively high doses (above 2,000 International Units daily, or IU/d), for example, vitamin E may be associated with increased risk of bleeding, and patients taking anti-coagulant medications may be especially at risk.** Interactions with other medications commonly taken by older people are also of potential concern. People are advised to consult with their physicians before taking high doses of supplemental vitamin E or other antioxidants.

The **815 people** participating in the **Morris study** were part of the **Chicago Health and Aging Project (CHAP),** a study of a large, diverse community of people age 65 and older. Participants were free of dementia at the start of the study and followed for an average of 3.9 years. At an average of 1.7 years from their baseline assessment, participants completed a questionnaire, asking them in detail about the kinds and quantities of foods consumed in the previous year.

Some **131 participants** had been diagnosed with AD by the end of the study period, when researchers examined the relationship between intake of antioxidants, including dietary and supplemental vitamins E and C, beta carotene, and a multivitamin, and development of AD. The most significant protective effect was found among people in the top fifth of dietary vitamin E intake (averaging 11.4 IU/d), whose risk of AD was 67 percent lower when compared to people in the group with the lowest vitamin E consumption from food (averaging 6.2 IU/d). (The recommended dietary allowance of vitamin E is 22 IU/d.) **No significant change in risk of AD was found when the scientists looked at vitamin E supplements, the other antioxidants and**

their supplements, or a general multivitamin. There was some evidence, though not statistically significant, that increased intake of dietary vitamin C and beta carotene was moving in a "protective direction," the researchers said.

The data were also analyzed to see if age, gender, race, education, or possible genetic risk for AD would influence the findings. **Only the presence or lack of apoE-e4, one form of a protein associated with increased risk of late-onset AD, seemed to matter: the protective effect of vitamin E from food was strongest among people who did not have the apoE-e4 risk factor allele.** "Dietary vitamin E may protect against Alzheimer's disease," says Morris, "but **the protection may only occur among people without the apoE-e4 allele."**

Morris suggests that further study in key areas is needed to confirm and explain some of the study's findings, including the link with apoE status and the study's striking distinction between dietary intake of vitamin E and use of supplements. For example, **the lack of a protective effect for the supplements could be explained by several factors.** Some participants in the study started taking supplements only recently and there may not have been sufficient time for the supplement to be found effective. Also, **people who believe they have memory problems could be more likely to take the supplements in the first place.** Another possible explanation might be variations in the forms of vitamin E, scientists note. **Most vitamin E supplements consist of alpha tocopherol while foods are generally more rich in gamma tocopherol.** These forms of vitamin E scavenge different types of free radicals, with one possibly more important than another in potentially reducing risk of cognitive decline.

A 2009 study also lends support to vitamin E in reducing AD

A 2009 study reported by Reuters Health found that an analysis of "real-world" clinical data indicated that **vitamin E, and drugs that reduce generalized inflammation, may slow the decline of mental and physical abilities in people with Alzheimer's disease (AD) over the long term.**

"Our results are consistent for **a potential benefit** of vitamin E on slowing functional decline and a smaller possible benefit of anti-inflammatory medications on slowing cognitive decline in patients suffering from Alzheimer's disease," Dr. Alireza Atri told Reuters Health.

Atri, at Massachusetts General Hospital (MGH), the VA Bedford Medical Center, and Harvard Medical School, Boston, led the National Institutes of Health-sponsored research. The findings, reported at the annual meeting of the American Geriatrics

Society in Chicago, stem from data on **540 patients** treated at the MGH Memory Disorders Unit.

All of the patients were receiving standard-of-care treatment with a drug intended to help patients with Alzheimer's. As part of their clinical care, 208 patients also took vitamin E but no anti-inflammatory, 49 took an anti-inflammatory but no vitamin E, 177 took both vitamin E and an anti-inflammatory, and 106 took neither.

While the daily dose of vitamin E ranged from 200 to 2000 units, the majority of patients were given high doses that ranged from 800 units daily to 1000 units twice daily.

Each patient's performance on cognitive tests and their ability to carry out daily functions such as dressing and personal care were assessed every 6 months. After **an average of 3 years,** "there was a **modest slowing of decline in function in those patients taking vitamin E,**" study investigator Michael R. Flaherty noted in a telephone interview with Reuters Health.

Flaherty, a second-year student at the University of New England College of Osteopathic Medicine in Biddeford, Maine, presented the findings at the meeting. He added that **the treatment benefit from vitamin E was "small to medium" but increased with time.**

Taking an anti-inflammatory medication was associated with "very consistent but **generally only small effects on slowing long-term decline in cognitive functioning,**" Atri told Reuters Health.

However, in patients who took both vitamin E and anti-inflammatory medications, **there appeared to be an additive effect in terms of slowing overall decline.**

Given that past studies on vitamin E have produced equivocal results, the investigators conclude that further studies are needed to assess the long-term balance of risks versus benefits for people with Alzheimer's disease from taking vitamin E and anti-inflammatory drugs. (Dr. Alireza Atri, Massachusetts General Hospital (MGH), 2009)

Group of drugs might cut AD risk by a quarter, maybe

In May of 2008, it was reported that **aspirin and related painkillers called non-steroidal anti-inflammatory drugs all seem to work equally well to**

cut a person's risk of developing Alzheimer's disease, researchers said on Wednesday.

The researchers examined data from **six studies involving 13,499 people** to gauge the protective effect from these commonly used drugs, called NSAIDs, on Alzheimer's risk.

Over the course of the studies, 820 of the people in the studies developed the disease.

Those who used NSAIDs, a class of pain-relieving drugs including aspirin, ibuprofen (Advil, Motrin and other brands) and naproxen (Aleve and other brands), collectively had a 23 percent lower risk for Alzheimer's in comparison to people who did not use these drugs.

But even though different types of NSAIDs have different properties, they delivered essentially the same level of risk reduction, the researchers wrote in the journal Neurology.

"When we looked at different sub-groups (of NSAIDs), we found no evidence that there was any difference in the reduction in risk," Peter Zandi of Johns Hopkins University in Baltimore said in a telephone interview.

Alzheimer's disease is the most common form of dementia among older people, and researchers have been working to understand its causes and risk factors and ways to reduce a person's chance of developing it.

It has been linked with inflammation, the process particularly targeted by NSAIDS. But they also have other, broad effects on the body.

Zandi said some previous research had suggested that ibuprofen may be provide a particular protective effect because it might guard against a type of plaque found in the brains of people with Alzheimer's disease.

"But that's not what we found," Zandi said, noting that ibuprofen delivered protection no better or worse than the others in this class of drugs.

"It's left us with a little bit of a mystery," Zandi said.

INCONSISTENT RESULTS

Researchers in the field have been cautioning people against taking these drugs specifically to ward of Alzheimer's until further studies are done to clarify the effects.

Zandi noted that previous research has delivered inconsistent results on the question of whether these drugs offer any protection against Alzheimer's.

Earlier this month, researchers including Dr. Steven Vlad of Boston University School of Medicine reported the results of a different study finding that **people who took ibuprofen had a 40 percent lower risk of Alzheimer's disease, while those who took other NSAIDs cut their risk by about 25 percent.**

Those findings were based on data on about **49,000 U.S. military** veterans who developed Alzheimer's and nearly 200,000 who had no form of dementia.

But another study published earlier led by Barbara Martin of Johns Hopkins found that NSAIDs did not appear to ward off the mental decline associated with the onset of Alzheimer's disease.

Alzheimer's disease starts out with mild memory loss and confusion, but escalates into profound memory loss and an inability to care for oneself. It is incurable and fatal.

Painkillers do not slow elder mental decline (Celebrex & Aleve)

In May of 2008, researchers reported results from a large government experiment which are dimming hopes **that two common painkillers can prevent Alzheimer's disease or slow mental decline in older people.**

The arthritis drug **Celebrex and the over-the-counter painkiller Aleve showed no benefit on thinking skills, new findings show. Earlier results from the same research showed the two drugs didn't prevent Alzheimer's, at least in the short term.**

The experiment was halted several years early in 2004 when heart risks turned up in a separate study on Celebrex. Researchers also had noticed more heart attacks and strokes in the people taking Aleve in the Alzheimer's prevention study.

Despite the study's early end, there was still enough data to hint at how the drugs act on thinking and memory. The findings were posted online 5/12/08 and will appear in July's *Archives of Neurology*.

"These were not the results we were hoping for," said co-author Barbara Martin of the Johns Hopkins Bloomberg School of Public Health. "We designed this study hoping we would see a protective effect of these drugs."

Researchers hope to continue monitoring the participants to see if they find any delayed benefit.

Scientists have speculated that non-steroidal anti-inflammatories, such as Aleve and Celebrex, might prevent Alzheimer's by reducing inflammation in the brain or by other means.

"The drugs have several effects in the brain and the different effects could be important at different stages in the illness," said study co-author Dr. John Breitner of the University of Washington in Seattle.

Previous studies had found that people who took the drugs ran a lower risk of developing Alzheimer's. But those were observational studies, meaning they observed people's behavior and health. The people who took the pills may have had other healthy habits that lowered their risk.

The halted study included more than **2,000 people** ages 70 and older with a family history of Alzheimer's but no thinking problems themselves. People were **randomly** assigned to take standard daily doses of either Celebrex, Aleve, also known as naproxen, or a dummy pill.

At the start and annually for up to three years, they took a battery of tests. In one, they named as many grocery items as they could in one minute.

All three groups scored about the same at the start. But **over time, the Aleve takers scored on average slightly lower than the people who took placebos. The Celebrex takers scored slightly lower than the placebo takers on most, but not all, of the tests.**

"**There's no evidence that people should be on these drugs (Celebrex & Aleve) to prevent Alzheimer's disease,**" said Dr. David Bennett of Chicago's Rush University Medical Center, who was not involved in the study but does similar research. "**With the side effects of these drugs, people shouldn't be taking them for this reason.**"

Both products now carry warnings about heart risks. Anti-inflammatory drugs also can cause serious gastrointestinal bleeding. Experts advise patients to ask their doctors about how long to take the drugs for pain.

The study was funded by the National Institute on Aging. Pfizer Inc. and Bayer Healthcare provided the drugs and matching dummy pills for the study, but did not participate in the research. Some of the authors reported receiving speaking or consulting fees from drug companies, including Pfizer.

"Unfortunately, as this paper demonstrates, research doesn't always translate into successful new treatments," said Dr. Gail Cawkwell of Pfizer in an e-mail. Cawkwell pointed out that the study did not find increased heart risks for Celebrex.

Bayer spokeswoman Tricia McKernan said the early end to the experiment reduces the relevance of the data. She said the findings don't apply to the intended use of Aleve as a short-term pain reliever.

Long-term ibuprofen use may cut AD risk

People who took the painkiller ibuprofen for more than five years had a 40 percent lower risk of developing Alzheimer's disease, U.S. researchers said.

They also found that **certain other medicines in the same class, known as non-steroidal anti-inflammatory drugs, or NSAIDs, reduced the risk of developing the illness by 25 percent**.

"Some of these medications taken long-term decrease the risk of Alzheimer's disease, but it's very dependent on the exact drugs used. **It doesn't appear that all NSAIDs decrease the risk at the same rate**," Dr. Steven Vlad of Boston University School of Medicine, whose study appears in the journal Neurology, said in a statement.

The study involved more than **49,000 U.S. veterans aged 55 and older who developed Alzheimer's and nearly 200,000 who had no form of dementia**. The researchers looked at more than **five years of** prescription data from the U.S. Veterans Affairs health care system, and at several different NSAIDs.

They found **those who were prescribed ibuprofen for more than five years were 40 percent less likely to develop Alzheimer's disease than those who did not.** The longer they used ibuprofen -- sold under many brand names, including **Motrin and Advil** -- the lower their risk.

The study also found that while some NSAIDs, **such as indomethacin, were associated with lower risks of Alzheimer's, other drugs in the class, such as Pfizer Inc's celecoxib, or Celebrex, were not.**

DOCTOR: DON'T START TAKING IBUPROFEN

Alzheimer's disease has been linked with inflammation, and researchers believe that anti-inflammatory drugs might help delay onset of the disease.

"What's new here is that where other studies have shown that NSAIDs as a class are associated with a lower risk of Alzheimer's disease, we have shown that **the risk varies by the individual drug," Vlad said by e-mail.**

"This kind of individual drug effect has been suggested before only in animal and other lab studies to date. Because our numbers were so big, we were actually able to find differences between individual drugs in humans," he said.

Despite the benefits, **Vlad does not recommend that people start taking ibuprofen in the hopes of staving off Alzheimer's disease.**

"All NSAIDs have significant risks including ulcers, gastrointestinal bleeding, kidney dysfunction, elevated blood pressure and, certainly in the case of COX-II inhibitors like (Merck Inc's withdrawn drug) Vioxx, a cardiovascular risk," he said.

"I think the major implications of this study are more in the direction of prompting further research: a trial of ibuprofen to prevent Alzheimer's disease might be reasonable," he said.

An estimated 5.2 million Americans have Alzheimer's disease, which is the most common form of dementia. The disease starts out with mild memory loss and confusion, but escalates into complete memory loss and an inability to care for oneself.

Alzheimer's disease has no cure and few effective treatments.

CHAPTER FOURTEEN

Short limbs linked with higher risk of memory loss. What?

Having short arms and legs may raise a person's risk of developing memory problems later in life, U.S. researchers said May of 2008.

They said **women with the shortest arm spans were 50 percent more likely to develop dementia and Alzheimer's disease than women with longer arm spans.** And the longer a woman's leg from floor to knee, the lower her risk for dementia.

In men, only a shorter arm span was linked with higher dementia risk, according to the study, which was published in the journal Neurology.

The researchers said several studies have suggested that early life environment plays a role in susceptibility to chronic disease in later life. Short limbs may be a sign of nutritional deficits early in life that ultimately play a role in brain development.

"Body measures such as knee height and arm span are often used as biological indicators of early life deficits, such as a lack of nutrients," said Tina Huang of Tufts University in Boston, who led the study.

Other studies have found a link between limb length and dementia in populations in Asia, and Huang wanted to see if the trend would hold true in a U.S. population, **where 80 percent of height is thought to be inherited.**

She and colleagues studied 2,798 people for an average of five years and took knee height and arm span measurements. Most people in the study were white, with an average age of 72.

By the end of the study, 480 had developed dementia.

"We found that shorter knee heights and arm spans were associated with an increased risk of dementia," Huang and colleagues wrote.

"Overall, our findings suggest that as they do in the Korean populations, anthropometric measures of short stature, even as defined by Western standards, similarly predict risk for dementia," they wrote.

Alzheimer's study links brain size to mental decline

Scientists in the US discovered that **elderly people who had no mental decline had larger brains than Alzheimer's patients**, even though their brain tissue showed signs normally associated with the disease.

The discovery presented at the American Academy of Neurology meeting in Chicago, by researchers from the Oregon Health and Science University (OHSU) in Portland.

The researchers working at the OHSU Layton Aging & Alzheimer's Disease Center discovered that brain volume and the occurrence of mental decline are linked in people with Alzheimer's.

Autopsy examinations of elderly deceased patients showed that the volume of the whole brain, and particularly the hippocampus (a region that sits at the base of the brain and is thought to be involved with encoding long term memory and emotions) tended to be larger in those patients who had not suffered cognitive impairment when they lived.

But the brains of these "healthy" patients still had the characteristic large clusters of protein plaques and tangles normally associated with Alzheimer's.

As co-investigator Dr Deniz Erten-Lyons, an assistant professor of neurology in the OHSU School of Medicine and a staff neurologist at the Portland Veterans Affairs Medical Center explained:

"Prior to death, these people did not suffer from mental decline. We also noted that these healthy study subjects had brain volumes that were on average, larger than the brain volumes of the Alzheimer's subjects we studied."

The researchers examined the brains of **36 deceased patients**, comprising 12 people who did not have symptoms of Alzheimer's before they died (no cognitive impairment) and 24 who did.

Using MRI (magnetic resonance imaging), they found the brains of the "healthy" subjects were about 10 per cent larger by volume than those of the Alzheimer's patients.

Senior scientist on the study, Dr Jeffrey Kaye, who is director of the Layton Aging and Alzheimer's Disease Center and a professor of neurology in the OHSU School of Medicine said:

"We are hopeful that this research will help us further understand the structural and genetic ties to Alzheimer's disease and perhaps offer clues that may help us develop new drugs or therapies."

"**We should caution that at this point we do not believe brain volume is an accurate tool for diagnosing the disease**. However, in the future, this correlation could be helpful to doctors and researchers alike," he added.

Although the study is quite small, it was well received in some quarters.

Professor Clive Ballard from the Alzheimer's Society in the UK, told the BBC the discovery "exciting" and needed "more exploration".

Ballard said it was consistent with other studies that showed "people with higher levels of education or cognitive reserve may be protected from some of the effects of dementia"

Big belly boosts risk of later dementia

AP Science writer, Malcolm Ritter wrote that **having a big belly in your 40s can boost your risk of getting Alzheimer's disease or other dementia decades later**, a new study suggests.

It's not just about your weight. While previous research has found evidence that obesity in middle age raises the chances of developing dementia later, the new work found a separate risk from storing a lot of fat in the abdomen. Even people who weren't overweight were susceptible.

That abdominal fat, sometimes described as making people apple-shaped rather than pear-shaped, has already been linked to higher risk of developing diabetes, stroke and heart disease. This is my ROSI syndrome of clustering of diseases.

"Now we can add dementia to that," said study author Rachel Whitmer of the Kaiser Permanente Division of Research in Oakland, Calif. She and others report the findings in 3/26/08 online issue of the journal Neurology.

The study involved **6,583 men and women who were ages 40 to 45 when they had checkups between 1964 and 1973**. As part of the exam, their belly size was measured by using a caliper to find the distance between their backs and the surface of their upper abdomens. For the study, a distance of about 10 inches or more was considered high. The researchers checked medical records to see who had developed Alzheimer's or another form of dementia by an average of 36 years later. At that point the participants were ages 73 to 87. There were 1,049 cases.

Analysis found that compared to people in the study with normal body weight and a low belly measurement:

• **Participants with normal body weight and high belly measurements were 89 percent more likely to have dementia.**

• Overweight people were 82 percent more likely if they had a low belly measurement, but more than twice as likely if they had a high belly measurement. ????

• Obese people were 81 percent more likely if they had a low belly measurement, but more than three times as likely if they had a high measurement.

Whitmer said there's no precise way to translate belly measurements into waist circumference. But most people have a sense of whether they have a big belly, she said. And if they do, the new study suggests they should get rid of it, she said.

It's not clear why abdominal fat would promote dementia, but it may pump out substances that harm the brain, she said.

I believe that the double bonded fats trap EMODs and help create an insufficiency state. Also, fat cells produce the antioxidant, estrogen, which could exacerbate the EMOD insufficiency.

Dr. Jose Luchsinger of the Columbia University Medical Center in New York, who studies the connection between obesity and Alzheimer's disease but didn't participate in the new work, cautioned that **such a study cannot prove abdominal fat promotes dementia**.

But the study results are "highly plausible" and "I'm not surprised at all," he said. **High insulin levels might help explain them, he said.**

Dr. Samuel Gandy, who chairs the medical and scientific advisory council of the Alzheimer's Association, said the results fit in with previous work that indicates **a person's characteristics in middle age can affect the risk of dementia in later life. And it's another example of how traits associated with the risk of developing heart disease are also linked to later dementia**, he said.

Increased level of magnetic iron oxides found in AD

A team of scientists, in 2008, led by Professor Jon Dobson, of Keele University in Staffordshire, UK, **have found, for the first time, raised levels of magnetic iron oxides in the part of the brain affected by Alzheimer's Disease** (AD).

Their research has also shown that this association was particularly strong in females compared to males. The group speculates that this may be a result of gender differences in the way the body handles and stores iron.

Though the results are based on a small number of samples, they give an indication that iron accumulation associated with Alzheimer's appears to involve the formation of strongly magnetic iron compounds. As these compounds have a strong effect on MRI signal intensity, with further study, it may be possible to use this as a biomarker for the development of an MRI-based Alzheimer's diagnostic technique.

The research team also included Quentin Pankhurst, London Centre for Nanotechnology and Department of Physics & Astronomy, University College, London; Dimitri Hautot, Institute of Science and Technology in Medicine, Keele University, and Nadeem Khan, Department of Neuropathology, Institute of Psychiatry, King's College London.

The study looked at brain tissue from 11 Alzheimer's Disease and 11 age-matched control subjects. It showed, for the first time, that **the total concentration of biogenic magnetite is generally higher in the Alzheimer brain (in some cases as much as 15 times greater than controls) and that there are gender-based differences, with Alzheimer's Disease with female subjects having significantly higher concentrations than all other groups.**

Professor Dobson said: **"Iron accumulation and dysregulation of iron transport and storage has been found to be associated with many other neurodegenerative conditions, such as Parkinson's disease, Huntington's disease (HD), multiple sclerosis and Amyotrophic Lateral Sclerosis.** In recent years, a hereditary neurodegenerative disease, neuroferritinopathy, has been linked to a mutation in the gene encoding for the ferritn light polypeptide. This direct link between neurodegeneration in the basal ganglia and ferritin, the body's primary iron storage protein, results in the accumulation of iron in the brain and symptoms similar to HD.

"There is still little known about the chemical form of iron associated with these diseases, its role in neurodegeneration (if any) and its origin. Investigations of brain iron based on histochemical staining techniques have generally ignored its chemical state."

This study shows a clear correlation in the concentration and the size of the biogenic magnetite in both the Alzheimer disease and control groups. It is also notable that **the largest magnetite concentrations and smallest particles are all from Alzheimer disease** subjects, and that **the data from the control subjects follow the same trend.** This implies that the genesis of the biogenic magnetite may be the same in all cases, but that in Alzheimer Disease it may be more indicative of an accelerated process.

Professor Dobson added: "We speculate that magnetite formation within the ferritin core may occur generally in the brain, perhaps associated with aging, and that the process may become abnormal and uncontrolled in the Alzheimer brain. At this stage, this should be considered a working hypothesis and needs to be examined in larger studies. It appears, however, that elevated levels of magnetic iron oxides, which include **reactive Fe2+,** are present in AD tissue, a finding that lends weight to **the suggestion that redox-active iron may play a role in neurodegenerative disease."** A paper on the study, Increased Levels of Magnetic Compunds in Alzheimer's Disease, was scheduled for publication in the Journal of Alzheimer's Disease. 2008 (Volume 13:1).

Scientists discover link between AD and copper

Copper can damage a molecule that escorts out of the brain a substance called amyloid beta that builds up in toxic quantities in the brains of people with Alzheimer's disease. The new findings demonstrate one way in which copper might contribute to the development of the disease, though scientists say much more research needs to be done to clarify what role, **if any**, copper ultimately plays.

The research by neuroscientists at the University of Rochester Medical Center was presented at the annual meeting of the Society for Neuroscience in San Diego Nov. 3-7, 2007. The work was highlighted as part of a press conference on potential environmental influences on Alzheimer's disease.

For decades, many scientists have hypothesized that a variety of metals, including aluminum, iron, zinc and copper, might play a role in Alzheimer's disease, but no link has ever been proven. In the past few years, several scientists have reported that copper is one component of the amyloid beta clumps -- tiny trash heaps filled with all sorts of molecules and substances -- that speckle the brains of people with Alzheimer's disease.

The new results go much further, showing that copper damages the major known system the brain uses to get rid of amyloid beta. The find marks perhaps the first time that scientists have found a specific way -- a "molecular mechanism" -- that a metal could contribute to the disease process in Alzheimer's disease.

"Metals like aluminum have been suspected for years, but the mechanism through which metals might act has been unclear," said Rashid Deane, Ph.D., the lead author of the work who presented the results in San Diego. "We've demonstrated one mechanism through which copper increases levels of amyloid beta in the brain, by damaging the molecule that gets rid of the substance."

The team found that copper damages a molecule known as LRP (low-density lipoprotein receptor-related protein), a molecule that acts like an escort service in the brain, shuttling amyloid-beta out of the brain and into the body. The molecule's role in Alzheimer's was revealed more than a decade ago by another author of the work, Berislav Zlokovic, M.D., Ph.D., professor of Neurosurgery and Neurology and director of the Frank P. Smith Laboratory for Neuroscience and Neurosurgery Research. **Zlokovic is widely recognized for demonstrating that blood vessels, blood flow, and the blood-brain barrier are central to the development of Alzheimer's disease.**

The study was done in mice as well as on cells from the brains of people who died from Alzheimer's disease. Deane's team compared mice that drank water containing trace amounts of copper (.12 milligrams per liter, less than one-tenth the 1.3 mg/l level of copper allowed in drinking water by the Environmental Protection Agency), to mice that drank distilled water.

Mice that drank water with trace levels of copper had about twice as much copper in the cells lining the blood vessels of the brain as the mice that did not. They also had about one-third fewer LRP molecules in those blood vessels and about one-third more amyloid beta in their brains than the control mice, after 10 weeks.

Using human cells, the team discovered that copper damages the protein LRP to such an extent that it stops working. The team has shown previously that having fewer functioning LRP molecules results in higher levels of amyloid beta, which ultimately aggregates together and kills brain cells.

"We all have some amyloid beta in the brain normally," said Deane, associate professor of Neurological Surgery. "When you age, a little bit more accumulates in the brain naturally. But the process is greatly accelerated in people with Alzheimer's disease."

While it's clear from the study that copper can damage LRP, Deane says **it's preliminary to draw the conclusion that copper causes Alzheimer's disease based on the study.**

"There's a great deal more work that needs to be done to fully understand the role that copper may play in Alzheimer's disease," said Deane. "We need to explore the mechanism of how copper breaks down LRP much more fully. Then, of course, we must see if the same is true in people. There are different ways to measure copper in the blood, and indeed, **there is some research linking low levels of copper to Alzheimer's, while there is other research linking high levels of copper to the disease.**"

Right?

Deane emphasizes that having **appropriate levels of copper in our body is crucial for our health.** Copper helps keep our bones our strong and our skin toned, and it helps our nerves fire crisply and our cells to generate the energy we need to live. It helps keep our blood healthy so we can get the oxygen we need to all our organs. And it plays a role in keeping our immune system strong.

While drinking water is the most obvious source of copper in our diet, because of copper pipes, the substance is also quite common in red meat, nuts, shellfish, and many fruits and vegetables.

The research highlights the importance of the **blood-brain barrier, an intricate filtering mechanism that lines the inside of blood vessels inside the brain and is designed to keep toxic substances out.** It's as if the ultra-sensitive brain is designed to be isolated from the common blood supply. Thousands of molecules act as sentries, decided exactly which substances are allowed into and out of the brain, and which aren't allowed to cross the barrier. LRP is one such sentry, specializing in the removal of amyloid beta from the brain.

I ask, " if oxygen is toxic, then why does the blood brain barrier selectively allow such large quantities to flood the brain?" The answer is that oxygen is not toxic and that it is essential to normal brain functioning.

"The body needs to maintain the environment of the brain pristinely so that our brain cells stay healthy and are able to function effectively," said Deane. "It's the job of the blood-brain barrier to keep the brain safe and healthy. It may very well be a breakdown with the barrier that is at the root of Alzheimer's disease."

Copper protects against Alzheimer's

In 2009, research showed that there could be a protective role for copper in AD.

Two articles in a forthcoming issue of the Journal of Alzheimer's Disease by Dr Chris Exley, Reader in Bioinorganic Chemistry in the Research Institute for the Environment, Physical Sciences and Applied Mathematics at Keele University, UK, (**"Copper abolishes the beta-sheet secondary structure of preformed amyloid fibrils of Abeta42"**) and Dr Zhao-Feng Jiang, of Beijing Union University, Beijing, China ("Coordinating to three histidine residues: Cu(II) promoting oligomeric, fibril amyloid beta peptide to aggregate in a non-beta-sheeted way") **have confirmed a potentially protective role for copper in Alzheimer's Disease.**

Previous research has shown that **copper is one component of the amyloid beta plaques** which are found in the brains of people of Alzheimer's disease.

A central tenet of the **Amyloid Cascade Hypothesis of Alzheimer's disease** is the aberrant deposition in the brain of Abeta42 in beta-sheets in neuritic or senile plaques. The Keele team have shown in previous research in JAD (House et al., (2004) JAD 6, 291-301) that **copper (Cu(II)) prevents the deposition of Abeta42 in beta-sheets while in the current research they show that Cu(II) abolishes the beta-sheet structure of preformed amyloid fibrils of Abeta42.** A similar finding was made by the group of Jiang for the other form of beta amyloid, Abeta40, and **together these observations strongly suggest that copper prevents both the formation and the accumulation of plaques in the brain.**

Coincident with the copper-catalysed dissolution of beta-sheets of Abeta42, Exley's group made the first observation of the in vitro formation of spherulites of this peptide. These spherical globules of amyloid have only previously been observed in vitro for the other amyloid-forming proteins insulin and beta-lactoglobulin. Copper appeared to have a role in the formation of spherulites of Abeta42 and this will be investigated in future research. The role of metals in the formation, deposition and metabolism of Abeta in Alzheimer's disease is much debated and these new findings highlight a potential protective role for copper in Alzheimer's disease. **I believe that this is important because copper (the cupric oxidized elemental form) is a prooxidant, as are all heavy transition metals. I believe that the "dissolution of the amyloid sheets" was due to oxidation.**

Copper attacks free radicals. Copper (the cuprous reduced elemental form) is a strong antioxidant. It works by attaching itself to the enzyme Superoxide dismutase (SOD). Copper also binds to a protein to form ceruloplasmin, which is an antioxidant. Copper is a component of or a cofactor for approximately 50 different enzymes. **These enzymes need copper to function properly.**

CHAPTER FIFTEEN

AD and THC

THC inhibits major AD marker

Marijuana's Active Ingredient Shown to Inhibit Primary Marker of Alzheimer's Disease

Discovery Could Lead to More Effective Treatments

In August of 2006, scientists at The Scripps Research Institute found that **the active ingredient in marijuana, tetrahydrocannabinol or THC, inhibited the formation of amyloid plaque, the primary pathological marker for Alzheimer's disease**. In fact, the study said, **THC is "a considerably superior inhibitor of [amyloid plaque] aggregation" to several currently approved drugs for treating the disease.**

The study was published online August 9, 2006 in the journal **Molecular Pharmaceutics**, a publication of the American Chemical Society.

According to the new Scripps Research study, which used both computer modeling and biochemical assays, THC inhibits the enzyme acetylcholinesterase (AChE), which acts as a "molecular chaperone" to accelerate the formation of amyloid plaque in the brains of Alzheimer victims. **Although experts disagree on whether the presence of beta-amyloid plaques in those areas critical to memory and cognition is a symptom or cause, it remains a significant hallmark of the disease.**

With its strong inhibitory abilities, the study said, THC "may provide an improved therapeutic for Alzheimer's disease" that would treat "both the symptoms and progression" of the disease.

"While **we are certainly not advocating the use of illegal drugs**, these findings offer convincing evidence that THC possesses remarkable inhibitory qualities, especially when compared to AChE inhibitors currently available to patients," said Kim Janda, Ph.D., who is Ely R. Callaway, Jr. Professor of Chemistry at Scripps Research, a member of The Skaggs Institute for Chemical Biology, and director of the Worm Institute of Research and Medicine. "In a test against propidium, one of the most effective inhibitors reported to date, **THC blocked AChE-induced aggregation completely**, while the propidium did not. Although our study is far from final, it does show that **there is a previously unrecognized molecular mechanism through which THC may directly affect the progression of Alzheimer's disease.**"

As the new study points out, any new treatment that could halt or even slow the progression of Alzheimer's disease would have a major impact on the quality of life for patients, as well as reducing the staggering health care costs associated with the disease.

Alzheimer's disease is the leading cause of dementia among the elderly, and the numbers are growing. The Alzheimer's Association estimates 5.5 million Americans have the disease, a figure that could reach as high as 16 million by 2050. A survey by the National Center for Health Statistics noted that **half of all nursing home residents have Alzheimer's disease or a related disorder.** The costs of caring for Alzheimer's patients are at least $100 billion annually, according to the National Institute on Aging.

Over the last two decades, the causes of Alzheimer's disease have been clarified through extensive biochemical and neurobiological studies, leading to an assortment of possible therapeutic strategies including interference with beta amyloid metabolism, the focus of the Scripps Research study.

The cholinergic system - the nerve cell system in the brain that uses acetylcholine (Ach) as a neurotransmitter - is the most dramatic of the neurotransmitter systems affected by Alzheimer's disease. **Levels of acetylcholine, which was first identified in 1914, are abnormally low in the brains of Alzheimer's patients**. Currently, there are four FDA-approved drugs that treat the symptoms of Alzheimer's disease by inhibiting the active site of acetylcholinesterase, the enzyme responsible for the degradation of acetylcholine.

"When we investigated the power of THC to inhibit the aggregation of beta-amyloid," Janda said, "we found that THC was a very effective inhibitor of acetylcholinesterase. In addition to propidium, **we also found that THC was considerably more effective than two of the approved drugs for Alzheimer's disease treatment, donepezil (Aricept ®) and tacrine (Cognex ®),** which reduced amyloid aggregation by only 22 percent and 7 percent, respectively, at twice the concentration used in our studies. Our results are conclusive enough to warrant further investigation."

Admitedly, this is just the opposite of what I expected. But, I remember that THC is a prooxidant and this may also be part of its mechanism of action.

Other authors of the study, titled "A Molecular Link Between the Active Component of Marijuana and Alzheimer's Disease Pathology," include Lisa M. Eubanks, Claude J. Rogers, and Tobin J. Dickerson of The Scripps Research Institute, the Skaggs Institute for Chemical Biology, and the Worm Institute for Research and Medicine; and Albert E. Beuscher IV, George F. Koob, and Arthur J. Olson of The Scripps Research Institute.

The study was supported by the Skaggs Institute for Chemical Biology at Scripps Research and the National Institutes of Health.

A molecular link between the active component of marijuana and Alzheimer's disease pathology

Alzheimer's disease is the leading cause of dementia among the elderly, and with the ever-increasing size of this population, cases of Alzheimer's disease are expected to triple over the next 50 years. Consequently, the development of treatments that slow or halt the disease progression have become imperative to both improve the quality of life for patients and reduce the health care costs attributable to Alzheimer's disease. Here, we demonstrate that **the active component of marijuana, Delta9-tetrahydrocannabinol (THC), competitively inhibits the enzyme acetylcholinesterase (AChE) as well as prevents AChE-induced amyloid beta-peptide (Abeta) aggregation, the key pathological marker of Alzheimer's disease.** Computational modeling of the THC-AChE interaction revealed that THC binds in the peripheral anionic site of AChE, the critical region involved in amyloidgenesis. **Compared to currently approved drugs prescribed for the treatment of Alzheimer's disease, THC is a considerably superior inhibitor of Abeta aggregation,** and this study provides a previously unrecognized molecular mechanism through which cannabinoid molecules may directly impact the progression of this debilitating disease. (Eubanks et al, 2006)

Alzheimer's disease: taking the edge off with cannabinoids?

Alzheimer's disease is an age-related neurodegenerative condition associated with cognitive decline. The pathological hallmarks of the disease are the deposition of beta-amyloid protein and hyperphosphorylation of tau, which evoke neuronal cell death and impair inter-neuronal communication. The disease is also associated with neuroinflammation, excitotoxicity and oxidative stress. In recent years the proclivity of cannabinoids to exert a neuroprotective influence has received substantial interest as a means to mitigate the symptoms of neurodegenerative conditions. In brains obtained from Alzheimer's patients alterations in components of the cannabinoid system have been reported, suggesting that the cannabinoid system either contributes to, or is altered by, the pathophysiology of the disease. **Certain cannabinoids can protect neurons from the deleterious effects of beta-amyloid and are capable of reducing tau phosphorylation**. The propensity of cannabinoids to reduce beta-amyloid-evoked oxidative stress and neurodegeneration, whilst stimulating neurotrophin expression neurogenesis, are interesting properties that may be beneficial in the treatment of Alzheimer's disease. **Delta 9-tetrahydrocannabinol can also inhibit acetylcholinesterase activity and limit amyloidogenesis** which may improve cholinergic transmission and delay disease progression. Targeting cannabinoid receptors on microglia may reduce the neuroinflammation that is a feature of Alzheimer's disease, without causing psychoactive effects. Thus, **cannabinoids offer a multi-faceted approach for the treatment of Alzheimer's disease by providing neuroprotection and reducing neuroinflammation, whilst simultaneously supporting the brain's intrinsic repair mechanisms by augmenting neurotrophin expression and enhancing neurogenesis**. (Campbell, Gowran, 2007)

Shockingly, THC offers more hope than all of the other potential therapeutics for AD that I have reviewed.

And, yes, you guessed it: "I didn't inhale."

THC is a prooxidant (or maybe an antioxidant)

Oxidative stress is produced by marijuana smoke.

Marijuana (MJ) smoking produces inflammation, edema, and cell injury in the tracheobronchial mucosa of smokers and may be a risk factor for lung cancer. Because oxidative stress may mediate some of these effects, this study was designed to test the hypothesis that cannabinoids in MJ smoke contribute to cellular oxidative stress. Oxidative stress was evaluated in an endothelial cell line (ECV 304) following exposure to smoke produced from MJ cigarettes containing either 0, 1.77, or 3.95% Δ^9-tetrahydrocannabinol (Δ^9-THC). **Brief exposure to smoke from 3.95% MJ cigarettes stimulated the formation of reactive oxygen species (ROS) by 80% over control levels** and lowered intracellular glutathione levels by 81%. Smoke-induced ROS generation increased in a dose- and time-dependent manner. **In contrast, exposure to smoke from MJ containing 0% Δ^9-THC produced no increase in ROS** despite a 70% decline in glutathione levels. Smoke from MJ containing 1.77% Δ^9-THC stimulated intermediate levels of ROS. A brief, 30-min exposure to MJ smoke, regardless of the Δ^9-THC content, also induced necrotic cell death that increased steadily up to 48 h of observation. MJ smoke passed through a Cambridge filter that removed particulate matter was 3.4-fold more active in ROS production compared with unfiltered smoke, suggesting that most of the oxidative effects are produced by the gaseous phase. Alveolar macrophages obtained from habitual MJ smokers displayed low levels of glutathione compared with macrophages from nonsmokers. We conclude **that MJ smoke containing Δ^9-THC is a potent source of cellular oxidative stress** that could contribute significantly to cell injury and dysfunction in the lungs of smokers. (Sarafian, et al, 1999)

However, persistent efforts to legalize marijuana (MJ) and political movements advocating medicinal uses tend to promote the notion that little or no hazardous risk is associated with MJ smoking.

Approximately 60 different cannabinoids classified as C-21 terpenophenolic compounds can be found in the smoke derived from MJ, and the cannabinoid content of an MJ plant varies considerably depending on the type of plant and conditions of cultivation.

Some reports suggest that, over the past 10 to 20 yr, the cannabinoid content in MJ cigarettes may have increased severalfold. There is little information on toxicologic effects of individual constituents found in MJ smoke.

In the present studies Sarafian, et al examined the effects of whole MJ cigarette smoke with and without Δ^9-THC and of the gas phase of the smoke on the generation of reactive oxygen species (ROS) and on levels of antioxidants in the cultured human endothelial cell line, ECV 304. Cellular production of EMODs and reduced antioxidant activity were considered to be toxicologic markers of oxidative stress. Human alveolar macrophages collected from the lungs of habitual MJ smokers were also evaluated for evidence of *in situ* exposure to oxidative stress, and were compared with findings in macrophages from control nonsmokers.

Clearly, the AD antagonist, THC, is a prooxidant.

On the other hand, direct measurement of oxidative stress revealed that cannabinoids prevented serum-deprived cell death by antioxidation. The antioxidative property of cannabinoids was confirmed by their ability to antagonize oxidative stress and consequent cell death induced by the retinoid anhydroretinol.

Therefore, **cannabinoids act as antioxidants** to modulate cell survival and growth of B lymphocytes and fibroblasts. (Chen, Buck, 2000)

Cannabinoids have been used to treat cancer, nausea, inhibit appetite and inhibit pain.

Yet, most interesting is the section titled Antitumour effects of cannabinoids, where author Manuel Guzmán shows that cannabinoids destroy many forms of tumors and cancer cells.

Guzmán claims that "cannabinoids are selective antitumor compounds, as they can kill tumor cells without affecting their non-transformed counterparts." In fact, instead of harming normal cells, cannabinoids "might even protect them from cell death."

Citing over 100 references of research from scientific and medicinal journals, this article compiles all major studies into how cannabinoids affect cancerous tumors and cancer patients.

In 2000, Manuel Guzmán led a study which showed that application of THC destroyed otherwise incurable brain cancer tumors in rats.

Interesting studies on THC killing cancer include:

A study published in the July 2002 edition of the medical journal Blood, which found that THC and some other cannabinoids produced "programmed cell death" in different varieties of human leukemia and lymphoma cell lines, thereby destroying the cancerous cells but leaving other cells unharmed.

A study published in a 1975 edition of the Journal of the National Cancer Institute, which showed that THC slowed the growth of lung cancer, breast cancer and virus-induced leukemia in rats.

A 1994 study, which documented that THC may protect against malignant cancers, and which was buried by the US government. The $2 million study, funded by the US Department of Health and Human Services, sought to show that large doses of THC produced cancer in rats. Instead, researchers found that massive doses of THC had a positive effect, actually slowing the growth of stomach cancers. The rats given THC lived longer than their non-exposed counterparts.

It appears to me that the tumoricidal character of THC must be acting via EMOD-induced apoptosis.

Alzheimer's memory loss faster among well-educated

Will Dunham reported that **having more years of formal education delays the memory loss linked to Alzheimer's disease, but once the condition begins to take hold, better-educated people decline more rapidly**, researchers said in October 2007.

Their study, published in the journal Neurology, tracked memory loss in a group of elderly people from New York City's Bronx borough before they were diagnosed with Alzheimer's or another form of old-age dementia.

Every year of education delayed the accelerated memory decline that precedes dementia by about 2-1/2 months, according to the researchers at Yeshiva University's Albert Einstein College of Medicine in New York.

But once this memory loss began, the rate of decline unfolded 4 percent more quickly for each additional year of education, the researchers said.

Someone with 16 years of schooling might experience memory decline 50 percent more quickly than another person with just four years education, based on the findings.

Alzheimer's disease is a degenerative brain malady that is the most common form of dementia among the elderly.

"An elderly person who starts to see memory loss might well deteriorate fairly rapidly, particularly if he or she has a high education or high IQ," Charles Hall, a professor of epidemiology at Albert Einstein College of Medicine who led the study, said in a telephone interview.

"And this is important to clinicians to know so they can advise their patients that things might well get very bad very fast, whereas in a lot of other people the decline is relatively gradual over a long period of time," Hall added.

People with more years of formal education appear to have a greater "cognitive reserve," Hall said, referring to the brain's ability to keep working despite damage.

While better-educated people may be diagnosed with Alzheimer's later than people with less education, it appears they have suffered brain damage but their "cognitive reserve" was able to hide and delay the effects, the researchers said.

The study started in the 1980s, tracking **488 people** born from 1894 and 1908 and giving them periodic memory tests. The findings published were based on 117 of them who eventually developed Alzheimer's or another dementia.

Most of the participants were followed until either death or diagnosis of dementia. Those diagnosed with dementia were followed for up to about 16 years, with an average of six years.

The study included people with postgraduate education as well as others with fewer than three years of elementary school. Hall noted that levels of education that people received varied much more in the early part of the 20th century than they do now.

Hall said the study was valuable in part because it examined memory loss before a formal diagnosis of Alzheimer's. Other studies have detected quicker memory loss among more highly educated people after diagnosis of Alzheimer's.

Cold sore virus 'increases Alzheimer's risk'

HSV-1 virus: spread by kissing

The virus that causes cold sores when passed on through kissing could help trigger Alzheimer's, scientists say.

Researchers found brain **cells exposed to the herpes simplex virus-1 (HSV-1) produce large quantities of a chemical that builds up and prevents the transmission of messages in the brains of Alzheimer's sufferers.**

Previous studies suggest the virus is much more active in people with a variant of a gene carried by 30 per cent of the population and half of Alzheimer's patients.

As antiviral drugs can be used to treat herpes infections, the findings could ultimately lead to those with the gene defect being vaccinated in childhood to significantly reduce their risk of developing the disease.

HSV-1 is present in 80 per cent of the adult population. It is passed on mainly through saliva, but also through sexual contact. The virus usually remains dormant in the body, but can become more active and cause cold sores in response to other factors such as ill health or stress.

I believe that an EMOD insufficiency "allows" the virus to manifest itself as a coldsore. If EMOD levels were high enough, it would result in the oxidative inactivation of the virus or the oxidative breakdown of the virus.

Prof Ruth Itzhaki and colleagues at the University of Manchester, whose work is highlighted in Nov. 2007, New Scientist, **exposed human brain cells with HSV-1 in laboratory experiments. They found this caused a dramatic increase within the cells in levels of amyloid beta protein** – a substance that makes up the main constituent of the plaques that form in the brains of people with Alzheimer's.

The researchers saw similar increases in the chemical in the brains of mice they infected with HSV-1. They also examined brain sections from deceased Alzheimer's patients and found DNA from the HSV-1 virus attached to the plaques.

US researchers showed that **HSV-1 was more active in mice with a genetic variant called ApoE4 than those with the normal form of the gene.**

Prof Itzhaki added: "I think there's enough evidence to begin treating people with ApoE4 antiviral drugs to slow the progression of the disease." **I do not agree because there is still inadequate data to justify treatment.**

Approximately 350,000 people in the UK have Alzheimer's, including one in 10 people aged over 65. The degenerative disease undermines brain cells and their ability to communicate - leading to memory loss and changes to behaviour and mood.

Prof Clive Ballard, director of research at the Alzheimer's Society, said further research would be needed to prove a link between the virus and the disease. "If this link could be investigated further researchers have suggested anti-viral drugs used on herpes, may have an impact on treatment targets for Alzheimer's disease.

"This latest work is based on cell culture experiments and more research is needed before we can establish how relevant it may be to people with Alzheimer's disease and the emergence of possible new treatment targets." (Science Correspondent By Nic Fleming.

Last Updated: 2:37PM GMT 07 Nov 2007).

New link between Alzheimers and herpes virus

In December of 2008, Science Daily reported that **the virus behind cold sores is a major cause of the insoluble protein plaques found in the brains of Alzheimer's disease sufferers,** University of Manchester researchers have revealed.

They believe the herpes simplex virus is a significant factor in developing the debilitating disease and **could be treated by antiviral agents such as acyclovir,** which is already used to treat cold sores and other diseases caused by the herpes virus. Another future possibility is vaccination against the virus to prevent the development of the disease in the first place.

Alzheimer's disease (AD) is characterized by progressive memory loss and severe cognitive impairment. **It affects over 20 million people world-wide,** and the numbers will rise with increasing longevity. However, despite enormous investment into research on the characteristic abnormalities of AD brain - amyloid plaques and neu-rofibrillary tangles - **the underlying causes are unknown and current treatments are ineffectual.**

Professor Ruth Itzhaki and her team at the University's Faculty of Life Sciences have investigated the role of herpes simplex virus type 1 (HSV1) in AD, publishing their very recent, highly significant findings in the **Journal of Pathology in December of 2008**.

Most people are infected with this virus, which then remains life-long in the peripheral nervous system, and in 20-40% of those infected it causes cold sores. Evidence of a viral role in AD would point to the use of antiviral agents to stop progression of the disease.

The team discovered that the HSV1 DNA is located very specifically in amyloid plaques: 90% of plaques in Alzheimer's disease sufferers' brains contain HSV1 DNA, and most of the viral DNA is located within amyloid plaques.

The team had previously shown that HSV1 infection of nerve-type cells induces deposition of the main component, beta amyloid, of amyloid plaques. Together, these findings strongly implicate HSV1 as a major factor in the formation of amyloid deposits and plaques, abnormalities thought by many in the field to be major contributors to Alzheimer's disease.

The team had discovered much earlier that **the virus is present in brains of many elderly people and that in those people with a specific genetic factor, there is a high risk of developing Alzheimer's disease.**

The team's data strongly suggest that HSV1 has a major role in Alzheimer's disease and point to the usage of antiviral agents for treating the disease, and in fact, in preliminary experiments they have shown that **acyclovir reduces the amyloid deposition and reduces also certain other feature of the disease which they have found are caused by HSV1 infection.**

Professor Itzhaki explains: "We suggest that **HSV1 enters the brain in the elderly as their immune systems decline** and then establishes a dormant infection from which it is repeatedly activated by events such as stress, immunosuppression, and various infections.

"The ensuing active HSV1 infection causes severe damage in brain cells, most of which die and then disintegrate, thereby releasing **amyloid aggregates** which develop into **amyloid plaques** after other components of dying cells are deposited on them."

Her colleague Dr Matthew Wozniak adds: "Antiviral agents would inhibit the harmful consequences of HSV1 action; in other words, inhibit a likely major cause of the disease irrespective of the actual damaging processes involved, whereas current treatments at best merely inhibit some of the symptoms of the disease."

They very much hope also that clinical trials will be set up to test the effect of antiviral agents on Alzheimer's disease patients.

I believe that EMOD insufficiency allows the HSV1 virus to locate in the brain and it also allows the formation of amyloid plaques. Oxidation would both kill the virus and break down the plaques. A lack of oxygen has been implicated in the formation of Alzheimer's.

Does curcumin have a role in AD

It is not known whether curcumin taken orally can cross the blood brain barrier or inhibit the progression of Alzheimer's disease in humans. However, curcumin has been found to inhibit amyloid beta oligomer formation in vitro. (Yang et al, 2005)

When injected peripherally, curcumin was found to cross the blood brain barrier in an animal model of Alzheimer's disease. **In animal models of Alzheimer's disease, dietary curcumin has decreased biomarkers of inflammation and oxidative damage, amyloid plaque burden in the brain, and amyloid beta-induced memory deficits.** (Pan et al, 2008)

A small 6-month pilot trial with 34 subjects with AD were randomized to placebo or two doses of the antioxidant, **curcumin. There was no cognitive decline in the placebo group, and no improvement was observed with curcumin.** (Baum et al, 2008)

Clinical trials of oral curcumin supplementation in patients with early Alzheimer's disease are under way and results of a 6-month trial in 27 patients with Alzheimer's disease found that oral supplementation with up to 4 g/day of curcumin was safe. We must await further results.

CHAPTER SIXTEEN

Diabetes in mid-life linked to increased risk of AD

Men who develop diabetes in mid-life appear to significantly increase their risk of developing Alzheimer's disease, according to a long-term study published in the **April 9, 2008, online issue of Neurology®,** the medical journal of the American Academy of Neurology.

"Our results have important public health implications given the increasing numbers of people developing diabetes and the need for more powerful interventions," said study author Elina Rönnemaa, MD, with Uppsala University in Uppsala, Sweden.

The study involved **2,269 men** in Sweden who underwent glucose testing at age 50 to test for diabetes, which is caused by abnormal insulin levels. During an average follow up of 32 years, **102 participants** were diagnosed with Alzheimer's disease, 57 with vascular dementia and 235 with other types of dementia or cognitive impairment.

The study found that the **men with low insulin secretion capacity at age 50 were nearly one-and-a-half times more likely to develop Alzheimer's disease** than people without insulin problems. The risk remained significant regardless of blood pressure, cholesterol, body mass index and education.

"Our results suggest a link between insulin problems and the origins of Alzheimer's disease and emphasize the importance of insulin in normal brain function," said Rönnemaa. "It's possible that insulin problems damage blood vessels in the brain, which leads to memory problems and Alzheimer's disease, but more research is needed to identify the exact mechanisms."

The study also found **the association between diabetes and risk of Alzheimer's disease was strongest in people who did not have the APOE4 gene, which is known to increase the risk of Alzheimer's disease.** Rönnemaa says this shows that insulin problems are an important risk factor for Alzheimer's disease when the high risk gene is missing.

Discovery supports theory of Alzheimer's disease as form of diabetes

In September of 2007, it was found that insulin, it turns out, may be as important for the mind as it is for the body. Research in the last few years has raised the possibility that Alzheimer's memory loss could be due to a novel "third form of diabetes."

Scientists at Northwestern University have discovered why **brain insulin signaling -- crucial for memory formation --** would stop working in Alzheimer's disease. They have shown that **a toxic protein found in the brains of individuals with Alzheimer's removes insulin receptors from nerve cells,** rendering those neurons insulin resistant. (The protein, known to attack memory-forming synapses, is called an **ADDL for "amyloid ß-derived diffusible ligand."**)

With other research showing that levels of brain insulin and its related receptors are lower in individuals with Alzheimer's disease, the Northwestern study sheds light on the **emerging idea of Alzheimer's being a "type 3" diabetes.**

The new findings, published online by the **FASEB Journal,** could help researchers determine which aspects of existing drugs now used to treat diabetic patients may protect neurons from ADDLs and improve insulin signaling in individuals with Alzheimer's. (The FASEB Journal is a publication of the Federation of American Societies for Experimental Biology.)

In the brain, insulin and insulin receptors are vital to learning and memory. When insulin binds to a receptor at a synapse, it turns on a mechanism necessary for nerve cells to survive and memories to form. That Alzheimer's disease may in part be caused by insulin resistance in the brain has scientists asking how that process gets initiated. **Please remember that hydrogen peroxide is an insulin mimetic.**

"We found the binding of ADDLs to synapses somehow prevents insulin receptors from accumulating at the synapses where they are needed," said William L. Klein, professor of neurobiology and physiology in the Weinberg College of Arts and Sciences, who led the research team. "Instead, they are piling up where they are made, in the cell body, near the nucleus. Insulin cannot reach receptors there. This finding is the first molecular evidence as to why nerve cells should become insulin resistant in Alzheimer's disease."

ADDLS are small, soluble aggregated proteins. The clinical data strongly support a theory in which **ADDLs accumulate at the beginning of Alzheimer's disease and block memory function by a process predicted to be reversible**.

In earlier research, Klein and colleagues found that ADDLs bind very specifically at synapses, initiating deterioration of synapse function and causing changes in synapse composition and shape. Now Klein and his team have shown that the molecules that make memories at synapses -- **insulin receptors -- are being removed by ADDLs from the surface membrane of nerve cells.**

Insulin protects brain from Alzheimer's toxins

As of February 2009 new research indicated that the hormone insulin shields the brain from toxic proteins associated with Alzheimer's disease. Researchers at Northwestern University in the United States and at the Federal University of Rio de Janiero in Brazil found that **cells taken from the brain's memory centers were protected by insulin from the toxic proteins that attacked them in Alzheimer's.**

The scientists involved say that sensitivity to insulin declines with age. In their view, **Alzheimer's is a form of brain diabetes** where brain cells become more vulnerable to damaging proteins as they lose the protection of insulin over time.

I believe that this means that hydrogen peroxide could be used to treat or prevent Alzheimer's disease.

A provocative new theory suggests that one root cause of Alzheimer's disease is linked to diabetes — **a theory about to be tested in thousands of Alzheimer's patients given the diabetes drug Avandia in hopes of slowing brain decay**.

It's a scary scenario: Alzheimer's already is expected to skyrocket as the population grays, rising from 4.5 million sufferers today to a staggering 14 million by 2050. If the new theory is right, the nation's current obesity-fueled epidemic of Type 2 diabetes could worsen that toll.

But proponents see potential good news: If diabetic-like changes in the way brain cells use sugar to generate energy truly trigger Alzheimer's in at least some patients, then maybe doctors could intervene early and slow down that degeneration

A preliminary experiment involving **511 Alzheimer's patients** found signals that Avandia might help — albeit in people who lack a gene that spurs more aggressive Alzheimer's.

Those results, combined with other evidence that the diabetes pathway is important, have Avandia maker GlaxoSmithKline poised to open three Phase III clinical trials to test whether the diabetes drug, also called **rosiglitazone**, might protect certain patients' brains.

Diabetes has long been listed a risk factor for Alzheimer's later in life because it damages blood vessels that supply the brain.

I believe that this indicates that oxygen to the brain can also be reduced.

The Avandia research suggests a more insidious connection: that **Alzheimer's can be silently triggered when brain cells can't properly use their main fuel, sugar** — just as Type 2 diabetes is triggered when insulin gradually loses its ability to process sugar body-wide. **"When they're in an insulin-resistant state, it does not just affect the body, it affects the brain as well,"** explains Suzanne Craft of the Veterans Affairs Puget Sound Health care System, who led the initial research.

Memory loss is slower in AD patients with diabetes surprises researchers

Researchers from France and the UK who set out to investigate whether people with Alzheimer's disease and diabetes have more rapid memory loss were surprised to find not only that they did not, but that their memory loss was actually slower than that of Alzheimer's patients without diabetes. Speculating on the reasons, they suggested it could be the effect of diabetes drugs, or that Alzheimer's patients with diabetes have different kinds of lesions in the brain.

The study was the work of first author Dr Caroline Sanz, of INSERM, the French National Institute for Health and Medical Research in Toulouse, and colleagues, and is published in the **27 October, 2009 print issue of *Neurology***, the medical journal of the American Academy of Neurology.

The researchers already knew from previous studies that diabetes increases the risk of Alzheimer's disease and the risk of memory loss in people who don't have Alzheimer's, but it was unclear whether people with both Alzheimer's and diabetes experienced more rapid memory loss.

Sanz told the press that their findings surprised them: **"Our initial hypothesis was that diabetes would increase the rate of cognitive decline in people with Alzheimer's disease."**

For the study, which was sponsored by the French Ministry of Health and the Toulouse University Hospital, the researchers followed **608 community-dwelling patients** with mild to moderate Alzheimer's disease for **4 years**, during which time they tested their thinking and memory skills twice a year with the commonly used MMSE (mini mental state examination) test of cognitive function.

63 of the 608 participants (10.4 per cent), also had diabetes.

The authors found that after applying a "mixed model" to take into account "sex, age, educational level, dementia severity, cholinesterase inhibitor use, and vascular factors (hypertension, atrial fibrillation, coronary heart disease, and hypercholesterolemia)", the results showed that:

At the start of the study period, both groups (Alzheimer's patients with and without diabetes) had the same average MMSE scores of 20. Over each six-month testing period, the overall group score went down by an average of 1.24 points. However, **those without diabetes declined by 0.38 points more per six-month period than those with diabetes. Sanz and colleagues concluded that:**

"In a cohort of community-dwelling patients with Alzheimer disease (AD), the presence of diabetes mellitus (DM) was associated with a lower rate of cognitive decline." "Future studies will need to address the potential impact of DM in the cerebral aging process and to assess the neuropathologic variations in patients with AD with DM," they added.

Speculating on the reasons why they found that the rate of cognitive decline was slower for the Alzheimer's patients in their study, Sanz suggested that: "One possible explanation is that diabetes in the elderly differs from that in younger people and in addition, elderly people with diabetes may be more likely to receive cardiovascular medications such as drugs for hugh blood pressure than people who don't have diabetes."

"These drugs have been reported to decrease the risk of developing Alzheimer's disease and also the rate of cognitive decline in people with Alzheimer's disease," she added, explaining that another reason for these findings could be due to: "Differences in brain lesions in those people with diabetes compared to those without diabetes." (Sanz et al, 2009)

Alzheimer's and diabetes facts: my conclusions

Here is how I now see the picture:

- Alzheimer's is considered to be diabetes of the brain.
- High blood glucose lowers EMOD levels
- Hydrogen peroxide is an insulin mimetic.
- Lower caloric intake improves memory.
- Gastric bypass decreases caloric intake and cures diabetes.
- Could gastric bypass improve memory?
- An adequate oxygen levels is critical to normal brain functioning.
- Strokes, CVD, COPD, etc all increase the risk of Alzheimer's and lower O_2 levels.
- Could increased O_2 and decreased caloric intake have a synergistic affect on dementia?

Don't panic if you're diabetic, stresses Dr. Ralph Nixon of New York University, vice chairman of the Alzheimer's Association's scientific advisory council. **Genetics still are the prime risk factor for dementia.**

"It by no means means that you're going to develop Alzheimer's disease, and certainly many people with Alzheimer's don't have diabetes," he cautions.

But the latest research strengthens the link, and has scientists asking if diabetes and its related "metabolic syndrome" increase risk solely by spurring brain changes that underlie Alzheimer's — or if they add an extra layer of injury to an already struggling brain, what Nixon calls "essentially a two-hit situation."

Among the findings:

Brain functioning subtly slows as Type 2 diabetics' blood-sugar rises, well before people have any obvious memory problems. **RMH Note: rising blood sugar also causes an EMOD insufficiency.**

In a major national study, doctors gave a battery of cognitive tests to nearly 3,000 diabetics. **Every 1 percentage point increase in their A1C score — an average of glucose control over a few months — meant small but meaningful drops in tests of memory**, the ability to multitask, and other cognitive tasks, Wake Forest University scientists wrote in the journal Diabetes Care.

The government-funded study is testing whether better treatment to lower those A1C scores in turn improves brain function.

_At Columbia, Stern is co-directing a powerful study: Hundreds of aging New York City residents agreed to regular testing while they were still healthy, allowing scientists to catch the earliest signs of dementia. **Stern tracked yearly changes in 156 who developed Alzheimer's, and found that those who had a history of diabetes and high cholesterol worsened faster,** he reports this month in a special issue of Archives of Neurology dedicated to the link.

_Type 2 diabetes occurs as a result of insulin resistance, as the body gradually loses sensitivity to this hormone that's essential for turning blood sugar into energy. A similar effect in the brain helps explain the dementia link, Dr. Suzanne Craft of the Veterans Affairs Puget Sound Health Care System concludes in a research review also published in that journal. Insulin influences memory in a variety of ways, and an insulin-resistant body in turn affects brain cells' insulin-related activity.

Other factors — such as brain inflammation and cell-damaging **oxidative stress — may play a role**, too. But clearly more affected is a silent dysfunction of glucose control, not something that suddenly begins after diabetes is diagnosed.

"You want to think of it more as a continuum than just whether or not you have diabetes," Stern says.

While scientists sort out exactly what's going on, the research does point to some common-sense protections: If you have diabetes, closely follow your doctor's advice for controlling it. **Try to lower high cholesterol and blood pressure that can harm the brain's blood supply and exacerbate memory problems.**

And if you're still healthy, **Nixon advises "hedging your bets against Alzheimer's" with the same steps that help prevent both diabetes and heart disease — a good diet and plenty of exercise.**

Blood sugar loss may trigger Alzheimer's

Exercise and controlling cholesterol may ward off degenerative disease.

In December of 2008, an article found that **a slow, chronic reduction of blood sugar to the brain could trigger some forms of Alzheimer's disease**, U.S. researchers said.

The study of human and mice brains suggests a reduction of blood flow deprives energy to the brain, setting off a process that ultimately produces the sticky clumps of protein researchers believe is a cause of the disease. The finding could lead to strategies such as exercise, reducing cholesterol and managing blood pressure to keep Alzheimer's at bay, Robert Vassar and colleagues at Northwestern University's Feinberg School of Medicine in Chicago reported.

"This finding is significant because it suggests that improving blood flow to the brain might be an effective therapeutic approach to prevent or treat Alzheimer's," Vassar, who led the study, said in a statement.

"If people start early enough, maybe they can dodge the bullet."

Alzheimer's disease is incurable and is the most common form of dementia among older people. **It affects the regions of the brain involving thought, memory and language**.

While the most advanced drugs have focused on removing clumps of beta amyloid protein that forms plaques in the brain, researchers also are looking at therapies to address the toxic tangles caused by an abnormal build-up of the protein tau.

Vassar and colleagues analyzed human and mice brains to discover that **a protein called eIF2alpha is altered when the brain does not get enough energy**. This boosts production of an enzyme that in turn flips a switch to produce the sticky protein clumps.

The finding published in the journal Dec. 2008 issue of **Neuron** could lead to drugs designed to block the eIF2alpha production that begins the formation of the **protein clumps, also known as amyloid plaques,** Vassar added.

"What we are talking about is a slow, insidious process over many years," he said. "It's so mild (people) don't even notice it, but it has an effect over time because it's producing a chronic reduction in the blood flow."

Research on mice links fast food to AD

A November 2008 article found that **mice fed junk food for nine months showed signs of developing the abnormal brain tangles** strongly associated with Alzheimer's disease, a Swedish researcher said.

The findings, which come from a series of published papers by a researcher at Sweden's Karolinska Institutet, show how **a diet rich in fat, sugar and cholesterol could increase the risk of the most common type of dementia**.

"On examining the brains of these mice, we found a chemical change not unlike that found in the Alzheimer brain," Susanne Akterin, a researcher at the Karolinska Institutet's Alzheimer's Disease Research Center, who led the study, said in a statement.

"We now suspect that **a high intake of fat and cholesterol in combination with genetic factors ... can adversely affect several brain substances**, which can be a contributory factor in the development of Alzheimer's."

While the most advanced drugs have focused on removing clumps of beta amyloid protein that forms plaques in the brain, researchers are also now looking at therapies to address **the toxic tangles caused by an abnormal build-up of the protein tau**.

In her research, Akterin focused on a gene variant called apoE4, found in 15 to 20 percent of people and which is a known risk factor for Alzheimer's. The gene is involved in the transport of cholesterol.

She studied mice genetically engineered to mimic the effect of the variant gene in humans, and which were fed a diet rich in fat, sugar and cholesterol for nine months -- meals representing the nutritional content of fast food.

These mice showed chemical changes in their brains, indicating an abnormal build-up of the protein tau as well as signs that cholesterol in food reduced levels of another protein called Arc involved in memory storage, Akterin said.

"All in all, **the results give some indication of how Alzheimer's can be prevented**, but more research in this field needs to be done before proper advice can be passed on to the general public," she said.

CHAPTER SEVENTEEN

Low SOD associated with diseases

Low SOD (superoxide dismutase) levels in humans have also been associated with a host of degenerative diseases, including:

- **fibromyalgia** (Bagis et al, 2005),
- **diabetes** (Abou-Seif et al, 2004),
- **cancer** (Cai et al, 2004) (Ough et al, 2004) (Manju et al, 2002),
- **multiple sclerosis** (Lund-Olesen, 2000),
- **Alzheimer's** (Choi et al, 2005),
- and **Parkinson's disease** (Choi et al, 2005) (Hattori, 2004).

I believe that the low SOD levels result in low peroxide levels, which allows for the manifestation of the above diseases. After all, the purpose of SOD is to generate hydrogen peroxide! It does so by adding an electron to superoxide (reducing it).

SOD levels in humans vary by as much as 50% owing to genetic differences, which may help to explain why some people are more prone to degenerative diseases while others lead long, disease-free lives. (Ueda, Ogata, 1978)

SOD and Human Health

The CuZnSOD gene, SOD1, is located on human Chromosome 21 at location 21q22.1. It has been associated with two specific medical conditions: Amyotrophic Lateral Sclerosis (ALS) and Down syndrome, also known as Trisomy-21.

ALS, also known as Lou Gehrig's disease, is a progressive, fatal disease where the motor neurons progressively degenerate. The disease usually starts out with muscle weakness, followed by progressive loss of muscle control and muscle wasting. **The**

actual cause of death is usually an infection, indicating an EMOD deficiency, due to the weakened condition of the body. The association of one form of ALS with mutations in the SOD1 gene was made in 1993. (Rosen et al, 1993)

This is consistent with my proposal that an EMOD insufficiency allows for infections and varying other diseases. Actually, I predicted that chronic granulomatous disease patients would have a higher level of dementia and lowered intellectual levels and that prediction was true. Our brains need EMODs.

This form of ALS is caused by inadequate activity by the mutated SOD, leaving the motor neurons open to oxidative damage and death. **I believe that this means that the body is not generating enough H_2O_2, which is needed in high quantities by the nervous system.**

Individuals with Down syndrome suffer the exact opposite fate. Down syndrome is caused by 3 copies of chromosome 21 being present in each (or most in the case of mosaic Trisomy-21) cell. **SOD1, being located on Chromosome 21, is therefore triplicated.** Measurements of SOD activity in individuals with Down syndrome show that **there is overexpression of this gene, with an activity level of about 150% of normal.** (Gulesserian et al, 2001)

There is a corresponding upregulation of either catalase or glutathione peroxidase in some tissues, but not in neurons. (Brooksbank et al, 1983)

While there is still some disagreement in the scientific community about the implication of this overexpression, **many scientists believe that the overexpression of SOD can be linked directly to the premature aging, neuronal degeneration, early-onset Alzheimer's disease, and other clinical features of Down syndrome.** (de Haan et al, 1997)

In fact, one case study identified a boy with a micro-duplication of SOD1 with many of the clinical features of Down syndrome, but without a duplication of any other part of chromosome 21. (Huret et al, 1987)

Another very interesting area of research into CuZnSOD is being done in the area of **Alzheimer's disease.** The brain lesions that are characteristic of Alzheimer's disease show evidence of oxidative processes as well as other damage, such as inflammation. Estevez et al. examined how **zinc-deficient CuZnSOD not only did not function as an antioxidant, but instead behaved like a pro-oxidant compound.** (Estevez et al, 1999)

I have been saying for years that SOD is not an antioxidant enzyme.

They observed that the loss of zinc from CuZnSOD which still had its copper was sufficient to induce apoptosis in cultured motor neurons. This finding is significant not only in the disease of ALS which has been directly tied to this enzyme, but also to Alzheimer's disease, where pathological behavior of this enzyme is suspected. (Bush, 2003)

I believe that the above data on SOD confirms my belief that SOD is indeed a prooxidant enzyme and NOT an antioxidant.

Hypoxia and Alzheimer's disease

There is a clear link between low oxygen levels in the brain and Alzheimer's disease, but the exact mechanisms behind this are not yet fully understood.

Lowered oxygen levels, or hypoxia, seems to increase the risk of dementia. Research has show that **reduced blood supply increases levels of amyloid precursor protein and beta-amyloid.** Researchers at the University of Leeds suggest that the underlying mechanism may involve **disruption of calcium channels and increased production of free radicals. Some of the extra calcium channels can, however, be closed down by antioxidants,** which may lead to new approaches to therapy.

A healthy brain needs a good supply of oxygen. Oxygen is delivered to the brain by blood, which travels through a network of arteries and blood vessels. If this network becomes damaged or blocked, or the blood supply itself is low in oxygen and insufficient oxygen will be delivered to the brain cells. A reduction in the supply of oxygen to any tissue, including the brain, is called hypoxia.

A person whose blood supply to the brain has been interrupted by a stroke is ten times more likely to develop dementia than someone who has not.

People with low blood oxygen levels caused by long-term respiratory disease are also at increased risk of developing dementia. However researchers do not fully understand which mechanisms within the brain cause this effect. This article is a review of the evidence that links Alzheimer's disease and low oxygen levels (hypoxia).

Beta-amyloid is main culprit for damage in AD

People who have Alzheimer's disease always develop what have become known as plaques and tangles in their brains. These are deposits of proteins that develop between brain cells. **The plaques are mostly made up of a protein called beta-amyloid, whilst a protein called tau forms the tangles.** There is much debate about the specific role of these deposits, but the majority of researchers agree that beta-amyloid is an important cause of the damage to neurones and other cells in the brain that occurs in Alzheimer's disease.

Beta-amyloid is made from amyloid precursor protein (also known as APP). APP is a long protein and betaamyloid is produced when two different enzymes chop down APP: beta secretase makes the first cut and then gamma secretase gets to work to produce beta-amyloid. Researchers are very interested in how beta-amyloid is produced, because if they can understand the production process they might be able to intervene and prevent the damaging protein from being produced.

However, despite the fact that high levels of betaamyloid are thought to be behind much of the damage that occurs in the brain in Alzheimer's disease, **it is interesting to note that completely stopping the production of beta-amyloid has been found to be lethal for brain cells.**

Beta-amyloid boosted after reduced blood flow

Research shows that **levels of amyloid precursor protein (APP) in the brain tend to increase after blood flow has been reduced.** This is probably a protective measure as APP can be turned into a substance that helps to protect brain cells (known as soluble alpha APP). However, having increased levels of APP also means that more of the damaging beta amyloid can be produced, research has shown that **this happens after both mild and severe reductions in blood to the brain.**

Neurotoxicity of beta-amyloid

It's not yet clear to researchers how beta-amyloid damages brain cells. This is because it involves a complex series of processes, but also because it is difficult to accurately recreate Alzheimer's disease in the laboratory. It is after all a disease that takes many years to develop. Experiments in the laboratory have to rely on a much cruder model of the disease, with cells being exposed to unrealistically high concentrations of beta-amyloid.

Using genetically altered animals, particularly mice, has provided a valuable new way of modelling Alzheimer's disease. This has enabled unique advances in understanding the condition, but the transgenic animal models are still far from perfect.

A further complicating factor in improving understanding of how beta-amyloid damages neurones is the fact that it's looking more and more likely that **most of the**

damage is done at a very early stage of the protein accumulating in the brain, when the protein is smaller and chemically different to the version of beta-amyloid that ends up forming into plaques.

Despite the difficulties of pinning down exactly how the damage to the brain seen in Alzheimer's disease is done, the evidence to date indicates that **the damage caused to neurones by beta-amyloid involves the disruption of calcium levels in the brain and the creation of damaging free radicals due to oxidative stress.**

Understanding the role of calcium channels

Research carried out by Professor Chris Peers and colleagues at the University of Leeds has shown that neurones that are deprived of oxygen increase their production of free radicals and beta-amyloid and also open up more of their calcium channels, which leads to an increased chance of apoptosis or cell suicide. **This research clearly establishes that reducing the oxygen supply to neurones creates the same causes of damage as those that occur when people develop Alzheimer's disease.**

Free radicals are a chemical by-product of some of the oxygen that we breathe. They are unstable and can cause damage to proteins, cell membranes and even our DNA.

It is **paradoxical** that reducing the amount of oxygen to cells leads to the creation of something that requires oxygen, but this comes about because when cells are under stress, due to lack of oxygen, they become inefficient at using the remaining oxygen, enabling damaging free radicals to form. **(RMH Note: This is not proven.)**

Hypoxia increases levels of free radicals in the neurones, which in turn increases the amount of beta-amyloid and opens up extra calcium pathways. The research teams have shown that **certain calcium pathways can be closed down again by the introduction of antioxidants.**

This work is part of ongoing research to fully understand how neurones and their supporting cells are affected by hypoxia and how these effects interact with beta-amyloid to cause the type of damage that can lead to Alzheimer's disease. Gaining understanding of these mechanisms is vital in being able to design ways of preventing this common form of dementia. (Peers et al, 2009)

Alzheimer's Society research- snoring linked to Alzheimer's

A report in June of 2007 found that research funded by the Alzheimer's Society hit the headlines as journalists seized on studies analysing the **impact of oxygen and the** brain. **A potential link between snoring and Alzheimer's disease captured the imagination of both journalists and the public**, helping to raise the Society's research profile.

The link emerged as University of Leeds scientists released a study into the impact of levels of oxygen to the brain. The team were investigating how stroke victims could be more vulnerable to Alzheimer's disease - years or even decades after making a full recovery.

It has been known for some time that **strokes and Alzheimer's disease are linked**, but the Leeds team has shown how an incident of reduced oxygen to the brain - caused by the stroke - can leave the patient vulnerable to the gradual build-up of toxic chemicals which can cause Alzheimer's disease.

Professor Chris Peers, lead researcher says, 'Our research is looking into what happens when **oxygen levels in the brain are reduced by a number of factors, from long-term conditions to sudden incidents such as a heart attack, stroke or even head trauma**. Even though the patient may outwardly recover, the hidden cell damage may be irreversible.

It could even be an issue for people who snore heavily, whose sleep patterns are such that there will be times in the night when their brain is deprived of sufficient oxygen.'

The research centered on the damage done by low-oxygen incidents to a group of brain cells called **astrocytes**. When the brain is functioning normally, it makes connections through the release of tiny amounts of chemical across the synapses. Once the chemical has been transmitted, it is "mopped up" by the astrocytes.

Dr Susanne Sorensen, head of research at the Alzheimer's Society, says, 'The team examined the role of cells that support neurones in the brain. This is exciting because rather than focussing on neurones they looked at processes in the brain, which until now have not be researched in so much detail.'

Brain's oxygen supply key to Alzheimer's risk-

In Novemver of 2006, HealthDay News reported **less oxygenated blood to the brain may mean a bigger build-up of the protein plaques that are so closely tied to Alzheimer's disease**. The Canadian team says a specific gene may be key to this process. (HealthDay News, 2006)

"If you have less oxygen, you turn up this gene and obviously generate more beta-amyloid [protein]. If you have a higher level of beta-amyloid, you form more plaque. If you have this plaque, then you will have dementia," explained lead researcher Weihong Song, a professor of psychiatry who holds a Canada Research Chair in Alzheimer's disease at the University of British Columbia in Vancouver.

His team described the findings in the Nov. 20, 2006 issue of the *Proceedings of the National Academy of Sciences*. Experts have long known that **lowered brain-oxygen levels, caused by reduced blood flow, increase the risk of Alzheimer's disease**. For example, Song said, "**If you have a stroke, you have a two or three times increased risk of dementia.**" (PNAS, 2006)

The link between low oxygen and plaque formation may be a gene called BACE 1, he added. This gene encodes a protein that converts the precursor amyloid molecule to the more dangerous beta-amyloid form. In their studies with mice, Song's group found that **lower oxygen levels increased the activity of the gene, BACE 1**.

But its not quite that simple, added Dr. Ralph A Nixon, professor of psychiatry and cell biology at New York University and a spokesman for the Alzheimer's Association.

To start with, there is an ongoing debate about whether the amyloid plaques cause the loss of mental function seen in Alzheimer's disease, Nixon said. "What this paper does is add to a hypothesis that relates to amyloid overproduction and accumulation in the brain," he said. "Whether it establishes an association is the issue."

Hypoxia -- low blood-oxygen levels -- "does a lot of things to the brain," Nixon said. "It has a lot of effects on brain function other than what is being described here. There should be at least some consideration of the broader context -- that **hypoxia itself is a cause of impairment.**" Nevertheless, Nixon said, the report "is an interesting additional link that has not been appreciated before between hypoxia and this metabolic pathway."

Nixon and Song did agree on one point.

"The study reinforces another message that has emerged in recent years -- that **the health of the cardiovascular system is very important for the health of the brain**," Nixon said. "The things one does to promote the health of the cardiovascular system are going to help the brain when it is challenged in Alzheimer's disease. Lifestyle factors such as diet and exercise are also an edge against hypoxia."

Song concurred. "**If we can improve blood flow to the brain, maybe we can help slow Alzheimer's progression**. This report provides the mechanics for that. Increasing blood flow for the heart also helps slow Alzheimer's disease," he said. **I believe that this is saying that increased blood flow increases oxygen levels,**

which increases EMOD levels and in turn decreases the incidence of dementia. (Song, 2006)

Low brain oxygen ups Alzheimer's risk

In 2006, it was reported that **low levels of brain oxygen may boost Alzheimer's risk** in mice. Researchers included Weihong Song, MD, PhD, of the psychiatry department and Brain Research Centre at Canada's University of British Columbia.

Song's team studied mice that had a gene tied to Alzheimer's disease.

The researchers kept some mice in cages with low-oxygen air for 16 hours a day for a month. They kept the other mice in cages with normal oxygen levels. In humans, conditions such as **stroke that hamper blood flow in the brain can limit the brain's oxygen supply.**

After the month, the researchers tested both sets of mice on a memory test in which they were timed while swimming through a water maze to reach a hidden platform.

The mice that had lived in low oxygen performed worse. Those mice also had more amyloid beta plaque -- a hallmark of Alzheimer's disease -- in their brains, compared to the mice with normal brain oxygen levels.

Song and colleagues also studied the mice's genes.

Under the influence of low brain oxygen levels, the BACE1 gene upped production of amyloid beta, the key protein in Alzheimer's brain plaque. Even a "slight" rise in BACE1 activity "could lead to a dramatic increase in [amyloid beta] production," the researchers write. Low brain oxygen levels might also affect other genes and may spur brain cell death, worsening memory in Alzheimer's disease, Song's team notes.

Boosting brain oxygen levels may benefit Alzheimer's patients, the researchers say. However, their study did not test that theory.

The report appeared in *Proceedings of the National Academy of Sciences*.

If you have less oxygen, you turn up this gene and obviously generate more beta-amyloid [protein]. If you have a higher level of beta-amyloid, you form more plaque. If you have this plaque, then you will have dementia," explained lead researcher Weihong Song, a professor of psychiatry who holds a Canada Research Chair in Alzheimer's disease at the University of British Columbia in Vancouver.

His team described the findings in a 2006 issue of the *Proceedings of the National Academy of Sciences.*

Experts have long known that lowered brain-oxygen levels, caused by reduced blood flow, increase the risk of Alzheimer's disease. For example, Song said, "If you have a stroke, you have a two or three times increased risk of dementia."

The link between low oxygen and plaque formation may be a gene called BACE 1, he added. This gene encodes a protein that converts the precursor amyloid molecule to the more dangerous beta-amyloid form.

In their studies with mice, Song's group found that lower oxygen levels increased the activity of the gene.

But its not quite that simple, added Dr. Ralph A Nixon, professor of psychiatry and cell biology at New York University and a spokesman for the Alzheimer's Association.

To start with, there is an ongoing debate about whether the amyloid plaques cause the loss of mental function seen in Alzheimer's disease, Nixon said.

"What this paper does is add to a hypothesis that relates to amyloid overproduction and accumulation in the brain," he said. "Whether it establishes an association is the issue."

Hypoxia -- low blood-oxygen levels -- "does a lot of things to the brain," Nixon said. "It has a lot of effects on brain function other than what is being described here. There should be at least some consideration of the broader context -- that **hypoxia itself is a cause of impairment**."

Nevertheless, Nixon said, the report "is an interesting additional link that has not been appreciated before between hypoxia and this metabloic pathway."

Anesthesia, Alzheimer's and low oxygen

Studies of human brain cells around April of 2008 showed that **the widely-used anesthetic desflurane does not contribute to increased production of amyloid-beta protein; however, when combined with low oxygen conditions, it can produce more of this Alzheimer's associated protein.**

Over 200 million people undergo surgery each year, and there has been concern that anesthetic use may contribute to Alzheimer's and other brain disorders. Bin Zhang, Yuanlin Dong, Rudolph Tanzi, Zhongcong Xie, and colleagues examined this possibility with commonly used inhalation anesthetics isoflurane previously and desflurane more recently.

They subjected human brain cells to 12% desflurane for **six hours** (mimicking a surgery condition) and observed no changes in either the production of amyloid-beta protein or the rate of cell death. However, when combined with **low oxygen levels (18%),** desflurane could stimulate these cellular changes associated with Alzheimer's **(hypoxia by itself did not induce any changes). (RMH Note: This is a very short term experiment.)** The results with desflurane are contrary to the researchers' previous work, which found isoflurane by itself could stimulate both amyloid production and cell death.

The researchers do emphasize that the current findings are from cell culture experiments, and the next critical step will be to confirm these findings in animal models and test the effects of other anesthetic agents. But, **these early results suggest that it is important to ensure anesthetic patients maintain sufficient oxygen in their brain**.

Hypoxia may stimulate risk of AD

Christopher Patterson and colleagues reviewed the modifiable risk factors for Alzheimer disease but did not mention that **hypoxia may stimulate the development of this illness** (Patterson et al, 2008)

Cigarette smoking, severe head injury with loss of consciousness and systolic hypertension in older people are risk factors that may cause hypoxia directly or induce it via neuronal ischemia; the disruption of neurovascular coupling has been implicated in hypertension, ischemic stroke and Alzheimer disease. We are interested in the authors' views on this issue as many patients with Alzheimer disease also have vascular infarctions and these patients deteriorate faster. (Sheng et al, 2007)

Patients with chronic obstructive pulmonary disease and obstructive sleep apnea syndrome often complain of memory lapses, which may result from intermittent or chronic hypoxic injury to the forebrain. Sun and colleagues defined the molecular mechanism of hypoxia leading to dementia and showed that **hypoxia leads to increased** beta-**secretase activity and production of** beta-**amyloid protein.** Until specific therapy becomes available, simple measures to prevent chronic hypoxic injury to the brain may help to prevent Alzheimer disease or may benefit people who already have the condition. (Sun et al, 2006)

Decreased blood flow in AD

In a June 26, 2009 article, Dr. Jennifer C Palmer and colleagues at the University of Bristol discovered that endothelin converting enzyme-2 (ECE-2) may cause the **decrease in cerebral blood flow seen in Alzheimer's disease.** These results were presented in the July 2009 issue of the **American Journal of Pathology**.

Alzheimer's disease is the most common form of dementia. Abeta peptide, which accumulates in the brain of Alzheimer's disease patients, is thought to lead to tightening of the blood vessels and reduction of cerebral blood flood. ECE-2 may contribute to these symptoms by converting an inactive precursor to endothelin-1, which constricts blood vessels.

To determine if ECE-2 affects cerebral blood flow in Alzheimer's disease, Palmer et al examined the expression of ECE-2. They found that ECE-2 levels were elevated in patients with Alzheimer's disease and that Abeta could increase ECE-2 expression in vitro. These data indicate that ECE-2 levels are increased in response to Abeta and may cause **the decrease in cerebral blood flow seen in Alzheimer's disease.**

Palmer et al "suggest that [endothelin-1] receptor antagonists, already licensed for treating other diseases, could be of benefit in [Alzheimer's disease] therapies." (Palmer et al, 2009). **I believe that the decreased blood flow seen in Alzheimer's is consistent with the decreased oxygen levels in the demented brain.**

Oxidative stress hypothesis in AD

The major hurdle in understanding Alzheimer's disease (AD) is a **lack of knowledge** about the etiology and pathogenesis of selective neuron death. In recent years, considerable data have accrued indicating that the brain in AD is under increased oxidative stress and this may have a role in the pathogenesis of neuron degeneration and death in this disorder.

The direct evidence supporting increased oxidative stress in AD is: (1) increased brain Fe, Al, and Hg in AD, capable of stimulating free radical generation; (2) increased lipid peroxidation and decreased polyunsaturated fatty acids in the AD brain, and increased 4-hydroxynonenal, an aldehyde product of lipid peroxidation in AD ventricular fluid; (3) increased protein and DNA oxidation in the AD brain; (4) diminished energy metabolism and

decreased cytochrome c oxidase in the brain in AD; (5) advanced glycation end products (AGE), malondialdehyde, carbonyls, peroxynitrite, heme oxygenase-1 and SOD-1 in neurofibrillary tangles and AGE, heme oxygenase-1, SOD-1 in senile plaques; and (6) studies showing that amyloid beta peptide is capable of generating free radicals.

Supporting indirect evidence comes from a variety of in vitro studies showing that free radicals are capable of mediating neuron degeneration and death. Overall, these studies indicate that free radicals are possibly involved in the pathogenesis of neuron death in AD. Because tissue injury itself can induce reactive oxygen species (ROS) generation, **it is not known whether this is a primary or secondary event.** Even if free radical generation is secondary to other initiating causes, they are deleterious and part of a cascade of events that can lead to neuron death, suggesting that therapeutic efforts aimed at removal of ROS or prevention of their formation may be beneficial in AD (Markesbery, 1997). **Antioxidants studies have failed to reverse or prevent AD up to this point.**

The redox chemistry of the Alzheimer's disease amyloid beta peptide

There is a growing body of evidence to support a role for oxidative stress in Alzheimer's disease (AD), with increased levels of lipid peroxidation, DNA and protein oxidation products (HNE, 8-HO-guanidine and protein carbonyls respectively) in AD brains.

The brain is a highly oxidative organ consuming 20% of the body's oxygen despite accounting for only 2% of the total body weight. With normal ageing the brain accumulates metals ions such iron (Fe), zinc (Zn) and copper (Cu). Consequently the brain is abundant in antioxidants to control and prevent the detrimental formation of reactive oxygen species (ROS) generated via Fenton chemistry involving redox active metal ion reduction and activation of molecular oxygen. In AD there is an over accumulation of the **Amyloid beta peptide (Abeta)**, this is the result of either an elevated generation from amyloid precursor protein (APP) or inefficient clearance of Abeta from the brain.

Abeta can efficiently generate reactive oxygen species in the presence of the transition metals copper and iron in vitro. Under oxidative conditions Abeta will form stable dityrosine cross-linked dimers which are generated from free radical attack on the tyrosine residue at position 10. There are elevated levels of urea and SDS resistant stable linked Abeta oligomers as well as dityrosine cross-linked peptides and proteins in AD brain. Since soluble Abeta levels correlate best with the degree of degeneration. (McLean et al, 1999) They suggest that the toxic Abeta species corresponds to a soluble dityrosine cross-linked oligomer. Current therapeutic strategies using **metal chelators such as clioquinol and desferrioxamine have had some success in altering the progression of AD symptoms**. Similarly, **natural antioxidants curcumin and ginkgo extract have modest but positive effects in slowing AD development.**

Therefore, drugs that target the oxidative pathways in AD could have genuine therapeutic efficacy. (Smith et al, 2007). **I have found that curcumin is a good prooxidant and I believe that that is responsible for its protective effect.**

CHAPTER EIGHTEEN

EMODs and the brain

The brain is particularly vulnerable to oxidative stress due to its high consumption of oxygen and glucose, enrichment in unsaturated fatty acids that are subject to oxidation, and presence of regions enriched in iron and ascorbate that are potent pro-oxidants for brain membranes. Moreover, higher levels of glucose upregulate the neuroinflammatory process measured as induction of iNOS and NO production. Coupled with the relatively reduced antioxidant defenses in the brain, exposure of brain cells to reactive oxygen or nitrogen species can be detrimental and is thought to contribute to the pathogenesis of many brain disorders. (Floyd, 1999). **Yet, the brain can function normally for a century.**

All aerobic organisms are exposed to EMODs simply because semireduced oxygen species, superoxide and hydrogen peroxide, are produced by mitochondria during respiration. (Chance et al, 1979)

The exact amount of EMODs produced is considered to be about 2% of the total oxygen consumed during respiration, but it may vary depending on several parameters. **Brain is considered abnormally sensitive to oxidative damage** and, in fact, early studies demonstrating the ease of peroxidation of brain membranes supported this notion. (Zaleska, Floyd, 1985)

Brain is enriched in the more easily peroxidizable fatty acids (20:4 and 22:6), consumes an inordinate fraction (20%) of the total oxygen consumption for its relatively small weight (2%), and is not particularly enriched in antioxidant defenses. (Floyd, Carney, 1992)

In fact, **brain is lower in catalase activity, about 10% of liver.** (Marklund et al, 1982)

Additionally, **human brain has higher levels of iron (Fe) in certain regions and in general has high levels of ascorbate.** Thus, if tissue organizational disruption occurs, the Fe/ascorbate mixture is expected to be an abnormally potent pro-oxidant for brain membranes. (Zaleska et al, 1989)

H_2O_2 production from isolated brain mitochondria is 2% of O_2 consumed

Rigorous measurement of H_2O_2 production from isolated brain mitochondria shows that it amounts to about 2% of the total oxygen consumed when NADH supplies the reducing equivalents. (Hensley et al, 1998). **I believe this indicates that the brain should be undergoing constant and rapid lipid peroxidation but it does not.**

In addition to mitochondria, additional sources of EMODs include mixed function oxidases as well as other oxidative processes. **Of particular importance to brain is the H_2O_2 produced by oxidative deamination of catecholamines.** Relative to this point, the DATATOP clinical trial for Parkinson's disease, which included deprenyl, a monamine oxidase B inhibitor, along with vitamin E, was designed in part to arrest oxidative stress on two fronts. (Shoulson et al, 1993)

The brain is disproportionately metabolically active for its size, accounting for up to 30% of an organism's total basal energy expenditure, whilst comprising only around 2–3% of total body mass (Siebert et al. 1986; Krassner 1986). **The brain is remarkable in its dependence on the blood for its immediate and constant supply of oxygen** and other essential energy substrates (e.g. glucose). **There is no storage capacity for oxygen** with a disruption of supply having an almost instantaneous effect (Yamatoto et al. 1993). This means that oxygen delivery must be adjusted within seconds in response to changes in metabolic rate. Under normal conditions metabolic activity is limited by the rate of oxygen delivery.

The normal arterial concentration of glucose is 5.5mM/L, and the normal level of oxygen is equivalent to 0.12mM/L. As **6 molecules of oxygen are required to oxidize 1 molecule of glucose,** then from the standpoint of supplying these metabolic needs, **the concentration of glucose is 275 times greater than that of oxygen** in the extracellular fluid at the surface of the cell. Thus **oxygen turnover is the highest amongst the essential nutrients. Oxygen diffuses readily across the mitochondrial membrane.**

It is generally accepted that **altitudes above 10,000 ft.**, lead to profound effects on human cognitive performance, and that these effects result from hypoxia induced by the low levels of available oxygen. Limited evidence also suggests that such decrements in performance may be reversed through oxygen administration. It is well known that **cognitive decline goes hand in hand with advancing age. Human aging is also associated with decreased glucose metabolism.**

Glucose metabolism is reliant on a sufficient and continuous supply of oxygen, and any compromise in this delivery system may be responsible, at least in part, for any resultant cognitive decline.

EMODs are continuously being generated in neurons during normal metabolism and neuronal activity.

Antioxidant defense enzymes in the brain have been shown to vary during the estrous cycle, to be altered following gonadectomy and to differ between the sexes, suggesting involvement of gonadal hormones in the control of processes which protect cells and tissues against oxidative damage. **I believe that the effects are due to the antioxidant nature of estrogens and testosterone.**

I also believe that this may be responsible for the sex differences seen in Alzheimer's disease risk.

Factors incriminating EMODs in AD

A second look into the oxidant mechanisms in Alzheimer's disease

Oxidative damage is a major feature of Alzheimer's disease pathophysiology.

Instead of succumbing to these oxidative abnormalities, neurons upregulate antioxidant defenses, which suggest a novel balance in oxidant homeostasis in Alzheimer's disease.

Evidence indicates that in the initial phase of Alzheimer's disease development, **amyloid-beta deposition and hyperphosphorylated tau are consequences of oxidative stress and function as a primary line of antioxidant defense.**

RMH Note: Does this mean that AD is being driven by "reductive stress?"

However, during the progression of the disease, the antioxidant activity of both agents evolves into pro-oxidant, representing a typical gain-of-function transformation.

This transformation is due to an increase in reactive species and a decrease in clearance mechanisms. However, **the notion that amyloid-beta and hyperphosphorylated tau function as protective components in the early stages of Alzheimer's disease brings into serious question the rationale of current therapeutic strategies aimed to remove both amyloid-beta and hyperphosphorylated tau**. (Moreira et al, 2005)

Overall, a multi-drug approach for AD seems to emerge as a potential alternative as none of the available drug therapies are capable of altering the progression of the disease. A multimodal treatment capable of limiting inflammatory processes may lead to a slowing of the disease progression, and may also reduce some of the cognitive symptoms and thus burden on families and care-givers.

Is Alzheimer's disease a mitochondrial disorder?

Cell bodies of neurons at risk of death in Alzheimer's disease (AD) have increased lipid peroxidation, nitration, free carbonyls, and nucleic acid oxidation.

These oxidative changes occur in all vulnerable neurons and are reduced in neurons that contain neurofibrillary pathology. Mitochondrial abnormalities are allegedly involved as a source of reactive oxygen species that culminates in perikaryal oxidative damage. However, because **mitochondria in AD do not exhibit striking evidence of oxidative damage, as would be expected if they produced free radicals directly**, the authors suspected that abnormal mitochondria are responsible for supplying a key reactant, that once in the cytoplasm, releases radicals.

Because abnormal mitochondria, H_2O_2 and redox-active iron are juxtaposed in the same AD neuron, it has all the markings of a "radical factory." The proximal causes of mitochondrial abnormalities likely involve reentry into the cell cycle, where organellokinesis and proliferation results in an increase of mitochondria and intermediately differentiated cells, with a consequent increase in turnover. Supporting this, the authors have considerable in vivo and in vitro evidence for mitotic disturbances in AD. (Cash et al, 2002). **I believe that the brain mitochondria are normally "radical factories."**

Oxidative stress and Alzheimer disease

Research in the field of molecular biology has helped to provide a better understanding of both the cascade of biochemical events that occurs with Alzheimer disease (AD) and the heterogeneous nature of the disease. One hypothesis that accounts for both the heterogeneous nature of AD and the fact that aging is the most obvious risk factor is that free radicals are involved. The probability of this involvement is supported by the fact that neurons are extremely sensitive to attacks by destructive free radicals.

Furthermore, lesions are present in the brains of AD patients that are typically associated with attacks by free radicals (eg, damage to DNA, protein oxidation, lipid peroxidation, and advanced glycosylation end products), and metals (eg, iron, copper, zinc, and aluminum) are present that have catalytic activity that produce free radicals.

Beta-Amyloid is aggregated and produces more free radicals in the presence of free radicals; beta-amyloid toxicity is eliminated by free radical scavengers. Apolipoprotein E is subject to attacks by free radicals, and apolipoprotein E peroxidation has been correlated with AD. In contrast, apolipoprotein E can act as a free radical scavenger and this behavior is isoform dependent. AD has been linked to mitochondrial anomalies affecting cytochrome-c oxidase, and these anomalies may contribute to the abnormal production of free radicals.

Finally, many free radical scavengers (eg, vitamin E, selegeline, and Ginkgo biloba extract EGb 761) have produced promising results in relation to AD, as has desferrioxamine-an iron-chelating agent-and anti-inflammatory drugs and **estrogens**, which also have an antioxidant effect. (Christen, 2000) **This 2000 report has not been supported by subsequent experimentation. The premise sounded good, but the experiments failed to support their notions that oxidative stress is causative of AD.**

Also, **if estrogen decreases the risk of AD, I ask, why do women have a higher rate of AD?**

Alzheimer's disease and other neurodegenerative disorders

Alzheimer's disease, the cause of one of the most common types of dementia, is a brain disorder affecting the elderly and is characterized by the formation of two main protein aggregates: **senile plaques and neurofibrillary tangles**, which are involved in the process leading to progressive neuronal degeneration and death. Neurodegeneration in Alzheimer's disease is a pathologic condition of cells rather than an accelerated way of aging. The senile plaques are generated by a deposition in the human brain of fibrils of the beta-amyloid peptide (Abeta), a fragment derived from the proteolytic processing of the amyloid precursor protein (APP). Tau protein is the major component of paired helical filaments (PHFs), which form a compact filamentous network described as neurofibrillary tangles (NFTs). Experiments with hippocampal cells in culture have indicated a relationship between fibrillary amyloid and the cascade of molecular signals that trigger tau hyperphosphorylations. Two main protein kinases have been shown to be involved in anomalous tau phosphorylations: the cyclin-dependent kinase Cdk5 and glycogen synthase kinase GSK3beta. Cdk5 plays a critical role in brain development and is associated with neurogenesis as revealed by studies in brain cells in culture and neuroblastoma cells. Deregulation of this protein kinase as induced by extracellular amyloid loading results in tau hyperphosphorylations, thus triggering a sequence of molecular events that lead to neuronal degeneration. Inhibitors of Cdk5 and GSK3beta and antisense oligonucleotides exert protection against neuronal death. On the other hand, **there is cumulative evidence from studies in cultured brain cells and on brains that oxidative stress constitutes a main factor in the modification of normal signaling pathways in neuronal cells, leading to biochemical and structural abnormalities and neurodegeneration as related to the pathogenesis of Alzheimer's disease**. The analysis is extended to the action of neuroprotective factors including selective inhibitors of tau phosphorylating protein kinases, **estrogens, and antioxidants** among other molecules that apparently prevent neuronal degeneration. (Marccioni et al, 2001)

Again, this notion has been proved wrong.

Alzheimer disease: cellular and molecular aspects (vaccines)

A conclusive diagnosis of Alzheimer's disease (AD) can be made only by correlating clinical findings and neuropathological studies of post-mortem tissues.

Two leading neuropathological changes correlate with the diagnosis of AD:

First, the **neurofibrillary tangles (NFTs)** which accumulate in neuronal perikarya and are made of paired helical filaments (PHFs) containing the microtubule-associated protein **tau**;

Second, extracellular amyloid deposits in the form of diffuse or neuritic senile plaques which contain the amyloid peptide.

In AD, NFTs can be easily visualized using antibodies recognizing the microtubule associated protein tau and are composed of bundles of PHFs. In the autopsy-derived AD brain, tau is hyperphosphorylated and more than 30 phosphorylation sites have been identified in PHF-tau proteins. The formation of NFTs is thought to be associated with a collapse of the microtubule network, disturbances of axoplasmic transports, synapse loss, neuritic atrophy, and neuronal death.

Senile plaques are extracellular lesions which have been shown by electron microscopic studies to contain amyloid fibrils. Fibrils were isolated and a small 4.2 kDa polypeptide was purified from this material.

The amyloid peptide found in amyloid deposits of AD is designated Abeta. Since the Abeta peptide is small and unlikely to be a primary translational product, it was predicted to arise from a larger precursor.

In 1987, this amyloid peptide precursor (APP) was characterized from the analysis of a full-length cDNA encoding a primary translational product of 695 residues. This protein is synthesized by neurons as a 100-kDa glycosylated transmembrane protein with a single membrane spanning domain. The use of cellular models has clearly identified two catabolic pathways for APP. A non amyloidogenic pathway, in which APP is cleaved by beta-secretase within the sequence of the amyloid peptide. This cleavage precludes the formation of the full-length Abeta found in the amyloid core of senile plaques.

A second catabolic pathway of APP leads to the production of Abeta from its precursor. In this amyloidogenic pathway, APP is cleaved by beta-secretase at the N-terminus of Abeta. The C-terminal fragment of APP thus formed is in turn cleaved by beta-secretase to release the full-length amyloid peptide. In primary cultures of neurons over-expressing APP, the production of intraneuronal Abeta induces neuronal apoptosis.

This neurotoxicity, which is not observed in epithelial cells, seems to be related to the formation of intraneuronal aggregates of Abeta 1-42. In AD, the specific inhibition of beta- or beta-secretase activities would decrease the production of Abeta from its precursor, in such a way that its relative concentration could be low enough to avoid the formation of aggregates.

Molecules which can interact with Abeta in order to inhibit its aggregation are also being developed. **Immunization against Abeta has also been tested in both animal models and clinical studies. Although these clinical studies had to be interrupted due to the development of T-lymphocyte meningoencephalitis in some patients, very preliminary results indicate that antibodies against Abeta slow cognitive decline in AD, and generate areas of neocortex devoid of senile plaques.** (Octave, 2005)

Antioxidant free radical scavengers cause serious side effects and deaths

Tolerability of NXY-059 at higher target concentrations in patients with acute stroke (Lees, 2003) (#134)

NXY-059 is a nitrone-based free radical-trapping agent in development for acute stroke. **In patients with acute stroke, NXY-059 is well tolerated at concentrations known to be associated with neuroprotection in animal models of transient cerebral ischemia; however, higher target concentrations appear necessary on the basis of animal models of permanent ischemia. METHODS:** This was a randomized, double-blind, placebo-controlled, parallel-group, dose-escalation, multicenter study that evaluated safety, tolerability, and plasma concentrations of 2 NXY-059 dosing regimens within 24 hours of acute stroke. NXY-059 was administered as either 915 mg over 1 hour followed by 420 mg/h for 71 hours or 1820 mg for 1 hour followed by 844 mg/h for 71 hours; plasma concentrations were monitored. Neurological and functional outcomes were recorded for up to 30 days. RESULTS: One hundred thirty-five patients were recruited, of whom 134 received study treatment and completed assessments (844 mg/h, n=39; 420 mg/h, n=48; placebo, n=47). Mean age was 69 years (range, 34 to 92 years), and baseline National Institutes of Health Stroke Scale score was 8.5 (SD, 6.6). **Serious adverse events occurred in 3, 17, and 13 patients, respectively, with deaths in 0, 4, and 3 patients and treatment discontinuations because of adverse events in 0, 1, and 3 patients. Good outcome, defined by modified Rankin Scale score of 0 or 1, was seen in 53%, 29% and 40%, respectively.** No safety concern was identified in analysis of body temperature, blood pressure, or other laboratory parameters. **The unbound plasma concentration at steady state was 260+/-79 micromol/L, exceeding the target of 200 micromol/L in the high-dose group.** CONCLUSIONS: NXY-059 was well tolerated in patients with an acute stroke at and above concentrations shown to be neuroprotective in an animal model when initiated 4 hours after onset of permanent focal ischemia. (Lees, 2003)

Here are more "dead bodies" with antioxidant use.

Anti-psychotic drugs nearly doubles death rate in AD patients

Anti-psychotic drugs commonly used to treat Alzheimer's disease may double a patient's chance of dying within a few years, suggests a new study that adds to concerns already known about such medications.

"For the vast majority of Alzheimer's patients, taking these drugs is probably not a worthwhile risk," said Clive Ballard, the paper's lead author, of the Wolfson Centre for Age-Related Diseases at King's College London.

"Would I want to take a drug that slightly reduced my aggression but doubled my risk of dying? I'm not sure I would," Ballard said.

The research was published **January 2009** in the medical journal, **Lancet Neurology**.

There is a large increased long-term risk of mortality in patients with Alzheimer's disease (AD) who are prescribed antipsychotic medication. These results, from long-term follow-up of the **DART-AD study**, further highlight the need to seek less harmful treatments for neuropsychiatric symptoms in these patients. These are the conclusions of an article published in the February edition of *The Lancet Neurology*, written by Dr. Clive Ballard, Wolfson Centre for Age-Related Diseases, King's College London, UK, and colleagues. The study was funded by the UK Alzheimer's Research Trust.

While there is evidence of modest short term (6-12 weeks) benefits of antipsychotic treatment for the neuropsychiatric symptoms of AD, **there is also clear evidence of an increase in adverse effects, including parkinsonism, sedation, edema, chest infections, accelerated decline in brain function, stroke and mortality.**

However, all the data regarding mortality so far relate to short term follow-up of 12 weeks or less. The authors of this study have provided the first long-term follow-up data for AD patients given antipsychotic drugs.

Between 2001 and 2004, patients with AD aged between 67 and 100 years who resided in facilities in four UK areas were randomly assigned to continue with their antipsychotic treatment (thioridazine, chlorpromazine, haloperidol, trifluorperazine, or risperidone) for 12 months or to switch their medication to an oral placebo. The primary outcome was mortality at 12 months. An additional follow-up telephone assessment was done to establish whether each participant was still alive 24 months after the enrolment of the last participant (range 24-54 months). Causes of death were obtained from death certificates.

In total, **165 patients were randomised** and of these, 128 started treatment – 64 on antipsychotics, 64 on placebo. At 12 months, there was 70% survival in the antipsychotic group compared with 77% in placebo. However, longer term follow-up revealed bigger differences in survival. At 2 years, survival was 46% in the antipsychotic group and 71% in the placebo group, and at 36 months the difference was even greater: 30% antipsychotic versus 59% placebo. **Overall, across the whole study period, the risk of death was 42% lower in the placebo group than in the antipsychotic group.**

Ballard and colleagues followed 165 patients aged 67 to 100 years with moderate to severe Alzheimer's disease from 2001 to 2004 in Britain. Half continued taking their anti-psychotic drugs, which included Risperdal, Thorazine and Stelazine. The other half got placebos.

Of the 83 receiving drugs, 39 were dead after a year. Of the 82 taking fake pills, 27 were dead after a year. Most deaths in both groups were due to pneumonia.

After two years, 46 percent of Alzheimer's patients taking the anti-psychotics were alive, versus 71 percent of those not on the drugs. After three years, only 30 percent of patients on the drugs were alive, versus 59 percent of those not taking drugs.

The authors conclude: "Our data add further serious safety concerns about the long-term use of antipsychotics in this population, and clinicians should certainly try to replace antipsychotics with safer management approaches. Several studies have shown that psychological management can replace antipsychotic therapy without any appreciable worsening of neuropsychiatric symptoms; and although cholinesterase inhibitors do not seem to be an effective short-term pharmacological treatment for agitation, there is evidence that memantine or antidepressants such as citalopram might be safer and effective alternatives for some neuropsychiatric symptoms.

"Our opinion is that there is still an important but limited place for atypical antipsychotics in the treatment of severe neuropsychiatric manifestations, particularly aggression, of AD. However, the accumulating safety concerns, including the substantial increase in long-term mortality, emphasise the urgent need to put an end to unnecessary and prolonged prescribing."

The Leading Edge editorial in February's *Lancet Neurology*, also published Online first, concludes: "The risks and benefits of prescribing antipsychotics to patients with dementia need to be carefully balanced and these drugs should be used only if alternative strategies do not work. To protect the health and dignity of people with dementia and reduce the use of antipsychotic drugs, approaches that make the needs of patients central to decisions about care should be promoted."

What does the NHS Knowledge Service make of this study?

The advantages of this study are its randomised design and double blinding. However, it also has limitations that need to be considered.

- The study's main limitation was the high number of people who dropped out or died during follow up, particularly at 12 months. Because of this, it is not possible to be certain if the results in this very limited group of participants are representative of the results that would have been obtained in the whole group.

- The study was relatively small, and particularly so after many of the participants dropped out during follow up. As such, it may not have been large enough to detect clinically important differences between the groups.

- **BBC news reported that neuroleptics "were associated with a marked deterioration in verbal skills".** The researchers carried out several assessments on different measures of cognition: function, neuropsychiatric symptoms, and language. **The only assessment in which they found a statistically significant difference between antipsychotic and placebo groups was on an assessment of verbal fluency, with those continuing on antipsychotics having a slight drop in score compared to the placebo group.** However, the fact that this measure was not the primary outcome being assessed by the researchers, that only 40% of participants were assessed using this measure, and that multiple secondary outcomes were tested makes this result less reliable. It is also not possible to tell whether these differences in verbal score between the groups would result in clinically meaningful differences between the patients.

This study suggests that stopping, or continuing with, antipsychotics does not affect cognitive function in people with Alzheimer's disease.

CHAPTER NINETEEN

Megadoses of vitamin E fail to cure ALS

High dose vitamin E therapy in amyotrophic lateral sclerosis as add-on therapy to riluzole: results of a placebo-controlled double-blind study (Graf et al, 2005) (#160)

Increasing evidence has suggested that oxidative stress may be involved in the pathogenesis of amyotrophic lateral sclerosis (ALS). The antioxidant vitamin E (alpha-tocopherol) has been shown to slow down the onset and progression of the paralysis in transgenic mice expressing a mutation in the superoxide dismutase gene found in certain forms of familial ALS. The current study, **a double blind, placebo-controlled, randomised, stratified, parallel-group clinical trial**, was designed to determine **whether vitamin E (5000 mg per day)** may be efficacious in slowing down disease progression when added to riluzole. METHODS: **160 patients** in 6 German centers with either probable or definite ALS (according to the El Escorial Criteria) and a disease duration of less than 5 years, treated with riluzole, were included in this study and were randomly assigned to receive either alpha-tocopherol (5000 mg per day) or placebo for 18 months. The Primary outcome measure was survival, calculating time to death, tracheostomy or permanent assisted ventilation, according to the WFN-Criteria of clinical trials. Secondary outcome measures were the rate of deterioration of function assessed by the modified Norris limb and bulbar scales, manual muscle testing (BMRC), spasticity scale, ventilatory function and the Sickness Impact Profile (SIP ALS/19). Patients were assessed at entry and every 4 months thereafter during the study period until month 16 and at a final visit at month 18. Vitamin E samples were taken for compliance check and Quality Control of the trial. For Safety, a physical examination was performed at baseline and then every visit until the treatment discontinuation at month 18. Height and weight were recorded at baseline and weight alone at the follow-up visits. A neurological examination as well as vital signs (heart rate and blood pressure), an ECG and VEP's were recorded at each visit. Furthermore, spontaneously reported adverse experiences and serious adverse events were documented and standard laboratory tests including liver function tests performed. For Statistical Analysis, the population to be considered for the primary outcome measure was an "intent-to-treat" (ITT) population which included all randomised patients who had received at least one treatment dose (n = 160 patients). For the secondary outcome measures, a two way analysis of variance was performed on a patient population that included all randomised patients who had at least one assessment after inclusion. RESULTS: Concerning the primary endpoint, **no significant difference between placebo and treatment group** could be detected either with the stratified Logrank or the Wilcoxon test. The functional assessments showed a marginal trend in favor of vitamin E, without reaching significance. CONCLUSION: **Neither the primary nor the secondary outcome measures could determine whether a megadose of vitamin E is efficacious in slowing disease progression in ALS as an add-on therapy to riluzol.** Larger or longer studies might be needed. However, administration of this megadose does not seem to have any significant side effects in this patient population. (Graf et al, 2005). **This is just one more of the diseases that predictions for antioxidant therapy have failed to reverse or cure.**

Vitamin E plus selegiline fail in ALS study

The effect of selegiline and vitamin E in the treatment of ALS: an open randomized clinical trials (Kwiecinski et al, 2001) (#35)

A role for oxidative stress in the etiology or progression of amyotrophic lateral sclerosis (ALS) and other neurodegenerative diseases has been recently proposed. We conducted the 18-month, **randomized treatment trial with oral vitamin E (600 IU daily) and selegiline (10 mg daily) in 67 patients with sporadic ALS.** Thirty five patients were randomly assigned to receive antioxidative therapy (vitamin E plus selegiline) and the remaining 32 patients were the ALS controls who received symptomatic treatment. The primary end point was survival and functional status. At the end of 18-month study, 13 patients in the treatment group and 14 in the control group died or were tracheostomized. A decline in functional disability was also similar in both groups. **Long-term antioxidative treatment with vitamin E did not benefit patients with ALS.** (Kwiecinski et al, 2001)

Antioxidants fail to prolong survival of ALS patients

Survival in patients with amyotrophic lateral sclerosis, treated with an array of antioxidants (Vyth et al, 1996) (#36)

Between 1983 and 1988 we treated 36 patients with sporadic amyotrophic lateral sclerosis (**ALS) by an array of antioxidants** and added other drugs to the regimen whenever a patient reported deterioration. Our customary prescription sequence **was N-acetylcysteine (NAC); vitamins C and E; N-acetylmethionine (NAM); and dithiothreitol (DTT) or its isomer dithioerythritol (DTE).** Patients with a history of heavy exposure to metal were also given meso 2,3-dimercaptosuccinic acid (DMSA). NAC, NAM, DTT, and DTE were administered by subcutaneous injection or by mouth or by both routes, the other vitamins and DMSA by mouth alone. The hospital pharmacy supplied NAC and NAM injections fluid as 100 ml bottles of 5.0 and 5.85% solutions, respectively. DTT was delivered in special double-walled capsules of 200 mg. DTT/DTE injection fluid was added to the NAC and NAM bottles, the final DTT/DTE concentrations never exceeding 0.5%. DMSA was provided in 250 mg capsules. All of the 36 patients used NAC and DTT/DTE; 29 also used vitamins C and E; 21 also used NAM; and 7 also used DMSA, DMSA, NAM, vitamins C and E were tolerated well. **In many patients, DTT, DTE, NAC and NAM induced pain, redness and swelling at the injection sites in that order of decreasing frequency. DTT and DTE did often and NAC did sometimes cause gastric pain, nausea and other abdominal discomfort.** Comparison of survival in the treated group and in a cohort of untreated historical controls, disclosed a median survival of 3.4 years (95% confidence interval: 3.0-4.2) in the treated and of 2.8 (95% confidence interval 2.2-3.1) years in the control patients. This difference may be explained by self-selection of our highly motivated treated group and by its initial survival of diagnosis for an average of 8.5 months before onset of treatment. We conclude that **antioxidants neither seem to harm ALS patients, nor do they seem to prolong survival.** (Vyth et al, 1996)

SOD does not improve learning in young mice

Superoxide dismutase (SOD) is one of the most effective mechanisms in physiology for inactivating reactive oxygen species. Elevated SOD activity can be therapeutically useful by protecting against oxidative stress-induced neurotoxicity. Acutely increased extra-cellular-SOD (EC-SOD) activity protects against neurobehavioral impairment caused by acute ischemia. Chronically increased EC-SOD activity may also be therapeutically useful by protecting against chronic oxidative stress-induced neurobehavioral damage that accumulates during the aging process. We have found that mice **with genetic overexpression of EC-SOD do not show the aging-induced decline in learning and memory that control, wild type mice show.** From 14-22 months of age, the EC-SOD overexpressing mice have significantly better spatial learning working memory function than that of controls. This effect is specific to the aging period.

Young adult EC-SOD overexpressing mice do not have better learning and memory function than controls. The beneficial effects of increased EC-SOD activity with aging may be achieved without risk of impairment during younger ages by chronically administering EC-SOD mimetics from mature adulthood into the aging period. Novel EC-SOD mimetics may be useful in attenuating aging-induced cognitive impairments and other aspects of physiological decline with aging. (Levin, 2005)

A Phase I safety study of hyperbaric oxygen therapy for ALS

Vascular endothelial growth factor and mitochondrial abnormalities have been

described in ALS and its animal models. We have reported that **hyperbaric oxygen (HBO) treatment delayed the onset of weakness in the wobbler mouse.**

OBJECTIVE: To perform a Phase I safety study of HBO in patients with ALS.

METHODS: **Five patients with ALS** were treated for 60min with 100% oxygen at 2 atmospheres pressure daily for five days a week for four weeks. The patients reported any deterioration in their condition after each treatment, and their neurological condition was measured serially during the four weeks of the treatment, and for four further weeks.

RESULTS: **Four of five patients reported decreased fatigue**, while one patient dropped out at three weeks because of increased fatigue. **Maximum isometric voluntary contraction (MVIC) of all muscle groups except right hand grip improved significantly by up to 97%. Most improvement occurred during the four weeks after treatment**. It is possible that the improvement in muscle strength was a placebo or a learning effect, though no such effects have been detected in prior therapeutic trials in ALS using MVIC. No change was detected in other measures of neuromuscular function. CONCLUSIONS: A longer duration, placebo controlled trial in a larger number of patients is needed to determine the safety and efficacy of HBO. **Until that is completed, it is not recommended that ALS patients should be treated with HBO.** (Steele et al, 2004)

Ginkgo biloba for prevention of dementia. (DeKosky et al, 2008) (#3,069)

Ginkgo biloba is widely used for its potential effects on memory and cognition. To date, adequately powered clinical trials testing the effect of *G biloba* on dementia incidence are lacking. **Objective** To determine effectiveness of *G biloba* vs placebo in reducing the incidence of all-cause dementia and Alzheimer disease (AD) in elderly individuals with normal cognition and those with mild cognitive impairment (MCI). **Design, Setting, and Participants** Randomized, double-blind, placebo-controlled clinical trial conducted in 5 academic medical centers in the United States between 2000 and 2008 with a median follow-up of 6.1 years. Three thousand sixty-nine community volunteers aged 75 years or older with normal cognition (n = 2587) or MCI (n = 482) at study entry were assessed every 6 months for incident dementia. **Intervention** Twice-daily dose of 120-mg extract of *G biloba* (n = 1545) or placebo (n = 1524). **Main Outcome Measures** Incident dementia and AD determined by expert panel consensus. **Results** Five hundred twenty-three individuals developed dementia (246 receiving placebo and 277 receiving *G biloba*) with 92% of the dementia cases classified as possible or probable AD, or AD with evidence of vascular disease of the brain. Rates of dropout and loss to follow-up were low (6.3%), and the adverse effect profiles were similar for both groups. The overall dementia rate was 3.3 per 100 person-years in participants assigned to *G biloba* and 2.9 per 100 person-years in the placebo group. The hazard ratio (HR) for *G biloba* compared with placebo for all-cause dementia was 1.12 (95% confidence interval [CI], 0.94-1.33; $P = .21$) and for AD, 1.16 (95% CI, 0.97-1.39; $P = .11$). ***G biloba* also had no effect on the rate of progression to dementia in participants with MCI** (HR, 1.13; 95% CI, 0.85-1.50; $P = .39$). **Conclusions** In this study, ***G biloba* at 120 mg twice a day was not effective in reducing either the overall incidence rate of dementia or AD incidence in elderly individuals with normal cognition or those with MCI**. (DeKosky et al, 2008)

Ginkgo proves ineffective in preventing dementia, Alzheimer's disease

One of the most widely used herbal supplements, ginkgo, for improving memory and cognition has no impact on the development of dementia or Alzheimer's disease, according to new results from a $30 million, multi-center study.

The Ginkgo biloba for the Evaluation of Memory (GEM) Study was the largest clinical trial ever to evaluate the effects of the dietary supplement ginkgo biloba (ginkgo) on the occurrence of dementia. The study tested the effectiveness of 120 milligrams (mg) of ginkgo twice daily versus placebo in lowering the incidence of dementia and Alzheimer's in normal, elderly people and those with mild cognitive impairment.

Results from the Ginkgo biloba for the Evaluation of Memory (GEM) Study show that 240 mg of ginkgo daily has no effect on the onset of dementia or development of Alzheimer's. The study appears in the *Journal of the American Medical Association*. (DeKosky et al, 2008)

Many people today use ginkgo leaf extracts hoping to improve memory, to treat or help prevent Alzheimer's and other types of dementia, to decrease intermittent claudication (leg pain caused by narrowing arteries) and to treat sexual dysfunction, multiple sclerosis, tinnitus, and other health conditions.

In Europe and the United States, ginkgo supplements are among the best-selling herbal medications and it consistently ranks as a top medicine prescribed in France and Germany.

"Alzheimer's disease is a devastating disease affecting large numbers of older adults," said Gregory Burke, M.D., M.Sc., the lead investigator for the Wake Forest University Baptist Medical Center clinical site. "Our best strategy is to prevent dementia before it begins."

The study was conducted primarily to determine if ginkgo would decrease the incidence of all types of dementia and, more specifically, reduce the incidence of Alzheimer's. The study also aimed to evaluate ginkgo for its effects on overall cognitive decline, functional disability, incidence of cardiovascular disease and stroke, and total mortality.

The results were disappointing and surprising, said Burke and Jeff Williamson, M.D., M.H.S., principal investigator for the GEM Study Clinical Coordinating Center at Wake Forest Baptist. (DeKosky et al, 2008)

"In addition to its widespread use based on the belief that it helps memory function," Williamson said, "Ginkgo biloba had enough promising circumstantial evidence from laboratory and animal studies and enough safety information to warrant a full-scale test in humans."

Dementia is a form of brain disease that can seriously affect a person's ability to carry out daily activities. It is caused by many conditions, some of which are reversible. **Alzheimer's is one of the most common forms of dementia in older people, affecting nearly 4.5 million Americans**, according to the National Institute on Aging. It is an incurable disease with a slow progression beginning with mild memory loss and ending with severe brain damage and death.

The GEM Study was conducted at four clinical sites: Wake Forest Baptist, the University of Pittsburgh, Johns Hopkins University, and the University of California-Davis.

Investigators followed a total of **3,069 participants** age 75 or older, who had either normal cognition or mild cognitive impairment. Participants were randomized to receive twice-daily doses of either 120 mg of ginkgo extract or placebo. The dose of ginkgo was selected based on prior clinical study results that found 120 mg twice daily to be the most effective dose. The gingko product used in the study was supplied by Schwabe Pharmaceuticals and is sold in the United States as Ginkgold MaxTM, under the Nature's Way label.

Patients were followed for an average of about six years, with a maximum of just over seven years. During the study, 523 participants were diagnosed with dementia, 246 in the placebo group and 277 in the ginkgo group, leading researchers to declare that **ginkgo showed no overall effect for reducing all types of dementia or Alzheimer's.**

"It is very unlikely that ginkgo biloba is effective at any dose over a five-year period and in anyone over 75 years old," Williamson said. "It is also ineffective in people with signs of early memory loss. What is not known yet is whether the effect of ginkgo biloba might require taking the drug for many, many years, say 15 years, before there is even a sign of memory loss."

For the millions of people spending their money on over-the-counter ginkgo for the perceived promise of protection from dementia and Alzheimer's, Williamson suggests they spend their money elsewhere, while remaining mentally and physically active.

And though ginkgo failed to perform as hoped, Williamson explained that the trial was valuable in many ways to the scientific community. The study experience itself demonstrates the feasibility of conducting large dementia prevention trials in older adults, the researchers said.

"One of the most important findings from this study is that we can recruit and follow adequate numbers of volunteers for this purpose, even in the rapidly growing population of people over age 75," he said. "This will be critical for the most cost-effective use of scarce Medicare dollars in the future.

"Secondly, we are already learning a lot of new information from the GEMS volunteers about how dementia develops and how not all memory change is a sign of impending dementia," Williamson added.

The dietary supplement ginkgo, long promoted as an aid to memory, didn't help prevent dementia and Alzheimer's disease in the longest and largest test of the extract in older Americans.

"We don't think it (the antioxidant, gingko biloba) has a future as a powerful anti-dementia drug," said Dr. Steven DeKosky of the University of Virginia School of Medicine, who led the federally funded study.

Extracts from ginkgo tree leaves have antioxidant and anti-inflammatory effects, but earlier research on ginkgo and memory showed mixed results. Annual U.S. sales of the supplement reached $107 million in 2007, according to Nutrition Business Journal estimates.

Ginkgo has been believed to protect the brain by preventing the buildup of an Alzheimer's-related protein or by preventing cell-damaging oxidative stress. But, it doesn't.

It's been used for leg pain, ringing in the ears and sexual dysfunction. For the new study, appearing in the Journal of the American Medical Association, researchers recruited more than 3,000 people, ages 75 and older, from voter and mailing lists in Maryland, Pennsylvania, California and North Carolina.

Half were randomly assigned to take 120 milligrams of ginkgo biloba twice a day, a typical dose taken by people who think it may help memory. The others took identical dummy pills. Participants were screened for dementia every six months. After six years, dementia had been diagnosed at a similar rate in both groups; 277 in the ginkgo group and 246 in the group taking the dummy tablets. When the researchers looked only at Alzheimer's disease, that rate too was similar.

At the start, some people showed mild difficulties with thinking; ginkgo didn't work to prevent dementia in those people either. Ginkgo appears relatively safe, DeKosky said. There was no difference in the rate of adverse events such as heart attacks and gastrointestinal bleeding between the groups. There were 16 strokes from bleeding in the brain in the ginkgo group versus eight in the placebo group, a difference that wasn't statistically significant, he said, because the number of strokes was too small.

Would ginkgo work better to prevent dementia if people started taking it earlier, say, in middle age? The study didn't look at that, DeKosky acknowledged, adding that following people for 25 years from middle age to old age would be expensive research. The study also didn't test whether ginkgo improves thinking and memory in the short term. "It would have been terrific if this worked. It's inexpensive, available and relatively safe," said Paul Solomon, professor of neuroscience at Williams College in Williamstown, Mass., who wasn't involved in the new study but has studied ginko. "Now with this kind of evidence, you can confidently tell people it didn't show benefit in more than 3,000 people in six years of research," Solomon said.

There may still be a role for ginkgo in treating, rather than preventing, Alzheimer's disease, said Michael McGuffin, president of the American Herbal Products Association, a trade association. Some previous ginkgo trials have shown no benefit in Alzheimer's symptom treatment, while others have found it comparable to prescription drugs such as **Aricept, also known as donepezil**.

A four-month supply of ginkgo can cost less than $10. But not all brands contain what their labels claim. ConsumerLab.com, which tests the ingredients in supplements, reported Tuesday that of seven ginkgo products it reviewed, five failed to pass its tests. An eighth ginkgo product also passed the group's test in a voluntary certification program. The dementia study was funded by a grant from the National Institutes of Health's National Center for Complementary and Alternative Medicine, which is undertaking large, scientific tests of a number of commonly used dietary supplements. The agency said it's the largest-ever randomized trial of a botanical medicine. There have been larger studies of vitamins and minerals.

DeKosky reported receiving grants from and acting as a consultant for several drug companies, including some that make dementia drugs. Schwabe Pharmaceuticals of Karlsruhe, Germany, provided the ginkgo tablets and identical placebos.

People on the blood thinner warfarin shouldn't take ginkgo because of the risk of increased bleeding.

Once again, another antioxidant fails miserably.

***Ginkgo biloba* has been studied extensively for its effects on memory. It lacks predictable, clinically significant benefits in persons with acquired cognitive impairments, including dementia of any degree of severity.** (Birks et al, 2007)

The Ginkgo Evaluation of Memory Study (GEMS), a randomized controlled trial of *G. biloba* in elderly persons aged >75 y, found no effects on all-cause dementia, on AD, or on the rate of progression to dementia in elderly persons with mild cognitive impairment. (Dekosky et al, 2008)

Polypharmacy was common in GEMS; nearly 75% of participants used at least one prescription medication and one dietary supplement, and a third used ≥3 dietary supplements plus ≥3 prescription medications, posing risks of adverse drug interactions. (Nahin et al, 2006). For example, ***G. biloba* increases the risk of bleeding when taken with aspirin.** Another possible effect of polypharmacy on health behaviors is that use of multiple supplements may decrease adherence to prescription medications.

In summary, **the evidence suggests that dietary supplement use is unlikely to prevent cognitive impairment or AD, nor is e4+ status an indication for their use.** Behaviors that reduce cardiovascular disease risk are more promising. (Dwyer, Donoghue, 2010)

B vitamins fail in U.S. Alzheimer's disease study

An October 2008 study found that **high doses of B vitamins failed to slow cognitive decline in people with Alzheimer's disease,** dashing the hopes for a new weapon against the fatal, mind-robbing ailment, U.S. researchers said.

Experts had viewed B vitamins as a potential way to lower the risk of Alzheimer's disease or slow its progression because the vitamins can cut the amount of the amino acid homocysteine, found in high levels in the blood of Alzheimer's patients.

But when the researchers gave people with mild to moderate Alzheimer's disease **high-dose supplements of vitamins B6 and B12 and the B vitamin folic acid for 18 months, they did no better on tests assessing cognitive skills such as memory and language than similar patients who were given a placebo.**

And the people who got the vitamin supplements unexpectedly experienced greater amounts of depression, the researchers wrote in the Journal of the American Medical Association.

"Our results give a very clear answer that these vitamins should not be taken to treat Alzheimer's disease. They're ineffective," said Dr. Paul Aisen of the University of California San Diego, who led the study. (Aisen et al, 2008)

Alzheimer's is an incurable brain disease that worsens over time. It is the most common form of dementia in the elderly.

"Alzheimer's disease breeds a great deal of desperation. So people will go to the health food store and look on the shelf that says 'brain health' and take one of everything," said Bill Thies, vice president for medical and scientific relations at the Alzheimer's Association advocacy group.

"These B vitamins are included in there. But this data really suggests that they're probably not getting any benefit. **It is apparently a waste of money,**" Thies said.

The study involved 409 people with Alzheimer's disease at 40 sites throughout the United States. Some got daily doses of five milligrams of folic acid, one milligram of vitamin B12 and 25 milligrams of vitamin B6. The rest got daily placebo pills.

Those doses are far above the recommended daily allowance.

The people who took the B vitamins saw their homocysteine levels decline, but that did not translate into any benefits in terms of cognitive abilities compared to the placebo group.

This is the third study to question the benefits of reducing homocysteine levels. Two tests, also published in the New England Journal, showed that using B vitamins and folic acid to treat people with high homocysteine levels did not bring down their elevated risk of heart attack or stroke.

Dr. Lon Schneider of the Keck School of Medicine of the University of Southern California, another of the researchers, said the study did not look at whether lowering homocysteine much earlier in life would prevent or delay Alzheimer's.

Amyloid beta protein is toxic to brain cells and plays an important role in the disease. The researchers had hoped by reducing homocysteine, it could reduce the toxicity of amyloid beta protein, Schneider said.

People can get folic acid and other B vitamins in the diet through leafy green vegetables and fortified cereals or through vitamin supplements.

The study was part of an initiative funded by the U.S. National Institutes of Health testing promising ideas for Alzheimer's treatment not being pursued by drug companies.

"This is closing down one strategy, but we fortunately have many others," Aisen said. (Aisen et al, 2008)

CHAPTER TWENTY

Antioxidants in central nervous system diseases

Antioxidants in central nervous system diseases: preclinical promise and translational challenges (Kamat et al, 2008)

Oxidative damage is allegedly strongly implicated in the pathogenesis of neurodegenerative diseases including Alzheimer's disease, amyotrophic lateral sclerosis, Huntington's disease, Parkinson's disease and stroke (brain ischemia/reperfusion injury).

The availability of transgenic and toxin-inducible models of these conditions has facilitated the preclinical evaluation of putative antioxidant agents ranging from prototypic natural antioxidants such as vitamin E (alpha-tocopherol) to sophisticated synthetic free radical traps and catalytic oxidants. **Literature review shows that antioxidant therapies have enjoyed general success in preclinical studies across disparate animal models, but little benefit in human intervention studies or clinical trials.**

Recent high-profile failures of vitamin E trials in Parkinson's disease, and nitrone therapies in stroke, have diminished enthusiasm to pursue antioxidant neuroprotectants in the clinic. The translational disappointment of antioxidants likely arises from a combination of factors including failure to understand the drug candidate's mechanism of action in relationship to human disease, and failure to conduct preclinical studies using concentration and time parameters relevant to the clinical setting. This review discusses the rationale for using antioxidants in the prophylaxis or mitigation of human neurodiseases, with a critical discussion regarding ways in which future preclinical studies may be adjusted to offer more predictive value in selecting agents for translation into human trials. (Kamat et al, 2008)

EMODs: good and bad

EMODs, reactive oxygen species (ROS) and reactive nitrogen species (RNS, e.g. nitric oxide, NO(*)), are well recognized for playing a dual role as both deleterious and beneficial species. ROS and RNS are normally generated by tightly regulated enzymes, such as NO synthase (NOS) and NAD(P)H oxidase isoforms, respectively.

Beneficial effects of EMODs (e.g. superoxide radical and nitric oxide) occur at low/moderate concentrations and involve physiological roles in cellular responses to noxia (harmful agents), as for example in defense against infectious agents, in the function of a number of cellular signaling pathways, and the induction of a mitogenic response. Ironically, various EMOD-mediated actions in fact protect cells against EMOD-induced oxidative stress and re-establish or maintain "redox balance" termed also "redox homeostasis". The "two-faced" character of EMODs is clearly substantiated. For example, a growing body of evidence shows that EMODs within cells act as secondary messengers in intracellular signaling cascades which induce and maintain the oncogenic phenotype of cancer cells, however, **EMODs can also induce cellular senescence and apoptosis and can therefore function as anti-tumourigenic species.** (Valko et al, 2007)

Methylene blue

Methylene blue to treat Alzheimer's and Parkinson's diseases

An article in August of 2008 described a new study conducted by researchers at Children's Hospital & Research Center Oakland shows that a century-old drug, **methylene blue, may be able to slow or even cure Alzheimer's and Parkinson's disease.** Used at a very low concentration – about the equivalent of a few raindrops in four Olympic-sized swimming pools of water – the drug slows cellular aging and enhances mitochondrial function, potentially allowing those with the diseases to live longer, healthier lives. **I know that methylene blue is capable of producing singlet oxygen, when exposed to light and I believe that this is its mechanism of action or that it is combined with ascorbate and produces peroxide.**

A paper on the methylene blue study, conducted by Hani Atamna, PhD, and a his team at Children's, was published in the **March 2008 issue of the Federation of American Societies for Experimental Biology (FASEB)** Journal. Dr. Atamna's research found that **methylene blue can prevent or slow the decline of mitochondrial function, specifically an important enzyme called complex IV.**

Because mitochondria are the principal suppliers of energy to all animal and human cells, their healthy function is critical.

One of the key aspects of Alzheimer's disease is mitochondrial dysfunction, specifically complex IV dysfunction, which methylene blue improves. Our findings indicate that methylene blue, by enhancing mitochondrial function, expands the mitochondrial reserve of the brain. Adequate mitochondrial reserve is essential for preventing age-related disorders such as Alzheimer's disease."

Also impressed is one of Dr. Atamna's co-authors, **Bruce Ames, PhD, a senior scientist at Children's and world-renowned expert in nutrition and aging**. (Really?) **"What we potentially have is a wonder drug."** said Dr. Ames. "To find that such a common and inexpensive drug can be used to increase and prolong the quality of life by treating such serious diseases is truly exciting."

Methylene blue, first discovered in 1891, is now used to treat methemoglobinemia, a blood disorder. But because **high concentrations of methylene blue were known to damage the brain,** no one thought to experiment with low concentrations. Also, drugs such as methylene blue do not easily reach the brain.

Dr. Atamna's research is the first to show that **low concentrations of the drug have the ability to slow cellular aging in cultured cells in the laboratory and in live mice**. He believes methylene blue has the potential to become another commonplace low-cost treatment like aspirin, prescribed as a blood thinner for people with heart disorders.

Dr. Atamna's research, funded by the Bruce and Giovanna Ames Foundation, was conducted at Children's research institute and will continue when Dr. Atamna assumes a position as a professor of Neuroscience at The Commonwealth Medical College in Pennsylvania. (Atamna et al, 2007)

Methylene blue (MB) has been used clinically for about a century to treat numerous ailments. We show that **MB and other diaminophenothiazines** extend the life span of human IMR90 fibroblasts in tissue culture by >20 population doubling (PDLs). MB delays senescence at nM levels in IMR90 by enhancing mitochondrial function. **MB increases mitochondrial complex IV by 30%, enhances cellular oxygen consumption by 37–70%,** increases heme synthesis, and **reverses premature senescence caused by H_2O_2 or cadmium.**

MB also induces phase-2 antioxidant enzymes in hepG2 cells. Flavin-dependent enzymes are known to use NAD(P)H to reduce MB to leucomethylene blue (MBH$_2$), whereas cytochrome c reoxidizes MBH$_2$ to MB. Experiments on lysates from rat liver mitochondria suggest the ratio MB/cytochrome c is important for the protective actions of

MB. **We propose that the cellular senescence delay caused by MB is due to cycling between MB and MBH$_2$ in mitochondria**, which may partly explain the increase in specific mitochondrial activities.

Cycling of MB between oxidized and reduced forms may block oxidant production by mitochondria (RMH Note: Actually, it likely increases the prooxidant environment.). Mitochondrial dysfunction and oxidative stress are thought to be key aberrations that lead to cellular senescence and aging. MB may be useful to delay mitochondrial dysfunction with aging and the decrease in complex IV in Alzheimer disease. (Atamna et al, 2007)

Methylene blue produces hydrogen peroxide as a redox cycler (malaria)

Methylene blue (MB) has experienced a renaissance mainly as a component of drug combinations against Plasmodium falciparum malaria. Investigators reported biochemically relevant pharmacological data on MB such as rate constants for the uncatalyzed reaction of MB at pH 7.4 with cellular reductants like NAD(P)H (k = 4 M(-1) s(-1)), thioredoxins (k = 8.5 to 26 M(-1) s(-1)), dihydrolipoamide (k = 53 M(-1) s(-1)), and slowly reacting glutathione. As the disulfide reductases are prominent targets of MB, optical tests for enzymes reducing MB at the expense of NAD(P)H under aerobic conditions were developed. The product leucomethylene blue (leucoMB) is auto-oxidized back to MB at pH 7 but can be stabilized by enzymes at pH 5.0, which makes this colorless compound an interesting drug candidate. **MB was found to be an inhibitor and/or a redox-cycling substrate of mammalian and P. falciparum disulfide reductases**, with the kcat values ranging from 0.03 s(-1) to 10 s(-1) at 25 degrees C. Kinetic spectroscopy of mutagenized glutathione reductase indicates that MB reduction is conducted by enzyme-bound reduced flavin rather than by the active-site dithiol Cys58/Cys63. The enzyme-catalyzed reduction of MB and subsequent auto-oxidation of the product leucoMB mean that **MB is a redox-cycling agent which produces H$_2$O$_2$ at the expense of O$_2$ and of NAD(P)H in each cycle, turning the antioxidant disulfide reductases into pro-oxidant enzymes.** This explains the terms subversive substrate or turncoat inhibitor for MB. The results are discussed in cell-pathological and clinical contexts. (Buchholz et al, 2008). **I believe that this ties into other prooxidant methods of treating malaria, in that all effective methods utilize prooxidant systems.**

Malaria parasite has strong antioxidative defenses

The malaria parasite Plasmodium falciparum is highly adapted to cope with the oxidative stress to which it is exposed during the erythrocytic stages of its life cycle. This includes the defense against oxidative insults arising from the parasite's metabolism of hemoglobin which results in the formation of reactive oxygen species and the release of toxic ferriprotoporphyrin IX. Central to the parasite's defenses are superoxide dismutases and thioredoxin-dependent peroxidases; however, they lack catalase and glutathione peroxidases. The vital importance of the thioredoxin redox cycle (comprising NADPH, thioredoxin reductase and thioredoxin) is emphasized by the confirmation that thioredoxin reductase is essential for the survival of intraerythrocytic P. falciparum. The parasites also contain a fully functional glutathione redox system and the low-molecular-weight thiol glutathione is not only an important intracellular thiol redox buffer but also a cofactor for several redox active enzymes such as glutathione S-transferase and glutaredoxin. Recent findings have shown that in addition to these cytosolic redox systems the parasite also has an important mitochondrial antioxidant defense system and it is suggested that lipoic acid plays a pivotal part in defending the organelle from oxidative damage. (Muller, 2004). I believe that this confirms the need for defensive antioxidant systems for the viability of the malaria parasite. It is killed by increasing the oxidative capacity.

Methylene blue has syphilitic trypanocidal prooxidant activity

Methylene blue (MB) is known to have trypanocidal activity. They tested the interactions of MB with a number of trypanosomatid-specific molecules of the antioxidant metabolism. At pH 7, trypanothione and other (di)thiols were oxidized to disulfides by the phenothiazine drug. MB inhibited Trypanosoma cruzi trypanothione reductase (TR) (K(i)=1.9 microM), and served as a significant subversive substrate of this enzyme (K(M)=30 microM, k(cat)=4.9s(-1)). With lipoamide dehydrogenase, the second thiol-generating flavoenzyme of T. cruzi, the catalytic efficiency for MB reduction was found to be almost 10(6)M(-1)s(-1). When the system MB-enzyme-molecular oxygen acts as a NAD(P)H-driven redox cycler, a reactive oxygen species, H(2)O(2) or superoxide, is produced in each cycle. Since MB is an affordable, available, and accessible drug it might be tested--alone or in drug combinations--against trypanosomatid-caused diseases of animal and man. (Buchholz et al, July 2008). This shows that prooxidants are also capable of killing syphilitic trypanosomes. This is also why I recommend prooxidant methods to treat the scourges of mankind, such as malaria, HIV/AIDS, cancer, atherosclerosis, infections, etc.

Tropical diseases killed oxidatively

Trypanosomes and leishmania, the causative agents of several tropical diseases, possess a unique redox metabolism which is based on **trypanothione**. The bis(glutathionyl) spermidine is the central thiol that delivers electrons for the synthesis of DNA precursors, **the detoxification of hydroperoxides** and other trypanothione-dependent pathways. Many of the reactions are mediated by tryparedoxin, a distant member of the thioredoxin protein family. Trypanothione is kept reduced by the parasite-specific flavoenzyme trypanothione reductase. Since glutathione reductases and thioredoxin reductases are missing, the reaction catalyzed by trypanothione reductase represents the only connection between the NADPH- and the thiol-based redox metabolisms. Thus, cellular thiol redox homeostasis is maintained by the biosynthesis and reduction of trypanothione. Nearly all proteins of the parasite-specific trypanothione metabolism have proved to be essential. (Krauth-Siegel et al, 2008). **This indicates that antioxidants, like trypanothione, protect some disease causing organisms from oxidative death.**

Role of EMODs

Oxidative stress is a "privilege" of aerobic organisms. It can be induced by endogenous and exogenous factors. Most often, it is characterized by the production of free radicals and nonradical oxygen and nitrogen products, referred to under a single term "reactive species" (RS), EMODs. Reactive oxygen (ROS) and nitrogen species (RNS) are "two-faced" products. **Produced in low/moderate concentrations as molecular signals, ROS regulate a series of physiological processes, such as a defense against infectious agents, the maintenance of vascular tone, the control of ventilation and erythropoietin production, and signal transduction from membrane receptors in various physiological processes**. Many of EMOD-mediated responses protect cells against oxidative stress and maintain "redox homeostasis". Then, both reactive species are produced by strictly regulated enzymes, such as nitric oxide synthase (NOS), and isoforms of NADPH oxidase, or as by-products from not so well regulated sources, such as the mitochondrial electron-transport chain. An excessive increase in EMOD production has been implicated in the pathogenesis of atherosclerosis, cardiovascular diseases, hypertension, ischemia/reperfusion injury, diabetes mellitus, neurodegenerative and immuno-inflammatory diseases. **Within the cells, EMODs can act as secondary messengers in intracellular signaling cascades, which can induce the oncogenic phenotype of cancer cells, cellular senescence and apoptosis.** (Srp Arh Celok Lek. 2008)

EMODs, ROS and aging

At high concentrations, free radicals and radical-derived, nonradical reactive species are hazardous for living organisms and damage all major cellular constituents.

At moderate concentrations, however, nitric oxide (NO), superoxide anion, and related reactive oxygen species (ROS, EMODs) play an important role as regulatory mediators in signaling processes.

Many of the ROS-mediated responses actually protect the cells against oxidative stress and reestablish "redox homeostasis." Higher organisms, however, have evolved the use of NO and EMODs also as signaling molecules for other physiological functions. These include regulation of vascular tone, monitoring of oxygen tension in the control of ventilation and erythropoietin production, and signal transduction from membrane receptors in various physiological processes. NO and EMODs are typically generated in these cases by tightly regulated enzymes such as NO synthase (NOS) and NAD(P)H oxidase isoforms, respectively.

In a given signaling protein, oxidative attack induces either a loss of function, a gain of function, or a switch to a different function. Excessive amounts of ROS may arise either from excessive stimulation of NAD(P)H oxidases or from less well-regulated sources such as the mitochondrial electron-transport chain. In mitochondria, ROS are generated as undesirable side products of the oxidative energy metabolism. An excessive and/or sustained increase in ROS production has been implicated in the pathogenesis of cancer, diabetes mellitus, atherosclerosis, neurodegenerative diseases, rheumatoid arthritis, ischemia/reperfusion injury, obstructive sleep apnea, and other diseases. In addition, free radicals have been implicated in the mechanism of senescence. **That the process of aging may result, at least in part, from radical-mediated oxidative damage was proposed more than 40 years ago by Harman (J Gerontol 11: 298-300, 1956).** There is growing evidence that aging involves, in addition, progressive changes in free radical-mediated regulatory processes that result in altered gene expression. (Dröge, 2002)

Harman's free radical theory has repeatedly been invalidated due to its lack of predictability. Also, please read my book, *Anti-aging, Anti-oxidant Scams*.

Position statement on human aging by Quackwatch

In 2004, Quackwatch gave a position statement on human aging developed by 51 scientists. Their conclusion was as follows: "Since recorded history individuals have been, and are continuing to be, victimized by promises of extended youth or increased longevity by using unproven methods that allegedly slow, stop or reverse aging. Our language on this matter must be unambiguous: there are no lifestyle changes, surgical procedures, vitamins, antioxidants, hormones or techniques of genetic engineering available today that have been demonstrated to influence the processes of human aging. We strongly urge the general public to avoid buying or using products or other interventions from anyone claiming that they will slow, stop or reverse aging." The scientifically respected free-radical theory of aging serves as a basis for the prominent role that antioxidants have in the antiaging movement. The claim that ingesting supplements containing antioxidants can influence aging is often used to sell antiaging formulations. The logic used by their proponents reflects a misunderstanding of how cells detect and repair the damage caused by free radicals and the important role that free radicals play in normal physiological processes (such as the immune response and cell communication). Nevertheless, **there is little doubt that ingesting fruits and vegetables (which contain antioxidants) can reduce the risk of having various age-associated diseases, such as cancer, heart disease, macular degeneration and cataracts. At present there is relatively little evidence from human studies that supplements containing antioxidants lead to a reduction in either the risk of these conditions or the rate of aging,** but there are a number of ongoing randomized trials that address the possible role of supplements in a range of age-related conditions, the results of which will be reported in the coming years. In the meantime, possible adverse effects of single-dose supplements, such as beta-carotene, caution against their indiscriminate use. **As such, antioxidant supplements may have some health benefits for some people, but so far there is no scientific evidence to justify the claim that they have any effect on human aging.** (Olansky, Hayflick, 2004)

CHAPTER TWENTY ONE

I have repeated this study because of its importance.

Vitamin E for Alzheimer's disease and mild cognitive impairment (Isaac et al, 2008 CD002854) (#769) Vitamin E is a dietary compound that functions as an anti-oxidant scavenging toxic free radicals. Evidence that free radicals may contribute to the pathological processes of cognitive impairment including Alzheimer's disease (AD) has led to interest in the use of Vitamin E in the treatment of Alzheimer's disease and Mild Cognitivie Impairment (MCI). OBJECTIVES: To assess the efficacy of Vitamin E in the treatment of Alzheimer's disease and prevention of progression of Mild Cognitive Impairment to Alzheimer's disease. SEARCH STRATEGY: The Cochrane Dementia and Cognitive Improvement's Specialized Register was searched on 8 January 2007 using the following terms: "Vitamin E", vitamin-E, alpha-tocopherol. The CDCIG Registers contains records from major health care databases and ongoing trial databases and is updated regularly. SELECTION CRITERIA: **All unconfounded, double blind, randomized trials in which treatment with Vitamin E at any dose was compared with placebo for patients with Alzheimer's disease or Mild Cognitive Impairment**. DATA COLLECTION AND ANALYSIS: Two reviewers independently applied the selection criteria and assessed study quality and extracted and analysed the data. For each outcome measure data were sought on every patient randomized. Where such data were not available an analysis of patients who completed treatment was conducted. MAIN RESULTS: Only 2 studies met the inclusion criteria. The primary outcome used in the AD study was survival time to the first of 4 endpoints: death, institutionalisation, loss of 2 out of 3 basic activities of daily living and severe dementia (defined as a global Clinical Dementia Rating of 3). The investigators reported the total numbers in each group who reached the primary endpoint within two years for participants completing the study ("completers"). There appeared to be some benefit from Vitamin E with fewer participants reaching endpoint - 58% (45/77) of completers compared with 74% (58/78) - a Peto odds ratio of 0.49, 95% confidence interval 0.25 to 0.96. However, more participants taking Vitamin E suffered a fall (12/77 compared with 4/78; odds ratio 3.07, 95% CI 1.09 to 8.62). It was not possible to interpret the reported results for specific endpoints or for secondary outcomes of cognition, dependence, behavioral disturbance and activities of daily living. The primary outcome used in the MCI study which had 769 participants (257 in the Vitamin E group and 259 in the placebo group; a third Donepezil group of 253 was not included in this review) was the time to progression from MCI to possible or probable AD. A total of 214 of the 769 participants had progression to dementia, with 212 being classified as having possible or probable AD. **There was no significant difference in the probability of progression from MCI to AD between the Vitamin E group and the placebo group.** There was no significant difference between the placebo group and the Vitamin E group in adverse events. Five subjects died in each group and 72 discontinued treatment in the Vitamin E group and 66 in the placebo group. AUTHORS' CONCLUSIONS: **There is no evidence of efficacy of Vitamin E in the prevention or treatment of people with AD or MCI.** More research is needed to identify the role of Vitamin E, if any, in the management of cognitive impairment. (Isaac et al, 2008 CD002854)

There is little evidence that dietary supplements can prevent or treat AD. Multivitamins do not reduce the risk of dementia. (Huang et al, 2006)

Large doses of vitamin E have little effect in slowing progression to AD among those with mild cognitive impairment. (Isaac et al, 2008)

Combinations of vitamin B-12 and folic acid in very large doses reduce homocysteine concentrations (a risk factor for cerebrovascular disease) but **fail to improve cognitive function in elderly persons with no or moderate cognitive impairment.** (Eussen et al, 2006), **nor do they slow cognitive decline in those with mild to moderate AD.** (Aisen et al, 2008)

Vitamin B-6, vitamin B-12, and folic acid either alone or in various combinations **do not improve cognitive function or dementia.** (Balk et al, 2007), **with the possible exception of folic acid alone or with vitamin B-12 among those with high homocysteine concentrations.** (Malouf et al, 2008)

There is inadequate evidence that fish oils or omega-3 fatty acids protect against decreases in cognitive functions and the incidence or clinical progression of dementias. (Lim et al, 2006)

Riboflavin, vitamin B-6, vitamin C, blueberry extract, α-lipoic acid, and the adrenal hormone dehydroepiandrosterone (DHEA) lack evidence of efficacy in humans.

Indictment of EMODs in AD

The following demonstrates the usual indictment of EMODs in disease causation, including Alzheimer's disease (AD).

Following the trend of the free radical theory to indict oxygen as the causative agent in most human pathophysiologies, papers such as this one by Mecocci were not uncommon.

Oxidative damage to mitochondrial DNA is increased in Alzheimer's disease

Oxidative damage to DNA may play a role in both normal aging and in neurodegenerative diseases. We examined whether Alzheimer's disease (AD) is associated with increased oxidative damage to both nDNA and mtDNA in postmortem brain tissue. We measured the oxidized nucleoside, 8-hydroxy-2'-deoxyguanosine (OH^{8}dG), in DNA isolated from three regions of cerebral cortex and cerebellum in 13 AD and 13 age-matched controls. There was a significant threefold increase in the amount of OH^{8}dG in mtDNA in parietal cortex of AD patients compared with controls. **In the entire group of samples there was a small significant increase in oxidative damage to nDNA and a highly significant threefold increase in oxidative damage to mtDNA in AD compared with age-matched controls.** These results confirm that mitochondrial DNA is particularly sensitive to oxidative damage, and they show that there is increased oxidative damage to DNA in AD, which may contribute to the neurodegenerative process. (Mecocci et al, 2004)

Alzheimer's disease and oxygen radicals: new insights

Alzheimer's disease (AD) is the most common form of neurodegenerative disease, with dementia, in the elderly. In addition to the presence of senile plaques and neurofibrillary tangles, **the AD brain exhibits evidence for oxygen radical-mediated damage, a situation commonly known as oxidative stress. However, the ability to directly implicate this mechanism in AD has been a difficult task** for several reasons.

First, **most of the analytical approaches used to investigate oxidative stress turned out to be unreliable.**

Second, **the majority of the published studies have been performed in postmortem tissues with advanced disease, leaving open the question as to**

whether oxidative stress is an early event or a common final step secondary to the degenerative process.

The discovery of the **isoprostanes, recent studies performed in living patients, and the development of transgenic animal models of AD-amyloidosis are three important factors that are helping us to better understand and define the role that oxygen radicals might play in AD pathogenesis.** Here we review some of the most recent works that have supported the importance of oxygen radical-mediated damage in AD. **The accumulated information points toward an earlier involvement than previously thought of oxidative stress in the pathogenesis of the disease,** making this a potential target for therapeutic intervention, especially in subjects at high risk for developing AD. (Pratico, 2002)

Studies continued with different oxidative markers and concluded the following:

Reactive oxygen-mediated processes are thought to contribute to the pathogenesis of Alzheimer's disease (AD). To investigate this hypothesis we studied autopsy tissue from 11 pairs of AD cases and control individuals matched for age, postmortem delay, and tissue storage time. **The temporal neocortex, which is severely involved by AD pathology, and the cerebellum, which is spared, were analyzed for tissue markers of lipid peroxidation (LPO).** The average chemiluminescence formed from bond breakage in tissue homogenates during a 3-h incubation, without the presence of catalysts such as metal ions or ascorbate, was significantly increased in the AD temporal cortex to 130% of matched controls. **Basal tissue content of LPO products (thiobarbituric acid reactive substances--TBARs) was not different between groups.**

However, TBARs were significantly elevated in AD temporal cortex to 135% of control after the incubation. In contrast, in the cerebellum there was no difference between AD and control tissue, indicating a disease-specific tissue effect. Because the use of oral antioxidants have received considerable attention in the last few years, **the results seen in the testing of an AD patient who took daily vitamin E supplements for 4 years is particularly interesting. The time course for CL reactivity in the temporal cortex was considerably delayed compared to all other samples.** This observation is consistent with the hypothesis that antioxidants within tissue will quench ROS-mediated reactions. This study indicates that **there is increased susceptibility to ROS in the AD temporal cortex that may contribute to the pathogenesis of the disease.** Furthermore, **our observation suggests that oral antioxidant supplementation may be protective against LPO in the human brain.** (McIntosh et al, 1997)

Studies then led to **predictions that antioxidants would curtail AD.**

There is a growing body of evidence to support a role for oxidative stress in Alzheimer's disease (AD), with increased levels of lipid peroxidation, DNA and protein oxidation products (HNE, 8-HO-guanidine and protein carbonyls respectively) in AD brains. The brain is a highly oxidative organ consuming 20% of the body's oxygen despite accounting for only 2% of the total body weight. With normal ageing the brain accumulates metals ions such iron (Fe), zinc (Zn) and copper (Cu). **Consequently the brain is abundant in antioxidants to control and prevent the detrimental formation of reactive oxygen species (ROS) generated via Fenton chemistry involving redox active metal ion reduction and activation of molecular oxygen.**

In AD there is an over accumulation of the Amyloid beta peptide (Abeta), this is the result of either an elevated generation from amyloid precursor protein (APP) or inefficient clearance of Abeta from the brain. **Abeta can efficiently generate reactive oxygen species in the presence of the transition metals copper and iron in vitro.** Under oxidative conditions Abeta will form stable dityrosine cross-linked dimers which are generated from free radical attack on the tyrosine residue at position 10. There are elevated levels of urea and SDS resistant stable linked Abeta oligomers as well as dityrosine cross-linked peptides and proteins in AD brain. Since soluble Abeta levels correlate best with the degree of degeneration, we suggest that the toxic Abeta species corresponds to a soluble dityrosine cross-linked oligomer. (McLean et al, 1999)

I believe that the accumulation of the antioxidant, Abeta, is one of the primary causes of AD and EMOD insufficiency. But, we must remember that it can also generate EMODs.

Current therapeutic strategies using metal chelators such as clioquinol (an antioxidant) and desferrioxamine have had some success in altering the progression of AD symptoms. Similarly, natural antioxidants curcumin and ginkgo extract have modest but positive effects in slowing AD development. Therefore, **drugs that target the oxidative pathways in AD could have genuine therapeutic efficacy.** (Smith et al, 2007)

Confusion about the role of EMODs and antioxidants continue today.

Amyloid beta peptide (Abeta) acts as antioxidant

Oxidative stress plays a key role in Alzheimer's disease (AD). In addition, the **abnormally high Cu(2+) ion concentrations present in senile plaques** has provoked a substantial interest in the relationship between the amyloid beta peptide (Abeta) found within plaques and redox-active copper ions. There have been a number of studies monitoring reactive oxygen species (ROS) generation by copper and ascorbate that suggest that **Abeta acts as a prooxidant producing H_2O_2. However, others have indicated Abeta acts as an antioxidant,** but to date most cell-free studies directly monitoring ROS have not supported this hypothesis. We therefore chose to look again at ROS generation by both monomeric and fibrillar forms of Abeta under aerobic conditions in the presence of Cu(2+) with/without the biological reductant ascorbate in a cell-free system. We used a variety of fluorescence and absorption based assays to monitor the production of ROS, as well as Cu(2+) reduction. **In contrast to previous studies, we show here that Abeta does not generate any more ROS than controls of Cu(2+) and ascorbate.** Abeta does not silence the redox activity of Cu(2+/+) via chelation, but rather hydroxyl radicals produced as a result of Fenton-Haber Weiss reactions of ascorbate and Cu(2+) **rapidly react with Abeta; thus the potentially harmful radicals are quenched. RMH Note: I believe that this indicates that Abeta is an antioxidant.** In support of this, chemical modification of the Abeta peptide was examined using (1)H NMR, and specific oxidation sites within the peptide were identified at the histidine and methionine residues. Our studies add significant weight to a modified amyloid cascade hypothesis in which sporadic AD is the result of **Abeta being upregulated as a response to oxidative stress.** However, our results do not preclude the possibility that Abeta in an oligomeric form may concentrate the redox-active copper at neuronal membranes and so cause lipid peroxidation. (Nadal et al, 2008)

Abeta aggregates generate toxic EMODs

Aggregation of the beta-amyloid peptide (Abeta) to amyloid plaques is a key event in Alzheimer's disease. According to the amyloid-cascade hypothesis, **Abeta aggregates are toxic to neurons through the production of reactive oxygen species (ROS).**

Copper ions play an important role, because they are able to bind to Abeta and influence its aggregation properties. Moreover, **Cu-Abeta is supposed to be directly involved in ROS production.** To get a better understanding of these reactions, we measured the production of HO(.) and the redox potential of Cu-Abeta. The results were compared to other biological copper-peptide complexes in order to get an insight into the biological relevance. Cu-Abeta produced more HO(.) than the complex of copper with Asp-Ala-His-Lys (Cu-DAHK), but less than with Gly-His-Lys (Cu-GHK). Cyclic voltammetry revealed that the order for reduction potential is Cu-GHK>Cu-Abeta>Cu-DAHK, but for the oxidation potential the order is reversed. Thus, easier copper redox cycling correlated to higher HO(.) production. The copper complex of the form Abeta1-42 showed a HO(.) production five-times higher than that of the form Abeta1-40. Time-dependence and aggregation studies suggest that an aggregation intermediate is responsible for this increased HO(.) production. (Guilloreau et al, 2007)

Abeta-(CuI) acts as an antioxidant and reduces oxygen to peroxide

The binding stoichiometry between Cu(II) and the full-length beta-amyloid Abeta(1-42) and the oxidation state of copper in the resultant complex were determined by electrospray ionization-Fourier transform ion cyclotron resonance mass spectrometry (ESI-FTICR-MS) and cyclic voltammetry. The same approach was extended to the copper complexes of Abeta(1-16) and Abeta(1-28). A stoichiometric ratio of 1:1 was directly observed, and the oxidation state of copper was deduced to be 2+ for all of the complexes, and residues tyrosine-10 and methionine-35 are not oxidized in the Abeta(1-42)-Cu(II) complex. The stoichiometric ratio remains the same in the presence of more than a 10-fold excess of Cu(II). Redox potentials of the sole tyrosine residue and the Cu(II) center were determined to be ca. 0.75 and 0.08 V vs Ag/AgCl [or 0.95 and 0.28 V vs normal hydrogen electrode (NHE)], respectively. More importantly, **for the first time, the Abeta-Cu(I) complex has been generated electrochemically and was found to catalyze the reduction of oxygen to produce hydrogen peroxide (like an antioxidant)**. The voltammetric behaviors of the three Abeta segments suggest that diffusion of oxygen to the metal center can be affected by the length and hydrophobicity of the Abeta peptide. The determination and assignment of the redox potentials clarify some misconceptions in the redox reactions involving Abeta and provide new insight into the possible roles of redox metal ions in the Alzheimer's disease (AD) pathogenesis.

In cellular environments, the reduction potential of the Abeta-Cu(II) complex is sufficiently high to react with antioxidants (e.g., ascorbic acid) and cellular redox buffers (e.g., glutathione), and the Abeta-Cu(I) complex produced could subsequently reduce oxygen to form hydrogen peroxide via a catalytic cycle.

Using voltammetry, the Abeta-Cu(II) complex formed in solution was found to be readily reduced by ascorbic acid. **Hydrogen peroxide produced, in addition to its role in damaging DNA, protein, and lipid molecules, can also be involved in the further consumption of antioxidants, causing their depletion in neurons and eventually damaging the neuronal defense system.** Another possibility is that Abeta-Cu(II) could react with species involved in the cascade of electron transfer events of mitochondria and might potentially sidetrack the electron transfer processes in the respiratory chain, leading to mitochondrial dysfunction. (Jiang et al,

2007). **I believe that this clearly demonstrates the antioxidant nature of Abeta-(CuI) complex.**

Some past nonsense went as follows:

Alzheimer's disease (AD) is the tragic brain-robbing disease of aging. It can be recognized by the progressive loss of memory and other aspects of cognitive functioning. **Its characteristic pathological features include tangles of nerve fibers, senile plaques (which contain aluminum, iron, and calcium) and the loss of brain cells.** (Lovell et al, 1995)

Oxidative damage has been implicated in AD, for a number of reasons.

High oxygen consumption and low antioxidant levels

First, **the brain has the highest oxygen consumption rate of any organ in the body, high concentrations of easily-oxidizable lipids, and a relative deficiency of antioxidant enzymes** (compared to other tissues). (Lovell et al, 1995)

High iron concentrations

Second, **iron, which plays an important role in free radical generation, has been found in high concentrations in the brain in AD.** (Lovell et al, 1995)

Past studies show antioxidants improve memory performance

Third, **antioxidant supplementation often improves memory performance in aged individuals.** (Perrig et al, 1997)

Down's syndrome, dementia and EMODs: refutation of the free radical theory

Some of the following was excerpted, abstracted or modified from: (Cocchi et al, 1988)

The reduced inactivation of oxygen's free radicals is one of the hypotheses put forward to account for the onset of Alzheimer's dementia. **However, scarce conclusive**

experimental data may exists to support this theory regarding human species and its refutation has not been established with any certainty either.

Subjects affected by **Down's syndrome have a documented increase in the enzyme superoxide-dismutase-1 (SOD) and about 30% increase in the enzyme glutathione-peroxidase**, both scavengers of oxygen's free radicals.

Thus, Down's have increased SOD and GPx, which can lead to an EMOD insufficiency.

For this reason Down subjects, who are less prone to cerebral palsy from prematurity and low birthweight (Cocchi, 1987; Cocchi and Branchesi, 1988), should also show a retardation in the onset of dementia, compared to normal individuals. This is not however the case, as on the contrary it is regularly found that **Down subjects anticipate by an average of 15 years roughly the onset of an Alzheimer type of dementia**.

The metabolic use of oxygen, by organic tissues in mammals, provokes normally an initial production of the radical anion superoxide ($O_2 \cdot$) which, if in excess, can alone damage the cellular DNA, oxidize the thiolic groups of the proteins and cause other toxic events such as lipidic peroxidation. (Brown, Fridovich, 1981) (Fridovich, Porter, 1981)

Anion superoxide is usually inactivated by its transformation into hydrogen peroxide (H_2O_2). This transformation comes about through two metabolic reactions. First, the divalent reduction of $O_2 \cdot$; catalysed by enzymes such as **urate- and D-amino-oxidase**; and second by spontaneous or enzymatic dismutation in the presence of the enzyme superoxide-dismutase (SOD). (Freeman, Crapo, 1984)

Hydrogen peroxide has been **alleged** to produce cytotoxicity. (Cutler, 1985), but **this is a debatable result in vivo**, and it is possible that cellular toxic effects are rather due to the formation of other reactive compounds.

Hydrogen peroxide normally becomes inactivated by at least two protective enzymatic mechanisms: Either reduced to $H_2 + O_2$, by the **catalase (CAT)** of the intercellular peroxisomes, or again reduced to H_2O, this time by means of **glutathione-peroxidase (GPx)**.

If for any reason, usually contingent and acute, and prevalently anoxic-ischemic, this inactivation system becomes inadequate, either the combination of superoxide and hydrogen peroxide derived from the dismutation, or Fenton-type reactions by the hydrogen peroxide in the presence of copper or iron salts can produce the hydroxyl radical (OH $\cdot$) which is extremely reactive with any type of organic molecule, so as to cause irreversible cellular damage.

Down's link cancer, Alzheimer's disease, cataracts, etc.

The following March 21, 2010 USA Today article was excerpted from **http://www.usatoday.com/news/health/2010-03-22-down22_CV_N.htm?csp=34&utm_source=feedburner&utm_medium=feed&utm_campaign=Feed%3A+usatoday-NewsTopStories+%28News+-+Top+Stories%29&utm_content=My+Yahoo**

In 1950, when Marybeth Solinski was born, a diagnosis of Down syndrome was practically a death sentence. Children with the condition often died before their 10th birthday. Yet Solinski, at 59, has outlived her parents. She has even joined AARP.

Her longevity illustrates the dramatic progress for people with Down syndrome. Thanks to better medical care, **the average life expectancy for a child with Down syndrome is now 60 years, according to the National Down Syndrome Society**, which estimates that about 400,000 people are living with the condition in the USA.

As they live longer, adults with Down syndrome — who have an extra copy of chromosome 21 — are teaching scientists about the genetic roots of aging, says Ira Lott, head of pediatric neurology at the University of California-Irvine School of Medicine. **Scientists today are searching this chromosome, which contains only about 200 of the body's roughly 20,000 genes,** to learn why **people with Down syndrome suffer disproportionately from some health problems, such as Alzheimer's disease, but are spared many others, such as heart attacks, strokes and certain types of cancer**.

9-18-11 I do not believe that it is merely coincidence that these are the same 3 conditions made worse by snythetic antioxidant vitamins: i.e., increased risk of cancer, heart disease and strokes.

By studying adults with Down syndrome, researchers hope to find new ways to combat diseases of aging in the larger population as well, Lott says. "It's an interesting detective story," says Lott, head of the science advisory board of the National Down Syndrome Society. "People with Down syndrome are unique when it comes to many aspects of aging."

Aging troubles start early

People with Down syndrome tend to age prematurely as they develop conditions such as menopause, brittle bones, arthritis, hearing loss, wrinkles and sagging skin about two decades earlier than usual, says Brian Chicoine, medical director of the adult Down syndrome center at Advocate Lutheran General Hospital in Park Ridge, Ill., the leading center of its kind.

Perhaps, these conditions are due to hormones whereas cancer, CVD and strokes are redox related. RMH 9-18-11

"People say they seem to age overnight," says Dennis McGuire, director of psychosocial services at the same center. "They suddenly develop wrinkles and gray hair." Solinski, for example, wears a brace on one leg and hearing aids in both ears, and she has had two corneal transplants. "She's more like a 79-year-old than a 59-year-old," says her sister, Lee Cornell of Illinois. Yet researchers suspect that this unique genetic profile also protects people with Down syndrome from many common ailments. A growing number of researchers are asking:

• What protects their hearts?

Half of babies with Down syndrome are born with correctable heart defects, and most adults with Down syndrome are overweight with high cholesterol. Despite these risks, however, **people with Down syndrome virtually never develop high blood pressure, heart attacks or hardening of the arteries,** Lott says. Doctors are still trying to learn why.

9-18-11 I believe that the high EMOD levels secondary to increased SOD reduces hypertension, MIs and atherosclerosis. My research has shown that excessive antioxidants can cause hypertension, increase MIs and atherosclerosis.

• Why don't they get cancer?

Doctors once believed that people with Down syndrome didn't live long enough to develop cancer, says Sandra Ryeom, a researcher at University of Pennsylvania School of Medicine in Philadelphia. **Yet, with the exception of a rare pediatric leukemia, even elderly adults with Down syndrome rarely develop solid tumors, such as those of the breast or lung.**

Again, I believe that this is due to the increased SOD and hydrogen peroxide levels which kill cancer.

Last May, **Ryeom and her colleagues found genes on the 21st chromosome that inhibit the growth of blood vessels necessary for tumor growth.** Getting an extra copy of these genes, and possibly others, may help the body keep cancers in check by depriving them of blood, she says.

Researchers already are trying to develop anti-cancer treatments based on genes found on chromosome 21, says Roger Reeves of Johns Hopkins University School of Medicine.

• What protects their eyes?

Although people with Down syndrome are at higher risk for cataracts, they rarely develop a form of blindness called macular degeneration, caused by an overgrowth of blood vessels in the retina, Ryeom says. Doctors suspect that the same genes that restrict blood vessel growth in tumors may also prevent abnormal blood vessel growth in the eye.

A link to Alzheimer's?

• Why do Down syndrome patients develop early Alzheimer's disease?

Adults with Down syndrome appear to develop the brain plaques and tangles characteristic of Alzheimer's disease very early in life — even as young as 3 or 4 years old. For decades, **however, their brains also appear to repair and compensate for the damage,** says scientist Elizabeth Head of the University of Kentucky's Sanders-Brown Center on Aging.

"Their brains may be clearing the plaques," says Head, who is now recruiting Down syndrome patients for a study on biomarkers of Alzheimer's. "As they get older, this protective process slows down." **I believe that they are clearing their plaques oxidatively due to the trisomy 21 and increased SOD and peroxide activity.**

By age 40 to 45, virtually everyone with Down syndrome has these plaques and tangles, although only 12% have dementia, Lott says. By age 65, up to 75% of people with Down syndrome have dementia.

Significantly, **doctors have found a gene that increases the risk of Alzheimer's, called APP, on the 21st chromosome**, Lott says. The gene, called **amyloid precursor protein**, is involved in the creation of the brain plaques seen in Alzheimer's patients. **People who inherit mutated copies of these genes may develop Alzheimer's disease decades earlier than usual,** says William Mobley, a neuroscience professor at the University of California-San Diego. Yet not all people with Down syndrome succumb. One of Chicoine's patients lived to 83 without dementia.

Solinski, of Chicago, loves learning so much that she takes flash cards on vacation. She pores over children's encyclopedias and Nancy Drew novels. She is learning to cook, she says, to follow in the footsteps of her mother, who died in August at 92. And, she says, "I want to be a great reader like my father." And Brooklyn resident Edward Barsky is still healthy and independent at 73, living in a group home and navigating public transportation on his own, says his sister, Vicki Ploscowe. "He's still going strong," says Ploscowe, of Manhattan.

If researchers could learn what protects certain people, they might be able to develop a therapy to prevent Alzheimer's — both in those with and those without Down syndrome, Head says.

'No other population' like this

People with Down syndrome present doctors with a rare opportunity to watch the disease progress, Lott says. "There's no other population where you can really study this," Lott says. Although some people without Down syndrome carry a gene that increases their risk of early dementia, "you don't know who in the general population is going to come down with sporadic Alzheimer's. **With Down syndrome, you know that virtually 100% of them will have plaques."**

For example, doctors don't yet know exactly how an extra copy of chromosome 21 causes or prevents disease, Lott says. It's possible that getting a 50% larger "dose" of a gene affects the body's susceptibility to a disease, he says. Or, it's possible that the extra genetic material simply makes the entire genome more unstable. Reeves says he's grateful to the Down syndrome community for teaching scientists so much. **"If it weren't for people with Down syndrome having fewer tumors,"** Reeves says, "we never would have thought to look for anything like this."

Summary for Down's:

high risk to develop: **age prematurely as they develop conditions such as menopause, brittle bones, arthritis, hearing loss, wrinkles and sagging skin about two decades earlier than usual. Cataracts. Alzheimer's disease, and a rare pediatric leukemia.**

low risk to develop: **macular degeneration, Down syndrome rarely develop solid tumors, such as those of the breast or lung. Virtually never develop high blood pressure, heart attacks or hardening of the arteries, strokes and certain types of cancer.**

LOW RISK: solid tumors, heart disease, atherosclerosis, stroke, macular degeneration

HIGH RISK: premature aging, arthritis, cataracts, Alzheimer's disease, a rare pediatric leukemia

It appears to me that the coexistence of diseases is still confirmed in the Down's patients, in that they get cancers, aging, arthritis, cataracts and Alzheimer's. This could be due to extra genes on the trisomy 21 chromosome.

The lower incidence for cancer, heart disease, strokes and macular degeneration could be due to the increased EMOD levels from the increased SOD levels.

The hypothesis of increased free radicals as the causal factor in dementia

One theory on aging attaches great importance to continuous and chronic cellular damage produced by oxygen free radicals, and tends to support this point of view by the report of lipofuscins build up, brought about by decay of the cellular membranes. (Harman, 1969) (Harman, 1978) (Miller, 1974) (Harman, 1981). **But the FRT is wrong!**

This build up (of lipofuscins) depends on oxygen and is age-related. (Cutler, 1985) (Mukai, Goldstein, 1976) (Clausen, 1984) (Cutler, 1984) (Votorica et al, 1984)

In actual fact the auto-oxidation of polyunsaturated fatty acids is a metabolic process which is able to form malondialdehyde and free radicals, both of which can react with essential cell components to give lipofuscins as a product of decay. Furthermore, free radicals can also directly damage the genes. Although, through the intervention of special enzymes, the cell tends to repair the damage done to DNA, the capacity to do so is strongest only in the mitotic phase. (Cleaver, 1978)

The free radicals can be formed by the oxidation of the cellular membranes of the cells belonging to the **CNS, which are highly sensitive to their toxic action, due to the fact that these are cells which do not reproduce themselves and lie in the post-mitotic stage,** when the activity is at its lowest. (Cleaver, 1978) (Johnson et al, 1986)

The accumulation of lipofuscins, which takes place particularly in the mito-chondria, is a process brought on by ageing and is not specific to Alzheimer's disease. (Miquel et al, 1977)

However, there is lots of aldehydes and ketones produced by the action of free radicals playing their part in the beginning of this process; in actual fact, **the formation of lipofuscins in an individual is a metabolic chain not yet fully understood.** It seems that malondialdehyde has a role in the formation of proteins and lipids, constituents of lipofuscins. On the other hand, CNS neurons also possess catalase, glutathione-peroxidase and superoxide-dismutase, being the scavengers against the action of the free radicals. (Clausen, 1984)

CHAPTER TWENTY TWO

MISCELLANEOUS ARTICLES ON AD

Data opposing the free radical hypothesis as cause of dementia

However interesting the hypothesis may be that the cytotoxic action of free radicals is the cause of dementia, it is based on questionable premises. Even though oxygen's free radicals are cytotoxic and can eventually lead to a build up of lipofuscins and although dementia and the accumulation of lipofuscins are two age-related processes, this does not necessarily mean, and it has yet to be demonstrated, that dementia is caused by the accumulation of lipofuscins.

It is quite true that a whole series of illnesses presenting an accumulation of lipofuscins (from neural ceroid lipofuscinoses to vitamin E deficiency and the effects of certain chronic intoxications) are also accompanied by mental deterioration. (Clausen, 1984) but **this is something common to all pathological thesaurismoses**.

It is known however that **in Alzheimer's disease, the most common form of dementia, an accumulation of lipofuscins in the mitochondria is present, but the same is true for non-dementia ageing.** (Miquel et al, 1977)

Research has been carried out to support this hypothesis. **No difference has been found between normal individuals and those with Alzheimer's type of dementia, regarding the activity of their brain SOD.** (Markiund et al, 1985)

Taking the erythrocyte as a model, outside of the CNS of a nerve cell, **the erythro-cytal activity of the SOD and GPx in patients affected by multi-infarctual dementia and Alzheimer's dementia has not been found to be different.** (Sulkava et al, 1986)

No significant differences in blood levels of 12 vitamins were found in a group of Alzheimer's disease patients and a control group of healthy, depressed or other-type-demented subjects. (Scileppi et al, 1984)

It should also be pointed out that neuropathological examination of cerebral lesions **in a patient with generalized glutathione deficiency, due to defective synthesis of glutathione (which might impair the cells antioxidant ability) revealed only selective atrophy of cells of the granular layer of the cerebellum and patchy loss of neurons in a laminar pattern of the visual cortex.**

No changes suggestive of senile dementia were noted. (Skullerud et al, 1960)

In addition to intravenous injections of liposome-entrapped catalase and superoxide dismutase against oxygen toxicity outside the CNS, intravenous injections of liposome-entrapped superoxide dismutase has also protective effects on post-traumatic brain edema. (Turrens et al, 1984) (Freeman et al, 1985) (Chan et al, 1987)

The fate of oxygen-free radicals in Down's syndrome subjects

There is however one important natural experiment which is able to question the hypothesis of the cytotoxic action of oxygen's free radicals as being the cause of dementia. It is well known that **Down subjects anticipate by an average of 10-15 years a form of dementia which is not distinguishable, either from a neuropathological point of view or a behavioral one, from Alzheimer's disease.** (Wisiewski, 1985)

Furthermore, **such a dementia is much more common in Downs than in the normal subjects, and affects over 40% of those who live beyond the age of 50 years.** (Dalton, Crapper, 1984)

It is interesting to note though that **in Down subjects, 50% increase is found in the enzymatic activity of the SOD-1, the control gene of which is allocated in chromosome 21, tripled in these individuals.** (Sinet et al, 1974) (Crosti et al, 1976) (Feaster et al, 1977) (Jezorowska et al, 1982) (Neve et al, 1983)

As well as this, **an adaptive increase of 30% has been revealed in the enzymatic activity of the GPx.** (Neve et al, 1983) (Sinet, 1975) (Brooksbank, Balasz, 1984) (Balasz, Brooksbank, 1985). **Here, I argue that the increase in the antioxidant enzyme is more so responsible for the dementia, due to its blocking the oxidation of the Abeta aggregate and to its creating an EMOD insufficiency.**

The increased presence of these two oxidant scavengers seems to be responsible for the reduced incidence of cerebral palsy (CP) from prematurity and low birthweight, the main risk factors for it. (Cocchi, 1987) (Cocchi, Branchesi, 1988)

These two conditions are quite frequent in Down's newborns and usually can lead to cerebral lesions by means of anoxic-ischemic mechanisms. (Cocchi, 1987) (Cocchi, Branchesi, 1988)

Being more able to inactivate the oxygen's free radicals, the Down's individuals should also therefore be protected from dementia, if this is due to the action of the free radicals.

The fact that this is not the case, but on the contrary, there is an anticipation and increase in the onset of demential evolutions, must be taken as a high probability disapproval of the theory that advances the chronic toxic action of the free radicals as the cause of Alzheimer's disease, at least for Down subjects.

Scientist tracks compounds formed when oxygen attacks

The compounds that form when "**oxygen turns from friend to foe**" are the focus of novel research that has garnered Dr. Jason D. Morrow a prestigious Burroughs Wellcome Fund Clinical Scientist Award in Translational Research.

Morrow, associate professor of Medicine and Pharmacology, and Dr. L. Jackson Roberts, professor of Pharmacology and Medicine, discovered the compounds, called **isoprostanes**, in 1990. **Isoprostanes are produced in cells when reactive molecules called free radicals interact with membrane lipids**. Excessive formation of free radicals is characteristic of oxidant stress.

"We look at the role of oxidant stress in human physiology and pathophysiology," Morrow said. "**The isoprostanes are the most accurate measure to assess oxidant stress in vivo in human beings, and a number of them possess potent bioactivity and likely mediate the pathophysiological consequences of oxidant stress.**"

I believe that isoprostanes are no better than a handful of other agents used to measure so-called oxidative stress. All of them lack concordance.

Morrow and his colleagues have focused on atherosclerosis and Alzheimer's disease. "We have been able to implicate oxidant stress in the pathophysiology of atherosclerosis," Morrow said. "High levels of isoprostanes are present, and we know they possess mitogenic activity that is consistent with the development of atherosclerotic plaques."

In fact, **of three accepted risk factors for atherosclerosis - heavy cigarette smoking, hypercholesterolemia, and hyperhomocysteinemia - all are associated with increased isoprostane formation**.

In **epidemiological studies**, antioxidants like vitamin C and vitamin E appear to decrease atherosclerosis, but it is unknown whether they decrease the production of isoprostanes. Morrow will address this question.

But, in randomized controlled trials (RCTs) the antioxidant vitamins fail to reverse or cure atherosclerosis. For years, we have been misled by observational and epidemiologic studies.

Morrow has collaborated with Dr. Thomas J. Montine, assistant professor of Pathology and Pharmacology, to study isoprostanes in Alzheimer's disease.

"We have shown that isoprostane levels in cerebrospinal fluid are significantly increased in living patients with an Alzheimer's disease diagnosis, and that the levels correlate with disease severity," Morrow said.

These findings support a theorized role for free radicals in Alzheimer's disease and have important implications for patients, Morrow said. Isoprostanes may serve as useful markers to assess and definitively diagnose the disease in living patients. Currently, Alzheimer's disease is a probable diagnosis that can only be confirmed by examining the brain after death.

"Isoprostanes **may** also be very useful for monitoring response to therapy, which for Alzheimer's disease is in its infancy," Morrow said. "One form of therapy is high dose vitamin E; but is it actually decreasing isoprostane levels? We don't know."

Isoprostanes are not formed only in association with disease. The body's cells produce these compounds at a fairly continuous and constant rate.

"I think their production is a consequence of free radical reactions that go on in the body all the time," Morrow said. "There are many sources of free radicals, including exogenous chemicals and endogenous enzyme systems."

And it's an unavoidable fact of life. Oxygen is constantly being breathed, and it participates in processes that produce free radicals. **Should we be taking vitamin E or C or other antioxidants all the time? That's an open question**, Morrow said.

My answer is a resounding, No!

"We have data that vitamin C deficiency is associated with increased oxidant stress. We now want to determine whether supplementation of vitamin C above normal levels decreases oxidant stress."

The body normally produces its own antioxidants that balance out the production of free radicals. No one really knows what throws the system out of whack and sparks disease.

The Burroughs Wellcome Fund (BWF), an independent private foundation, established this award program to address the shrinking number of physicians involved in biomedical research. Because physician-scientists are in a position to identify and implement advances in the basic sciences, a decrease in their presence within the research enterprise threatens the critical link between the bench and the bedside. The BWF Clinical Scientist Awards intend to strengthen that link.

BWF chose nine award recipients from a field of over 100 applicants. Each will receive $750,000 over the next five years, **with few strings attached**.

"The competition is incredibly stiff," said Dr. Eric G. Neilson, Hugh Jackson Morgan Professor and Chair of Medicine. "It is the pinnacle of achievement for a young investigator in Clinical Pharmacology to receive one of these awards.

Stroke: roles of B vitamins, homocysteine and antioxidants (Sanchez-Moreno et al, 2009)

In the present review concerning stroke, we evaluate the roles of B vitamins, - homocysteine and antioxidant vitamins. Stroke is a leading cause of death in developed countries. However, current therapeutic strategies for stroke have been largely unsuccessful. Several studies have reported important benefits on reducing the risk of stroke and improving the post-stroke-associated functional declines in patients who ate foods rich in micronutrients, including B vitamins and antioxidant vitamins E and C. Folic acid, vitamin B6 and vitamin B12 are all cofactors in homocysteine metabolism. Growing interest has been paid to hyperhomocysteinaemia as a risk factor for CVD. Hyperhomocysteinaemia has been linked to inadequate intake of vitamins, particularly to B-group vitamins and therefore may be amenable to nutritional intervention. Hence, poor dietary intake of folate, vitamin B6 and vitamin B12 are associated with increased risk of stroke. Elevated consumption of fruits and vegetables appears to protect against stroke. Antioxidant nutrients have important roles in cell function and have been implicated in processes associated with ageing, including vascular, inflammatory and neurological damage. Plasma vitamin E and C concentrations may serve as a biological marker of lifestyle or other factors associated with reduced stroke risk and may be useful in identifying those at high risk of stroke. After reviewing the observational and intervention studies, **there is an incomplete understanding of mechanisms and some conflicting findings; therefore the available evidence is insufficient to recommend the routine use of B vitamins, vitamin E and vitamin C for the prevention of stroke.** A better understanding of mechanisms, along with well-designed controlled clinical trials will allow further progress in this area. (Sanchez-Moreno et al, 2009)

Cognitive performance in relation to vitamin status in healthy elderly German women-the effect of 6-month multivitamin supplementation (Wolters et al, 2005) (#220)

Prior investigations have reported a link between poor status of antioxidants, folate, and cobalamin resulting in elevated total plasma homocysteine (tHcy) and methylmalonic acid (MMA) concentrations with an increased risk for reduced cognitive performance. The aim of the study was to evaluate the effect of a 6-month multivitamin supplementation on the cognitive performance of female seniors and to assess cognitive functioning in relation to vitamin status, tHcy, and MMA values at baseline. METHODS: The study was performed as a randomized placebo-controlled double-blind trial. **220 healthy, free-living women (aged 60-91 years) were included.** Blood drawings and cognitive tests were performed at the Institute of Food Science of the University of Hanover, Germany. Vitamin and cognitive status have been evaluated prior to and 6 months after supplementation. Plasma ascorbic acid, serum concentrations of alpha-tocopherol, beta-carotene, and coenzyme Q10, serum and erythrocyte folate as well as serum cobalamin, serum MMA, and plasma tHcy concentrations were measured. Activity coefficient of erythrocyte alpha aspartic aminotransferase was used as functional index for vitamin B(6) status. The cognitive performance was assessed by the Symbol Search test, a subtest of the Wechsler Adult Intelligence Scale (WAIS-III) and the pattern-recognition test. Intelligence as assessed by the 'Kurztest für Allgemeine Intelligenz' (KAI) was a further variable. RESULTS: **No significant differences in pattern-recognition and intelligence score were observed between vitamin and placebo group prior to and after multivitamin supplementation.** In the Symbol Search test, the vitamin group exhibited better test results than the placebo group at both measure points. One-way ANOVA showed a marginally significant linear trend between the baseline tHcy concentration and the pattern-recognition score (P = 0.051) in the total sample. Multiple backward regression revealed only a significant influence of the school graduation on baseline cognitive function test results. A general linear model showed that the changes in cognitive function scores could not be explained by the type of treatment or blood parameters. CONCLUSIONS: Our data indicate that **6 months supplementation of physiological dosages of antioxidants and B vitamins have no effect on cognitive performance in**

presumedly healthy and well-nourished female seniors. An intervention period of only 6 months may be too short for improving cognitive performance in well-educated elderly women without dementia. (Wolters et al, 2005)

Effect of multivitamin and multimineral supplementation on cognitive function in men and women aged 65 years and over: a randomised controlled trial (McNeill et al, 2007) (#910) Observational studies have frequently reported an association between cognitive function and nutrition in later life but randomised trials of B vitamins and antioxidant supplements have mostly found no beneficial effect. We examined the effect of daily supplementation with 11 vitamins and 5 minerals on cognitive function in older adults to assess the possibility that this could help to prevent cognitive decline. METHODS: The study was carried out as part of a randomised double blind placebo controlled trial of micronutrient supplementation based in six primary care health centres in North East Scotland. **910 men and women aged 65** years and over living in the community were recruited and **randomised**: 456 to active treatment and 454 to placebo. The active treatment consisted of a single tablet containing eleven vitamins and five minerals in amounts ranging from 50-210 % of the UK Reference Nutrient Intake or matching placebo tablet taken daily for 12 months. Digit span forward and verbal fluency tests, which assess immediate memory and executive functioning respectively, were conducted at the start and end of the intervention period. Risk of micronutrient deficiency at baseline was assessed by a simple risk questionnaire. RESULTS: **For digit span forward there was no evidence of an effect of supplements in all participants or in sub-groups defined by age or risk of deficiency.** For verbal fluency there was no evidence of a beneficial effect in the whole study population but there was weak evidence for a beneficial effect of supplementation in the two pre-specified sub-groups: in those aged 75 years and over (n 290; mean difference between supplemented and placebo groups 2.8 (95% CI -0.6, 6.2) units) and in those at increased risk of micronutrient deficiency assessed by the risk questionnaire (n 260; mean difference between supplemented and placebo groups 2.5 (95% CI -1.0, 6.1) units). CONCLUSION: **The results provide no evidence for a beneficial effect of daily multivitamin and multimineral supplements on these domains of cognitive function in community-living people over 65 years.** However, the possibility of beneficial effects in older people and those at greater risk of nutritional deficiency deserves further attention. (McNeill et al, 2007)

The suggestion that diet or nutrient supplements could delay or reduce cognitive decline in later life is consistent with the biological effects of B vitamins in lowering homocysteine levels and of antioxidant vitamins and minerals in protecting against tissue damage from reactive oxygen species. (Luchsinger et al, 2004)

Cross-sectional and longitudinal studies have provided some evidence in support of associations between nutrient intake or status and cognitive decline, **though the evidence is inconsistent.** (Luchsinger et al, 2004)

By contrast, intervention studies with antioxidant vitamins found no evidence for a beneficial effect of supplements. (Stott et al, 2005) (McMahon et al, 2006) (Eussen et al, 2006) (Heart Protection Study Collaborative Group MRC/BHF Heart Protection Study, 2002)

B vitamins also failed (McMahon et al, 2006) (Eussen et al, 2006) (Heart Protection Study Collaborative Group MRC/BHF Heart Protection Study, 2002) **given for 24 weeks or more in community-living older people have found no evidence for a beneficial effect of supplements, though a recent study of subjects with raised homocysteine levels found a significant benefit of folic acid supplementation for 3 years on global cognitive function and two of the five component cognitive domains.** (Durga et al, 2007)

Two randomised trials which used multivitamins for 24 weeks or more also found no evidence of a beneficial effect. (Cockle et al, 2000) (Wolters et al, 2005)

But a small trial of frail elderly people in residential care found a beneficial effect of multivitamin and multimineral supplementation in two of the five tests of cognitive function after six months. (Wouters-Wesseling et al, 2005)

Another trial of a multivitamin and multimineral supplement in healthy elderly subjects reported beneficial effects after one year in six of seven tests. (Chandra, 2001)

But, **these findings have recently been retracted in the light of concerns about the veracity of the data and possible conflicting commercial interest.** (Meguid, 2005)

The MAVIS (Mineral And Vitamin Intervention Study) trial was a large randomised, double-blind, placebo-controlled trial of multivitamin and multimineral supplementation designed to assess possible effects on infection in men and women aged 65 years or over, using a supplement containing eleven vitamins and five minerals. (Avenell et al, 2005)

In the MAVIS trial we also collected information on cognitive function to assess the possible effects of multivitamin and multimineral supplementation on cognition.

Overall, the McNeill et al results provide **no evidence for a beneficial effect of multivitamin and multimineral supplementation on cognitive function** in the majority of men and women 65 years and over living in the community. This result is consistent with all previous studies in non-selected elderly populations apart from the retracted Canadian study. In the McNeill et al present study the doses of the vitamins and minerals in the supplement ranged from 50–210% of the UK reference nutrient intake, i.e. levels which could be achieved by a well-balanced diet. Several other studies have used higher doses, particularly of B vitamins or **antioxidant vitamins but none of these found a beneficial effect.**

Does taking vitamin, mineral and fatty acid supplements prevent cognitive decline? A systematic review of randomized controlled trials (Jia et al, 2008) (#3,442) Observational studies have shown associations between nutritional status and cognition in later life but evidence from intervention studies is unclear. The present study systematically reviewed the evidence on the effect of nutrient supplementation on cognitive function in people aged >or=65 years. METHODS: Databases including MEDLINE and EMBASE were searched up to 1 September 2006. Randomized controlled trials using at least one kind of vitamin, mineral or omega-3 fatty acid, evaluating standardized neuropsychological test(s), were included. There were no restrictions on participants' baseline nutritional status or cognitive function. Quality assessment and data abstraction were conducted by one author and checked by another. RESULTS: Of 4229 articles retrieved, 22 trials **(3442 participants)** were identified. Many were small, short duration and of poor methodology. Only 16 out of 122 cognitive tests were significantly different between groups. **A meta-analysis showed no significant effect of taking B vitamins or antioxidant vitamins on global cognitive function.**

There was insufficient evidence to evaluate the effect of omega-3 fatty acids on any cognitive domains.

CONCLUSION: **There was little evidence of a beneficial effect from taking B vitamins or antioxidant supplements on global cognitive function in later life.** Larger-scale randomized controlled trials of longer duration in selected age groups are needed. (Jia et al, 2008)

Mitochondria and antioxidant targeted therapeutic strategies for Alzheimer's disease

Oxidative stress and mitochondrial dysfunction are important features present in Alzheimer's disease (AD). They appear early and contribute to disease progression, both in human postmortem AD brains as well as in transgenic AD mouse brains. For this reason, targeting oxidative stress and mitochondria in AD may lead to the development of promising therapeutic strategies. **Several exogenous antioxidant compounds have been tested and found beneficial in transgenic AD mice, such as vitamins and spices.** However, **their efficacy was much more modest in human trials.** More recently, new strategies have been elaborated to promote endogenous antioxidant systems. Different pathways involved in oxidative stress response have been identified. Compounds able to upregulate these pathways are being generated and tested in animal models of AD and in human patients. Upregulation of antioxidant gene expression was beneficial in mice, giving hope for future avenues in the treatment of AD and other neurodegenerative disorders. (Dumont et al, 2010)

The Dumont paper is used as a template for the following section.

Human patients

We turn now to a selective discussion of exogenous antioxidant drugs in human trials to treat or prevent AD or MCI. It should be noted at the outset that as yet no therapy, antioxidant or otherwise, has been shown to reverse, arrest, or even change the slope of decline in human trials.

One of the best studied antioxidants in AD is vitamin E (α-tocopherol). In 1997, the Alzheimer's Disease Cooperative Study (ADCS) published a double-blind, placebo-controlled, randomized, multicenter trial of deprenyl and vitamin E. (Sano et al, 1997)

Deprenyl inhibits the free-radical generating degradation of catecholamines by monoamine oxidase B. A total of 341 patients with AD of moderate severity were assigned to placebo, deprenyl, vitamin E, or both, and followed for an average of 2 years. **Unfortunately, the randomization failed, and at baseline the placebo group was significantly better cognitively than the other groups. No benefit of either deprenyl or vitamin E was seen without adjusting for this baseline difference**.

Beneficial delays in disease progression with vitamin E or deprenyl were seen when analyses were adjusted for baseline cognition, but the need for statistical adjustment leaves some doubt. This trial was similar to the earlier DATATOP (deprenyl and tocopherol antioxidative therapy of Parkinson's) trial, in which 800 subjects with Parkinson's disease were randomized to the same treatments, and the time to disability requiring L-dopa therapy was measured. (Shoulson, 1998)

No motor benefit was seen for vitamin E, and it remains unclear whether the benefit seen with deprenyl was due to augmentation of dopamine rather than an antioxidant effect. **There was no effect of either deprenyl or vitamin E on cognitive performance in early Parkinson's disease (PD)**. (Kieburtz et al, 1994)

A subsequent ADCS trial (The Alzheimer's Disease Cooperative Study) **of vitamin E in MCI showed no benefit on risk of progression to AD**. (Parnetti et al, 1995)

A total of 769 subjects randomly received vitamin E, the cholinesterase inhibitor donepezil, or placebo, and were followed for 3 years. **Donepezil** reduced the risk of

AD for 1 year in all patients, and for all 3 years in subjects with an apolipoprotein E ε4 allele, with a trend toward slowing of hippocampal atrophy. (Jack et al, 2008)

In contrast, there were no significant differences in rate of progression to AD between the vitamin E and placebo groups at any time point, either among all patients or among apolipoprotein E ε4 carriers. (Jack et al, 2008)

It is possible that vitamin E did not have an effect in AD or MCI because of kinetic issues. For an antioxidant to be effective, it must react with oxidants faster than the oxidants react with endogenous targets. The second order rate constant for the reaction of vitamin E with most oxidants is not robustly greater than the rate constant of the oxidants with their targets, which is typically greater than 10^6 M^{-1} s^{-1}. In addition, **it is not known whether supplementation with vitamin E significantly increases brain levels, although levels in CSF are increased**. (Vatassery et al, 1998)

Another reason that vitamin E may not have had an effect in AD or MCI could be that oxidative stress may be most important early in disease pathogenesis. **As noted above, vitamin E reduces amyloid levels and amyloid deposition in transgenic AD mice when started before plaque deposition, but not when started after plaques appear**. (Sung et al, 2004)

Even in clinically very mild AD (Clinical Dementia Rating 0.5), there are already sufficiently many plaques and tangles for a neuropathologic diagnosis of AD, and 50% decreases in entorhinal cortex layer II neurons.

This may be too late for antioxidants to be effective. Based on this hypothesis, antioxidants would be most efficacious in prevention.

In support of this hypothesis, several epidemiologic studies of antioxidant vitamin supplements suggest decreased risk of AD or dementia. In a prospective, population-based observational study of vitamin E and vitamin C use in 633 subjects, baseline use of any vitamins was determined for the preceding two weeks. (Morris et al, 1998). **After an average of 4.3 years, there were 91 incident cases of AD, none of which occurred in the 27 subjects who took vitamin E at baseline or the 23 subjects who took vitamin C at baseline.**

In the Honolulu-Asia Aging Study, vitamin E and vitamin C use was determined in 3,385 Japanese American men, and 3–10 years later cognitive status was classified as AD, vascular dementia, mixed/other dementia, low test scores without dementia, or cognitively intact. There was a significant protective effect of combined vitamin E and vitamin C for non-AD dementias

but not for AD. (Masaki et al, 2000). **However, among those without dementia, use of either vitamin E or vitamin C alone was associated with better cognitive performance.**

Similar results were found in the Canadian Study of Health and Aging. (Maxwell et al, 2005)

In the Rotterdam study, dietary intake of vitamin E, vitamin C, β-carotene, and flavonoids from food sources was assessed in 5,395 non-demented subjects who were then followed for an average of 6 years. The rate of incident AD was decreased by a factor of 0.82 for each 1 standard deviation increase in intake of vitamin C or vitamin E. Among current smokers, there were also significant protective effects for β-carotene and flavonoids. (Engelhart et al, 2002)

In the Nurses' Health Study, long term current users (14968 community-dwelling women) of vitamin E with vitamin C had significantly better global cognitive test scores than subjects who had never used either. (Grodstein et al, 2003)

In the Cache County study, vitamin E and vitamin C supplement use was determined in 4,408 subjects, of whom 200 had prevalent AD, and in whom 104 incident AD cases were identified during follow-up. **Combined use of vitamin E and vitamin C was associated with reduced AD prevalence and incidence.** (Zandi et al, 2004)

In follow-up from this study, increasing quartiles of vitamin C intake combined with vitamin E was associated with higher baseline Modified Mini-Mental State exam (3MS) scores, and **the effect was stronger for food sources than for supplements**]. (Wengreen et al, 2007)

Not all epidemiologic studies have shown positive results, though in general these studies have been smaller (< 1000 subjects).

NEGATIVE STUDIES

In the **Monongahela Valley Independent Elders Survey of 1,059 subjects,** intake of antioxidant supplements (vitamins A, C, E, β-carotene, zinc, and selenium) was initially associated with better cognitive performance in univariate analyses. However, women and persons with higher levels of education were more likely to take antioxidants, and in multivariate analyses including age, gender, and education, **there were no significant differences between antioxidant users and nonusers**. (Mendelsohn et al, 1998)

In a prospective, community-based study of 815 non-demented subjects, vitamin E from food, but **not from supplements**, was associated with decreased incidence of AD in the highest quintile of vitamin E intake, **a protective effect seen only among subjects not carrying an apolipoprotein E ε4 allele.** (Morris et al, 2002)

In the Washington Heights-Inwood Columbia Aging study of 980 non-demented subjects, intake of vitamin C and carotenes, or vitamin E in supplemental or dietary (nonsupplemental) forms, was not associated with decreased incidence of AD. (Luchsinger et al, 2003)

In the **Age-Related Eye Disease Study**, participants were randomly assigned to receive daily antioxidants (vitamin C, vitamin E, β-carotene), zinc and copper, antioxidants plus zinc and copper, or placebo, and a cognitive battery was administered to 2,166 elderly subjects after a median of 6.9 years of treatment. **There were no differences among the treatment groups in any of the cognitive tests.** (Yaffe et al, 2004)

In the Women's Health Study, a double-blind, randomized, placebo-controlled trial of vitamin E in 39,876 healthy women, 6,377 women 65 years or older participated in a cognitive sub-study. There were no differences between treatment groups in global composite scores at the first or last time points or in mean cognitive change over time. The failure of a potent antioxidant (vitamin E) to reduce cognitive decline substantially when used for almost a decade conveys a strong message. (Kang et al, 2006)

Kang et al **report no overall cognitive benefit of long-term vitamin E supplementation in a factorial design that also included low-dose aspirin.** They also found **no protection against substantial cognitive decline,** defined as the worst 10% of change between assessments averaging 4 years apart. (Kang et al, 2006)

Vitamin E increases mortality

The **American College of Physicians** performed a meta-analysis (combined data from published research studies) to see if there was a correlation between the amounts of vitamin E taken and the risk of all-cause mortality (death from any cause). Nineteen clinical trials (total of 135,967 patients) involving vitamin E were analyzed; the average intake of vitamin E in each of the trials was 400 IU per day. *(Annals of Internal Medicine, January 2005)*

The Results

The researchers found that patients taking as little as 150 IU vitamin E per day showed a significant increase in all-cause mortality.

To complicate matters, there have recently been **several large meta-analyses suggesting that high dose antioxidant vitamin supplementation may be associated with a slight increase in all-cause mortality.** One such analysis, focused on vitamin E, combined 19 clinical trials (135,967 participants). They found that in high dose vitamin E (> 400 IU/day) trials, the pooled all cause mortality risk difference was 39 per 10000 persons, whereas in low dose (≤ 400 IU/day) trials, the risk difference was about 16 per 10000. (Miller et al, 2005)

The **Cochrane Hepato-Biliary Group** attempted to analyze all randomized trials in adults involving β-carotene, vitamin A, vitamin C, vitamin E, and selenium. When all qualified randomized trials were included (68 trials, 232,606 participants), there was no significant effect on mortality. However, **in "low-bias" trials (180,938 participants), antioxidant supplementation was associated with a slight (~5%) but statistically significant increase in mortality. Specifically, there were slight but statistically significant increases in all-cause mortality with β-carotene (~7% increase), vitamin A (~16% increase), and vitamin E (~4% increase).** (Bjelakovic et al, 2007, JAMA) (Bjelakovic et al, 2008)

One potential explanation for a slight increase in mortality might be that antioxidants may also act as pro-oxidants under the right circumstances. For example, vitamin C combined with ferrous iron is a standard free-radical generating system.

I believe that it is preposterous for investigators to always assign bad results of studies to the possibility that they were acting like prooxidants. Their bias is so great that they can not bring themselves to say that excessive antioxidants are harmful, in and of themselves. So, any negative outcomes of their experiments must have been due to prooxidant-acting antioxidants. Such nonscience/nonsense is the result of their clinging to the invalidated teachings of the free radical theory.

An additional consideration is that antioxidant systems normally form a complex network. High dose supplementation with a single antioxidant vitamin in isolation could disrupt the balance of the network. The studies reviewed above, suggesting that antioxidant intake from food is superior to vitamin supplements, support the idea that the entire antioxidant network is important.

I believe that my prior results show that there are increased problems associated with supplement cocktails and the antioxidants tend to have a detrimental cumulative effect greater than that seen with single antioxidant supplements.

Other antioxidants

Several other antioxidant compounds have been examined in human AD trials with varying results. **Idebenone** is a water-soluble analog of ubiquinone. Early double-blind, placebo-controlled, randomized trials of idebenone in mild to moderate AD involved 92–450 subjects, and **suggested dose-dependent, beneficial effects on cognition and slowing of disease progression for up to 2 years**. (Bergamasco et al, 1994) (Weyer et al, 1997) (Gutzmann et al, 1998)

Idebenone was better tolerated and associated with less deterioration than the cholinesterase inhibitor tacrine. (Gutzmann et al, 2002)

In contrast, **the ADCS trial** (The Alzheimer's Disease Cooperative Study) **found no significant effect in 536 subjects randomized to placebo or 3 doses of the antioxidant, idebenone. There was a benefit in cognition when all 3 idebenone groups were combined, but this effect was deemed too small to be clinically significant.** (Thal et al, 2003)

Aggregation of $A\beta$ and $A\beta$-induced free radicals are dependent in part on binding of Cu and Zn ions. In a pilot Phase 2 clinical trial, 36 subjects with moderate AD were randomized to placebo or **clioquinol**, which inhibits Cu and Zn ions from binding to $A\beta$. (Ritchie et al, 2003)

Subjects more severely affected at baseline experienced significant worsening in the placebo group, compared with minimal deterioration in the clioquinol group. A subsequent trial of a second generation metal-binding compound, PBT2, involved 78 subjects with mild AD randomized to placebo or two doses of PBT2. **Compared to placebo, the higher dose was associated with decreased CSF $A\beta_{42}$ levels and improved performance in two tests of executive function.** (Lannfelt et al, 2008)

The curry spice **curcumin has antioxidant** (Lim et al, 2001), **anti-inflammatory, and amyloid-disaggregating properties** (Yang et al, 2005) *in vitro and in animal studies.*

In a small 6-month pilot trial, 34 subjects with AD were randomized to placebo or two doses of the antioxidant, **curcumin. There was no cognitive decline in the placebo group, and no improvement was observed with curcumin.** (Baum et al, 2008)

The Russian antihistamine latrepirdine (Dimebon) initially showed promise in a double-blind, placebo-controlled, randomized trial conducted in Russia, involving 183 subjects with mild to moderate AD. (Doody et al, 2008)

At 6 months and 1 year, **subjects on latrepirdine were significantly better than those in the placebo group with respect to all key outcomes – cognition, activities of daily living, behavior, and overall function**. Latrepirdine also improved MMSE scores in a trial of Huntington's disease. (Kieburtz et al, 2010)

The mechanism of these effects is obscure, but have been proposed to include interaction with glutamate receptors, blockade of voltage-dependent calcium channels, and inhibition of the mitochondrial permeability transition pore.

However, **the more recent CONNECTION trial, based in the US, Europe, and South America, showed no benefit for latrepirdine in any parameter for AD**. (ClinicalTrials.gov. A safety and efficacy study of oral Dimebon in patients with mild-to-moderate Alzheimer's disease (CONNECTION) [Accessed March 10, 2010];2009 July 14; http://clinicaltrials.gov/ct2/show/NCT00675623) (Alzheimer Research Forum. Dimebon disappoints in Phase 3 trial. [Accessed March 10, 2010];2010 March 4; http://www.alzforum.org/new/detail.asp?id=2387)

In summary, antioxidant/mitochondrial-based therapies have presented a mixed picture. **Many have not proved significantly effective in treatment of AD or MCI (mild cognitive impairment)**, though a few show promise. Efficacy may be greater in prevention of AD and reducing risk of cognitive decline with aging. Based on the studies reviewed here, future trials of antioxidants are likely to be more successful if focused on prevention or on very early stages of disease, and if a broad increase in the entire network of antioxidant defense systems is targeted. (Dumont et al, 2010)

Brain mitochondrial dysfunction in aging, neurodegeneration, and Parkinson's disease

Brain senescence and neurodegeneration occur with a mitochondrial dysfunction characterized by impaired electron transfer and by oxidative damage. Brain mitochondria of old animals show **decreased rates of electron transfer in complexes I and IV,** decreased membrane potential, **increased content of the oxidation products** of phospholipids and proteins and increased size and fragility. This impairment, with complex I inactivation and oxidative damage, is named "complex I syndrome" and is recognized as characteristic of mammalian brain aging and of neurodegenerative diseases. Mitochondrial dysfunction is more marked in brain areas as rat hippocampus and frontal cortex, in human cortex in Parkinson's disease and dementia with Lewy bodies, and in substantia nigra in Parkinson's disease. The molecular mechanisms involved in complex I inactivation include the synergistic inactivations produced by ONOO- mediated reactions, by reactions with free radical intermediates of lipid peroxidation and by amine-aldehyde adduction reactions. **The accumulation**

of oxidation products prompts the idea of antioxidant therapies. **High doses of vitamin E produce a significant protection of complex I activity and mitochondrial function in rats and mice, and with improvement of neurological functions and increased median life span in mice.**

Mitochondria-targeted antioxidants, as the Skulachev cations covalently attached to vitamin E, ubiquinone and PBN and the SS tetrapeptides, are negatively charged and accumulate in mitochondria where they exert their antioxidant effects. Activation of the cellular mechanisms that regulate mitochondrial biogenesis is another potential therapeutic strategy, since the process generates organelles devoid of oxidation products and with full enzymatic activity and capacity for ATP production. (Navarro, Boveris, 2010)

Here is my question: Since EMODs are believed to be produced at complex I, how does decreasing electron flow at this site increase oxidative products?

Accordingly, aged mammalian brain has a decreased capacity to produce ATP by oxidative phosphorylation and it is considered that this decreased capacity for energy production becomes limiting under physiological conditions in aged individuals. For instance, brain mitochondria isolated from mice at the time point of 50% survival (median life span) show about 50% of the activity at full adulthood of critical enzymes, such as complex I (NADH-ubiquinone reductase), complex IV (cytochrome oxidase) and mitochondrial nitric oxide synthase (mtNOS) (Navarro and Boveris, 2007).

Human neurodegenerative diseases are characterized by cumulative neuronal damage in specific brain areas that leads to neurological deficits when neuronal loss reaches a critical limit. For instance, Parkinson's disease evolves for years before typical motor signs appear with a loss of about 60% of the dopaminergic neurons of *substantia nigra pars compacta*. There is growing evidence that mitochondrial dysfunction and impairment of the respiratory complexes is associated with the neuronal loss in neurodegenerative diseases. Decreased complex IV activity has been reported in Alzheimer's disease (Chagnon et al., 1995) and decreased complex I activity is usually reported in the *substantia nigra* of *postmorten* samples in Parkinson's disease (Mizuno et al., 1989; Mann et al., 1992).

It is currently considered that the energy demands of brain and central nervous system are provided by very active glucose oxidation and aerobic metabolism; it is accepted than the O_2 uptake of brain and central nervous system accounts for about 20% of the O_2 uptake in basal metabolic conditions. It has been recently postulated that brain phospholipid oxidation products, as TBARS and organic hydroperoxides, reach systemic circulation and that the final product malonaldehyde (measured as TBARS) is increased by 21% in the plasma of patients with Parkinson's and Alzheimer's diseases and with vascular dementia (Serra et al., 2009). An estimation of the rate of brain lipid peroxidation in the mentioned neurodegenerative diseases indicates an about twice increased rate as compared to the normal condition.

It is becoming clear that mitochondria continuously and simultaneously respire, produce superoxide and NO, are subjected to free radical mediated processes that produce lipid peroxidation and protein oxidation and lose enzymatic activity. The loosing of enzymatic activity is also called the appearance of dysfunctional mitochondria. It is speculated that dysfunctional mitochondria, as they are defined by sub-normal or partially inactivated respiration, enzymatic activity, and ATP-production, have an extended time for mitochondrial turnover, which is associated with a higher level of mitochondrial oxidation products. It is also speculated that this high level of oxidation products is enough to trigger apoptosis, before *de novo* mitochondrial biogenesis takes the level of oxidized products to one half (non-oxidized phospholipids and proteins are incorporated in mitochondrial biogenesis)

It is expected that slowing down the processes of brain mitochondrial dysfunction that occurs upon aging will provide a decrease of the neurological deficits in aged humans. Antioxidants targeted to mitochondria are promising therapeutic agents for human neurodegenerative diseases, however a huge research has to be performed (Reddy, 2007).

The Skulachev cations attached to antioxidant molecules

(Note: I have included this rather confusing section only because it is appearing in some of the literature. Its inclusion does not mean that I agree with it or disagree with it.)

A new family of mitochondrial antioxidants is being developed. The new mitochondria-targeted antioxidants are covalent derivatives of vitamin E, ubiquinone, and PBN (α-phenyl-N-*tert*-butyl nitrone) that are covalently coupled to a triphenylphosphonium cationic group (Murphy and Smith, 2007). The phosphonium derivatives have been used for years in the determination of inner membrane potential and, following to the development and use by Russian bionergeticists, are commonly known as the **"Skulachev cations."** Lipophilic triphenyl-phosphonium cations are actively taken up by mitochondria due to the inner membrane potential (160–170 mV) with the inside negative, that according to the electrochemical potential (Guggenheim equation) produces an intramitochondrial accumulation of about 700 times (Skulachev, 2005, 2007).

The development and use of the phosphonium antioxidants takes advantage of the unique mitochondrial biophysical and biochemical characteristics that provide a negatively charged compartment and a reducing environment that allows regeneration of the free radical scavengers.

The molecule resulting from the coupling of triphenylphosphonium cation (TPP$^+$) with alpha-tocopherol, is called MitoVitE and was developed to prevent mitochondrial oxidative damage. Mitochondria incubated with 1–20 µM MitoVitE take up the phosphonium cations in about 15–30 min with accumulation ratios of up to 1000 times (Sheu et al., 2006). Higher levels of MitoVitE (50 µM) in the incubation medium are cytotoxic for Jurkat cells (Sheu et al., 2006). It is considered that MitoVitE is inserted in the lipid bilayer of the mitochondrial inner membrane and that the chroman group becomes redox active.

The semiquinone, formed after detoxifying a free radical by hydrogen donation, is reduced by electron transfer or tunneling from a reduced component of the respiratory chain. MitoVitE was reported to reduce H_2O_2-induced caspase activity (Hughes et al., 2005) and to prevent cell death in fibroblasts from patients with Friedrich ataxia, an inherited nervous system disease associated with decreased frataxin and increased iron-catalyzed oxidative damage (Jauslin et al., 2003), to inhibit cytochrome *c* release and caspase-3 activation, to inhibit complex I inactivation and to restore mitochondrial membrane potential in bovine aortic epithelial cells after oxidative stress (Reddy, 2006).

MitoQ$_{10}$ is a similar TPP$^+$ derivative with ubiquinone-50 (Q$_{10}$) that is similarly accumulated in mitochondria. Internalized MitoQ$_{10}$ is inmobilized by anchoring the isoprenoid chain into the lipid bilayer and becomes redox active: the oxidized form is readily reduced by complex II and is reduced by complex I. The ubiquinol molecule inserted in the mitochondrial inner membrane acts as a free radical trap and antioxidant preventing oxidative damage (Reddy, 2006). The electrical charge and the consequent superficial position of the TPP$^+$ moiety and the solubility of Q$_{10}$ in non-polar solvents indicate the isoprenoid chain of MitoQ$_{10}$ concentrates in the membrane core where it quenches fluorophors deep within the membrane. In isolated cells, MitoQ$_{10}$ protects from H_2O_2-induced apoptosis but not from the apoptosis induced by staurosporine or TNF-α (Murphy and Smith, 2007).

MitoPBN is another TPP$^+$ derivative, in this case with phenoxy-butyl-nitrone, that was designed to prevent mitochondrial lipid peroxidation and oxidative damage based on the well known and relatively selective PBN reaction with carbon-centered radicals (R.) and peroxyl radicals (ROO.) (Murphy et al., 2003). MitoPBN is rapidly taken up by mitochondria reaching intramitochondrial levels of 2.2–4.0 mM. MitoPBN was observed to block the oxygen-induced activation of uncoupling proteins (Murphy et al., 2003). An amphiphilic molecule derived from PBN and that is a nitronium cation (LPBNAH) shows a neuroprotective activity antagonizing oxidative damage of mitochondrial origin (Poeggeler et al., 2005).

Currently, other antioxidants of the phosphonium type are developed as effective mitochondria-targeted antioxidants (Kelso et al., 2001; James et al., 2007). For instance, the derivative with the selenium-containing ebselen shows hydroperoxide peroxidase activity (Mugesh et al., 2001).

Conclusion

The long standing concept of linking aging and an impaired mitochondrial energy supply is now receiving experimental support. It has been recognized that aging is associated with a decreased mitochondrial function, considered primarily as electron transfer and respiration, in a series of organs as brain, heart, liver, and kidney.

Brain mitochondria are more affected by the aging process than the mitochondria of other organs. This observation agrees with the general concept that the physiological functions that depend on the integrated response of the central nervous system are the most affected by aging.

The complex series of factors contributing to brain senescence and neurodegeneration in experimental animals, mice and rats, and humans converge to show a condition of brain mitochondrial dysfunction with two simultaneous conditions: impaired electron transfer and enzymatic activity and mitochondrial oxidative damage. **Brain dysfunctional mitochondria accumulate in aged rodents** and show marked decreases in the rates of active (+ADP) respiration, especially with malate–glutamate as substrate, marked decreases in the rates of electron transfer in complexes I and IV, decreased membrane potential, increased content of the oxidation products of phospholipids and proteins, and increased size and fragility.

In humans, data is starting to accumulate and shows about the same general picture dominated by complex I inactivation, with the corresponding impairment of mitochondrial respiration in the presence of NAD-linked substrates and the always present increased content of the oxidation products of phospholipids and proteins.

Interestingly, complex I and IV activities are consistently reported decreased in aged rats and mice. However in human neurodegenerative diseases the observations are consistent with complex I inactivation but not with complex IV inactivation. Both complexes are large molecules that are composed by a series of polypeptides and that are embedded in the phospholipid bilayer of the mitochondrial inner membrane. In both cases, phospholipids are necessary for enzyme activity; this can be easily understood as due to the hydrophobic bonding that holds together enzyme polypeptides and membrane phospholipids. Subtle differences in biological species phospholipid composition may account for the difference in complex IV sensitivity to aging in rats and mice and the complex IV insensitivity to neurodegenerative diseases in humans.

The oxidative mitochondrial partial inactivation of complex I accompanied by oxidative damage is a phenomenon, in short named **"complex I syndrome,"** that is being recognized as characteristic of mammalian brain aging and of human neurodegenerative diseases. Mitochondrial dysfunction has been recognized as a more marked phenomenon, in terms of complex I syndrome, in brain areas as hippocampus and frontal cortex in rats, human cortex in Parkinson's disease and dementia with Lewy bodies, and *substantia nigra* in Parkinson disease. The molecular mechanism involved in complex I inactivation is likely accounted for by the synergistic effects of $ONOO^{\square}$, by reactions with the free radical intermediates of the lipid peroxidation process, and by amine–aldehyde adduction reactions.

The accumulation of mitochondrial oxidation products in rodent aging and in neurodegenerative diseases prompted the idea of antioxidant therapies. High doses of vitamin E showed a highly significant protection of complex I activity and mitochondrial function, with improvement of neurological functions and with an increased median life span in mice. Other antioxidants showed similar effects. **Yet, human studies with vitamin E have failed in prevention or reversal of AD.**

Interestingly, a whole family of mitochondria-targeted antioxidants, as the Skulachev cations (derivatives of the phosphonium cation that covalently attached to either vitamin E, or ubiquinone or PBN) and the SS tetrapeptides, are under development and testing. These molecules are negatively charged and accumulate in mitochondria where they exert their antioxidant effects.

Activation of the cellular mechanisms that regulate mitochondrial biogenesis is another potential therapeutic strategy, considering that *de novo* generated mitochondria are devoid of oxidation products and show full enzymatic activity and full capacity for ATP production. Then, stimulation of mitochondrial biogenesis is a novel approach with a potential of beneficial effects in neurodegenerative diseases that are associated with mitochondrial dysfunction. (Navarro, Boveris, 2010)

CHAPTER TWENTY THREE

Traumatic brain injury (TBI) links to AD

The occurrence of TBI may be a risk factor for the development or early expression of neurodegenerative disorders such as AD and Parkinson's Disease (PD), although much remains to be learned about these potential associations. (Guskiewicz et al, 2005) (Bower et al, 2003) (Ramussen et al, 1995) (Schofield et al, 1997) (Van den Heuvel et al, 2007)

TBI and AD. Epidemiologic studies conducted during the past few decades have yielded **inconclusive findings** with regard to a relationship between TBI and AD. (Van den Heuvel et al, 2007)

Nonetheless, more recent evidence has supported the concept that the risk of subsequent development of AD is increased following repeated mild to moderate TBI or single occurrences of moderate to severe TBI. (Van den Heuvel et al, 2007)

In the Multi-Institutional Research in Alzheimer Genetic Epidemiology (MIRAGE) study, **the risk of AD was doubled when TBI was associated with loss of consciousness**, although even TBI without loss of consciousness significantly increased the risk compared to that with no head injury. (Guo et al, 2000)

In the aforementioned study of retired professional football players, no association was evident between recurrent concussion and AD, but **those who did develop AD had an earlier onset of disease than is seen in the general American male population**. (Guskiewicz et al, 2005)

As reported in *The New York Times* on September 29, 2009, a recent telephone survey of 1,063 retired National Football League players found that self-reported dementia-related diagnoses were reported significantly more often among the players than among the national population. **The study found that 1.9% of retired NFL play-**

ers aged 30-49 received a dementia related diagnosis, a figure that is 19 times the national average of adults aged 30-49.

The survey was commissioned by the NFL. Rates of concussions and other head traumas were not released by the NFL, so this report only hints at a connection between head trauma (which, presumably, accompanies NFL play) and later development of dementia. (Schwarz, Sept. 2009)

A long-term NFL-funded study of concussions in NFL players is currently under way. While the results will not be published for several years, critics have already pointed out flaws in the study design. Most criticism focuses on the fact that the study is run by NFL committee doctors and that all neurologic examinations will be conducted by one neurologist who has criticized any outside evidence of neurologic disability stemming from football play. (Schwarz, Oct. 2009)

This exchange of words over a scientific study that is years from completion highlights

the difficulties in assessing the long-term impact of an accumulation of neurologic insults in a specialized, and small, population.

Conflicting results have been reported concerning the possible impact of the *APOE*-e4 genotype on the risk of AD in patients with TBI. (Guo et al, 2000) (Schwarz, Oct. 2009) (O'Meara et al, 1997)

In the MIRAGE study, the magnitude of AD risk was actually higher among individuals with TBI who lacked the *APOE*-e4 allele. However, other investigations have documented an interaction between the *APOE*-e4 genotype and AD in TBI patients. (Mayeux et al, 1995) (Katzman et al, 1996)

In one study, the risk of AD was 10 times as high among patients with both *APOE*-e4 and TBI as in those who lacked both factors. (Mayeux et al, 1995)

This discrepancy may reflect differences in the populations studied, possibly suggesting

that an interaction between *APOE*-e4 and AD after TBI may vary by ethnicity. More work is needed to explore these issues. (Guo et al, 2000)

Actually, TBI is currently being studied in soccer players and has been studied in boxers for years. Most of the above material was excerpted from: http://www.neura.net/images/pdf/Neura_V913_Sports.pdf

In addition to the immediate post-injury complications discussed above, other long-term problems can develop after a TBI. These include Parkinson's disease and other motor problems, Alzheimer's disease, *dementia pugilistica* , and post-traumatic dementia.

Alzheimer's disease (AD) - Recent research suggests an association between head injury in early adulthood and the development of AD later in life; **the more severe the head injury, the greater the risk of developing AD**. Some evidence indicates that a head injury may interact with other factors to trigger the disease and may hasten the onset of the disease in individuals already at risk. For example, people who have a particular form of the protein apolipoprotein E (apoE4) and suffer a head injury fall into this increased risk category. (ApoE4 is a naturally occurring protein that helps transport cholesterol through the bloodstream.). However, there are inconsistencies in the data.

The NHL, National Hockey League, is becoming more aware of **chronic traumatic encephalopathy (CTE)**, following the recent deaths of three players called enforcers. Many players are making it known that concussions and brain damage is associated with repeated head trauma.

Only recently have pathologists started studying the brain structure of sports enthusiasts and those exposed to repeated blunt head trauma.

Viral mimics of AD

In the elderly, brain damage occurs in Alzheimer's disease and related neurodegenerative diseases. A condition known as Jacob-Creutzfeld disease can mimic Alzheimer's disease but is actually from a viral illness. Mad cow disease is a viral brain disease that is essentially the same as Jacob-Creutzfeld disease.

CHAPTER TWENTY FOUR

ADDENDUM

Additional 90 failed antioxidant studies to which can be combined with the 316 failed studies in *Antioxidants Failures and Dangers*, for a grand total of 406.

Total as of 9-25-11 is 90 for a grand total of 406

Total of harmful effects in studies as of 9-21-11 is 90 plus 20 for a grand total of 110 studies showing harmful adverse effects associated with antioxidants.

1985

Vitamins and endurance training. Food for running or faddish claims? (van der Beek, 1985)

The inter-relationship of food and physical performance, food is considered as a conglomerate of nutrients and man is depicted as a kind of organic pudding. This 'machine' concept of human performance in combination with the mysticism surrounding vitamins, has **led to the faddish belief that additional vitamins are necessary to improve physical performance by means of supercharging the metabolic processes in the body.** It is concluded that a marginal or subclinical deficiency state can be defined as an intermediate between optimal vitamin status and frank clinical deficiency. Marginal deficiency is characterized by biochemical values deviating from statistically derived reference limits as well as the absence of clinical signs and symptoms of vitamin deficiency. **An extensive historical review on depletion studies, epidemiological surveys and supplementation studies is presented.** It is concluded that a restricted intake of some B-complex vitamins-individually and in combination-of approximately less than 35 to 45% of the recommended dietary allowance may lead to decreased endurance capacity within a few weeks. **Studies on ascorbic acid (vitamin C) depletion and fat-soluble vitamin A deficiency have noted**

no decrease of endurance capacity. However, in a few recent epidemiological surveys, biochemical vitamin C deficiency was actually shown to decrease aerobic power. **With respect to the available evidence, it can be concluded that supplementation of diet with either single or multivitamin preparations containing B-complex vitamins, vitamin C or E does not improve physical performance in athletes with a normal biochemical vitamin balance resulting from a well-balanced diet.** (van der Beek, 1985)

1986

Studies on antioxidants: Their carcinogenic and modifying effects on chemical carcinogenesis (Ito et al, 1986)

Studies were conducted on the carcinogenic activity of butylated hydroxyanisole (BHA) in rats and hamsters. To obtain information concerning the mechanism of action of BHA on the forestomach, the following areas were examined: the effects of 12 phenolic compounds structurally related to BHA on the hamster forestomach, the effects of combinations of BHA and other antioxidants on the rat forestomach, and the metabolism of BHA in the forestomach. Also examined were the effects of several antioxidants on two-stage carcinogenesis in rats. *Squamous-cell carcinomas were induced in the forestomach of rats and hamsters fed BHA*. In a limited study, 1 of 13 hamsters developed a squamous-cell carcinoma. The tumorigenic action of crude BHA on the forestomach was largely due to the action of 3-*tert*-BHA. *p-tert*-Butylphenol and 2-*tert*-butyl-4-methylphenol induced pronounced hyperplasia and papillomas in the hamster forestomach. *BHA and other antioxidants, particularly propyl gallate and ethoxyquin, showed additive effects in inducing forestomach hyperplasia and cytotoxicity*. Neither BHA nor its metabolites were found in the forestomach epithelium, although small amounts of metabolites were detected in the stomach contents. Thus, a direct action on the stomach epithelium may be exerted by BHA itself or by metabolites formed on interaction of BHA with gastric juice. *BHA enhanced forestomach carcinogenesis initiated in rats by N-methyl-N'-nitro-N-nitrosoguanidine or N-methylnitrosourea (MNU) and enhanced urinary bladder carcinogenesis initiated by MNU or N-butyl-N-(4-hydroxybutyl)nitrosamine (BBN).* In contrast, it inhibited carcinogenesis initiated in the liver by either diethylnitrosamine or N-ethyl-N hydroxyethylnitrosamine (EHEN) and mammary carcinogenesis initiated by 7.12-dimethyl-benz[a]anthracene (DMBA). *BHT promoted urinary bladder carcinogenesis initiated by BBN or MNU and thyroid carcinogenesis initiated by MNU, but inhibited ear-duct carcinogenesis initiated by DMBA. Ethoxyquin promoted EHEN-initiated kidney carcinogenesis,* but inhibited both DMBA-initiated mammary and EHEN-initiated liver carcinogenesis. *Sodium ascorbate promoted forestomach and urinary bladder carcinogenesis, and sodium erythorbate also enhanced urinary bladder carcinogenesis.* α-Tocopherol inhibited ear-duct carcinogenesis. No antioxidants tested had any effect on glandular stomach carcinogenesis. Thus antioxidants have independent modifying (promoting or inhibitory) effects in different organs.

Abbreviations: BBN = *N*-butyl-*N*-(4-hydroxybutyl)nitrosamine; BHA = butylated hydroxyanisole; BHT = butylated hydroxytoluene; DEN = diethylnitrosamine; DMBA = 7,12-dimethylbenz[*a*]anthracene; EHEN = *N*-ethyl-*N*-hydroxyethylnitrosamine; GST-P = glutathione *S*-transferase, placental form; MNNG = *N*-methyl-*N'*-nitro-*N*-nitrosoguanidine; MNU = *N*-methylnitrosourea

(Ito et al, 1986) *Harmful effects of antioxidants*

Pathology of BHA- and BHT-induced lesions (Moch, 1986)

The pathology lesions from three studies, two with butylated hydroxyanisole (BHA) and one with butylated hydroxytoluene (BHT), are reviewed. When BHA was fed at 0.5 and 2.0% of the diet to F344 rats for two years, **there was an increase in epithelial hyperplasia of the forestomach at both treatment levels. Papilloma and squamous-cell carcinoma of the forestomach were increased at the 2.0% level.** When BHA was fed to beagle dogs at 1.0 and 1.3% of the diet for 180 days, no lesions/tumors of the distal esophagus or stomach could be identified either at gross necropsy or by light or electron microscopy. **The BHT was fed to Wistar rats at 0, 25, 100 and 250 mg/kg body weight. At the highest dose there was an increase in the number of rats with hepatocellular adenoma and with hepatocellular carcinoma.** (Moch, 1986)

1988

Vitamin and mineral supplementation: Effect on the running performance of trained athletes (Weight et al, 1998) (#)

There is limited scientific justification for the widespread use of vitamin and mineral supplements by athletes. We used a 9-mo, placebo-controlled crossover study design to determine whether a multivitamin and mineral supplement influenced the athletic performance of 30 competitive male athletes. At 0, 3, 6, and 9 mo the runners performed a progressive treadmill test to volitional exhaustion for measurement of maximal oxygen consumption, peak running speed, blood lactate turnpoint, and peak postexercise blood lactate level. Running time in a 15 km time trial was also measured.

None of these variables was influenced by 3 mo of active supplementation. We conclude that **3 mo of multivitamin and mineral supplementation was without any measurable ergogenic effect**. (Weight et al, 1998)

1992

Chronic multivitamin-mineral supplementation does not enhance physical performance (Singh et al, 1992) (#21)

The effects on physical performance of 90 d of supplementation with a high potency multivitamin-mineral supplement were studied in a double-blind, placebo-controlled design. **Twenty-two healthy**, physically active men were randomly assigned to a supplement (S) or placebo (P) group; both groups had similar physical characteristics. Performance was assessed from maximal aerobic capacity, endurance capacity, and isokinetic tests. Supplementation did not affect maximal aerobic capacity: pre and after approximately 12 wk of supplementation values for maximal oxygen consumption (48.5 +/- 1.3 vs 46.2 +/- 1.1 ml.kg-1.min-1), maximal heart rate (186 +/- 2 vs 187 +/- 2 beats.min-1) or treadmill time (19.96 +/- 0.48 vs 19.99 +/- 0.37 min) did not differ in the S group; similar findings were noted in the P group. Performance during the 90-min endurance run, as assessed from heart rates, rectal temperatures, and plasma glucose, lactate and adrenocorticotropin values, was not affected by treatment. Similarly, muscle strength and endurance were not affected. Thus, **supplementation did not affect physical performance in well-nourished men who maintained their physical activity**. (Singh et al, 1992)

The effect of 7 to 8 months of vitamin/mineral supplementation on athletic performance (Telford et al, 1992) (#82)

The effect of vitamin and mineral supplementation was studied over 7 to 8 months of training and competition in **82 athletes from four sports: basketball, gymnastics, rowing, and swimming.** Matched subgroups were formed and a double-blind design used, with subgroups being given either the supplementation or a placebo. All athletes were monitored to ensure that the recommended daily intakes (RDI) of vitamins and minerals were provided by diet alone. Sport-specific and some common tests of strength as well as aerobic and anaerobic fitness were performed. Coaches' assessment of improvement was also obtained. The only significant effect of supplementation was observed in the female basketball players, in which the supplementation was associated with increased body weight, skinfold sum, and jumping ability. A significant increase in skinfold sum was also demonstrated over the whole group as a result of supplementation. In general, however, **this study provided little evidence of any effect of supplementation to athletic performance for athletes consuming the dietary RDIs**. (Telford et al, 1992)

1995

Effects of vitamin E on susceptibility of low-density lipoprotein and low-density lipoprotein subfractions to oxidation and on protein glycation in NIDDM (Reaven et al, 1995) (#21)

OBJECTIVE: To evaluate the effect of vitamin E supplementation on the susceptibility of low-density lipoprotein (LDL) and LDL subfractions to oxidation and on protein glycation in non-insulin-dependent diabetes mellitus (NIDDM). RESEARCH DESIGN AND METHODS: **Twenty-one men with NIDDM** (HbA1c = 6-10%), ages 50-70, were randomly assigned to either 1,600 IU/day of vitamin E or placebo for 10 weeks after a 4-week placebo period. LDL and LDL subfractions were isolated after 4 weeks of placebo and after 6 and 10 weeks of therapy. Susceptibility of LDL to copper-mediated oxidation was measured by conjugated diene formation (lag time) and formation of thiobarbituric acid-reactive substances (TBARS). Fasting serum glucose, mean weekly blood glucose, HbA1c, and glycated plasma protein concentrations were also determined at these time points. RESULTS: Vitamin E content in plasma and LDL increased 4.0- and 3.7-fold, respectively, in the vitamin E-treated group. Vitamin E decreased the susceptibility of LDL to oxidation in comparison with placebo (lag time, 243 +/- 46 vs. 151 +/- 22 min, $P < 0.01$; 3 h TBARS, 24 +/- 12 vs. 66 +/- 18 nmol malondialdehyde/mg LDL, $P < 0.05$). Vitamin E content also increased significantly in both buoyant and dense LDL subfractions, and their oxidation was dramatically reduced. The lag time of LDL oxidation correlated well with the content of vitamin E in both LDL and its subfractions ($r = 0.69$-0.92). Glycemic indexes did not change significantly in either group during the study. Protein glycation, including glycated hemoglobin, glycated albumin, glycated total plasma proteins, and glycated LDL were unchanged in the vitamin E group. CONCLUSIONS: Supplementation of vitamin E in NIDDM leads to enrichment of LDL and LDL subfractions and reduced susceptibility to oxidation. **Despite a greater percentage increase in vitamin E content in small dense LDL, it remained substantially more susceptible to oxidation than was buoyant LDL.** This suggests that dense, LDL may gain less protection against oxidation from antioxidant supplementation than does larger, more buoyant LDL. In contrast to previous reports, vitamin E supplementation did not reduce glycation of intracellular or plasma proteins. **Daily supplementation with 1600 IU of α tocopherol for 10 weeks in a group of 21 diabetic men had no effect on HbA$_{1c}$, fasting blood glucose, or glycated plasma protein concentrations**, but had a beneficial effect on LDL oxidation. (Reaven et al, 1995)

However, in another trial of 15 diabetics and 10 control individuals, 4 months of daily supplementation with 1350 IU of α tocopherol significantly improved plasma glucose levels, triglycerides, total cholesterol levels, LDL, and HbA$_{1c}$, but **did not improve the response of β cells to glucose or FFAs.** (Paolisso et al, 1993)

Vitamin E status and response to exercise training (Tiidus, Houston, 1995)

Vitamin E is an important intra-membrane antioxidant and membrane stabilizer. Over the past 40 years, vitamin E supplementation has been advocated for athletes in the hope of improving performance, minimizing exercise-induced muscle damage and maximizing recovery. However, **there is currently a lack of conclusive evidence that exercise performance or recovery would benefit in any significant way from dietary vitamin E supplementation.** Exceeding current recommended intakes of vitamin E even by several orders of magnitude will result in relatively modest increases in tissue or serum vitamin E concentrations. **Most evidence suggests that there is no discernible effect of vitamin E supplementation on performance, training effect or rate of postexercise recovery in either recreational or elite athletes.** There is very little evidence, particularly involving humans, that exercise or training will significantly alter tissue or serum vitamin E levels. While there is some evidence that certain indices of tissue peroxidation may be reduced following dietary vitamin E supplementation, the physiological and performance consequences in humans of these relatively minor effects are unknown. Although there appears to be little reason for vitamin E supplementation among athletes, it does not appear that the practice of supplementation is harmful. (Tiidus, Houston, 1995)

1996

Survival in patients with amyotrophic lateral sclerosis, treated with an array of antioxidants (Vyth et al, 1996) (#36)

Between 1983 and 1988 we treated 36 patients with sporadic amyotrophic lateral sclerosis (**ALS) by an array of antioxidants** and added other drugs to the regimen whenever a patient reported deterioration. Our customary prescription sequence **was N-acetylcysteine (NAC); vitamins C and E; N-acetylmethionine (NAM); and dithiothreitol (DTT) or its isomer dithioerythritol (DTE).** Patients with a history of heavy exposure to metal were also given meso 2,3-dimercaptosuccinic acid (DMSA). NAC, NAM, DTT, and DTE were administered by subcutaneous injection or by mouth or by both routes, the other vitamins and DMSA by mouth alone. The hospital pharmacy supplied NAC and NAM injections fluid as 100 ml bottles of 5.0 and 5.85% solutions, respectively. DTT was delivered in special double-walled capsules of 200 mg. DTT/DTE injection fluid was added to the NAC and NAM bottles, the final DTT/DTE concentrations never exceeding 0.5%. DMSA was provided in 250 mg capsules. All of the 36 patients used NAC and DTT/DTE; 29 also used vitamins C and E; 21 also used NAM; and 7 also used DMSA, DMSA, NAM, vitamins C and E were tolerated well. **In many patients, DTT, DTE, NAC and NAM induced pain, redness and swelling at the injection sites in that order of decreasing** frequency. **DTT and DTE did often and NAC did sometimes cause gastric pain, nausea and other abdominal discomfort.** Comparison of survival in the treated group and in a cohort of untreated historical controls, disclosed a median survival of 3.4 years (95% confidence interval: 3.0-4.2) in the treated and of 2.8 (95% confidence interval 2.2-3.1) years in the control patients. This difference may be explained by self-selection of our highly motivated treated group and by its initial survival of diagnosis for an average of 8.5 months before onset of treatment. We conclude that **antioxidants neither seem to harm ALS patients, nor do they seem to prolong survival.** (Vyth et al, 1996)

1999

Antioxidants and exercise (Powers, Hamilton, 1999)

Muscular exercise results in an increased production of radicals and other forms of reactive oxygen species. Further more, growing evidence implicates cytotoxic ROS as an underlying cause in exercise-induced disturbances in muscle redox status that could result in muscle fatigue or injury. Muscle cells contain complex cellular defense mechanisms to minimize the risk for oxidative injury. Two major classes of endogenous protective mechanisms work together to reduce the harmful effects of oxidants in the cell: (1) enzymatic and (2) nonenzymatic antioxidants. Key antioxidant enzymes include superoxide dismutase, glutathione peroxidase, and catalase. These enzymes are responsible for removing superoxide radicals, hydrogen peroxide or organic hydroperoxides, and hydrogen peroxide, respectively. **Important nonenzymatic antioxidants include vitamins E and C, beta-carotene, GSH, uric acid, ubiquinone, and bilirubin. Vitamin E, beta-carotene, and ubiquinone are located in lipid regions of the cell, whereas uric acid, GSH, and bilirubin are in aqueous compartments of the cell.** Although numerous animal experiments have demonstrated that the addition of antioxidants can improve muscular performance, **to date, limited evidence shows that dietary supplementation with antioxidants improves human performance.** This is an important area for future research. (Powers, Hamilton, 1999)

2000

The effect of bilberry nutritional supplementation on night visual acuity and contrast sensitivity (Muth et al, 2000) (#15)

The purpose of this study was to investigate the effect of bilberry on night visual acuity (VA) and night contrast sensitivity (CS). METHODS: This study utilized a double-blind, placebo-controlled, crossover design. The subjects were young males with good vision; **eight received placebo and seven received active capsules for three weeks.** Active **capsules contained 160 mg of bilberry extract (25-percent**

anthocyanosides), and the placebo capsules contained only inactive ingredients. Subjects ingested one active or placebo capsule three times daily for 21 days. After the three-week treatment period, a one-month washout period was employed to allow any effect of bilberry on night vision to dissipate. In the second three-week treatment period, the eight subjects who first received placebo were given active capsules, and the seven who first received active capsules were given placebo. Night VA and night CS was tested throughout the three-month experiment. RESULTS: **There was no difference in night VA** during any of the measurement periods when examining the average night VA or the last night VA measurement during active and placebo treatments. In addition, there was no difference in night CS during any of the measurement periods when examining the average night CS or the last night CS measurement during active and placebo treatments. CONCLUSION: **The current study failed to find an effect of bilberry on night VA or night CS for a high dose of bilberry taken for a significant duration**. Hence, the current study casts doubt on the proposition that bilberry supplementation, in the forms currently available and in the doses recommended, is an effective treatment for the improvement of night vision in this population. (Muth et al, 2000)

Glutathione and hypotaurine in vitro: effects on human sperm motility, DNA integrity and production of reactive oxygen species (Donnelly et al, 2000)

Sperm DNA integrity is of paramount importance for the accurate conveyance of genetic material. DNA damage may be a major contributory factor in male infertility as DNA from sperm of infertile men has been found to be more susceptible to induced DNA damage in vitro than DNA from fertile men. Reactive oxygen species (ROS) are a significant source of DNA damage and human sperm are extremely sensitive to ROS attack due to their high content of polyunsaturated fatty acids and lack of capacity for DNA repair. Seminal plasma, which contains a wealth of antioxidants, provides sperm with crucial protection against oxidative insult. However, during preparation for use in assisted conception techniques, sperm are separated from seminal plasma and deprived of that essential protection. The aim of this study was to determine the effects of supplementation with glutathione and hypotaurine during sperm preparation on subsequent sperm motility, DNA integrity, induced DNA damage and ROS generation. Semen samples (n = 45) were divided into aliquots and prepared by Percoll density centrifugation (95.0-47.5%) using medium which had been supplemented with these antioxidants to a number of different concentrations all within physiological levels. Control aliquots were included which had no glutathione or hypotaurine added. Sperm motility was determined using computer-assisted semen analysis. DNA damage was induced using H_2O_2 and DNA integrity was determined using a modified alkaline single cell gel electrophoresis (Comet) assay, while ROS generation was measured using chemiluminescence. **Addition of glutathione and hypotaurine, either**

singly or in combination, to sperm preparation medium had no significant effect on sperm progressive motility or baseline DNA integrity. Despite this, sperm were still afforded significant protection against H(2)O(2)-induced damage and ROS generation. (Donnelly et al, 2000)

In general, antioxidants appear to be of limited value in protecting sperm DNA from gentle semen processing (e.g. incubation or density-gradient centrifugation). (Chi et al, 2008) (Donnelley et al, 1999) (Hughes et al, 1998) (Donnelly et al, 2000)

In some cases, antioxidant supplementation in vitro (e.g. combination of vitamins C and E) may cause sperm DNA damage. (Donnelly et al, 1999) (Hughes et al, 1998)

2001

Chronic administration of high doses of vitamin E appear to slow racing greyhounds (Hill et al, 2001)

We have also found that serum vitamin E declines and oxidative stress increases after a short sprint race but that *supplementation with high (1000 IU) but not moderate (100 IU) daily doses of vitamin E appears to slow racing greyhounds.* (Hill et al, 2001)

Oxidative stress in athletes during extreme endurance exercise

Despite the many known health benefits of exercise, there is a body of evidence suggesting that **endurance exercise is associated with oxidative stress.** To determine whether extreme endurance exercise induces lipid peroxidation, **11 athletes** (3 females, 8 males) were studied during a 50 km ultramarathon (trial 1) and during a sedentary protocol (trial 2) 1 month later. The evening before each trial, with dinner, subjects consumed 75 mg each d(3)-RRR and d(6)-all rac-alpha-tocopheryl acetates. Blood was obtained at baseline, 30 min pre-race, mid-race, post-race, 1 h post-race, 24 h post-race, and at corresponding times during trial 2. All 11 subjects completed the race; average run time was 391 +/- 23 min. Plasma F(2)-isoprostanes increased from 75 +/- 7 pg/ml at pre-race to 131 +/- 17 (p <.02) at post-race, then returned to baseline at 24 h post-race; F(2)-isoprostanes were unchanged during trial 2. Deuterated alpha-tocopherol disappearance rates were faster ($2.8 \times 10(-4)$ +/- $0.2 \times 10(-4)$) during the race compared to the sedentary trial ($2.3 \times 10(-4)$ +/- $0.2 \times 10(-4)$; p <.03). These data suggest that **extreme endurance exercise results in the generation of lipid peroxidation with a concomitant increase in vitamin E disappearance.**

(Mastaloudis et al, 2001). **Of course it increases oxidative stress, that is precisely why it is good for you. Why has this never occurred to others?**

The effect of selegiline and vitamin E in the treatment of ALS: an open randomized clinical trials (Kwiecinski et al, 2001) (#35)

A role for oxidative stress in the etiology or progression of amyotrophic lateral sclerosis (ALS) and other neurodegenerative diseases has been recently proposed. We conducted the 18-month, **randomized treatment trial with oral vitamin E (600 IU daily) and selegiline (10 mg daily) in 67 patients with sporadic ALS**. Thirty five patients were randomly assigned to receive antioxidative therapy (vitamin E plus selegiline) and the remaining 32 patients were the ALS controls who received symptomatic treatment. The primary end point was survival and functional status. At the end of 18-month study, 13 patients in the treatment group and 14 in the control group died or were tracheostomized. A decline in functional disability was also similar in both groups. **Long-term antioxidative treatment with vitamin E did not benefit patients with ALS.** (Kwiecinski et al, 2001)

2002

Supplemental vitamin C appears to slow racing Greyhounds

During strenuous exercise, markers of oxidation increase and antioxidant capacity decreases. Antioxidants such as vitamin C may combat this oxidation stress. The benefits of vitamin C to greyhounds undertaking intense sprint exercise has not been investigated. The objective of this experiment was to determine whether a large dose (1 g or 57 mmol) of ascorbic acid influences performance and oxidative stress in greyhounds. **Five** adult female, trained racing greyhounds were assigned to receive each of three treatments for 4 wk per treatment: 1) no supplemental ascorbate; 2) 1 g oral ascorbate daily, administered after racing; 3) 1 g oral ascorbate daily, administered 1 h before racing. Dogs raced 500 m twice weekly. At the end of each treatment period, blood was collected before and 5 min, 60 min and 24 h after racing. Plasma ascorbate, α-tocopherol, thiobarbituric acid-reducing substances (TBARS) and Trolox equivalent antioxidant capacity (TEAC) concentrations were measured and adjusted to compensate for hemoconcentration after racing. TBARS, TEAC and α-tocopherol concentrations were unaffected by supplemental vitamin C. Plasma ascorbic acid concentrations 60 min after racing were higher in dogs that received vitamin C before racing than in dogs that either received no vitamin C or received vitamin C after racing. **The dogs ran, on average, 0.2 s slower when supplemented with 1 g of vitamin C**, equivalent to a lead of 3 m at the finish of a 500-m race. *Supplementation with vitamin C, therefore, appeared to slow racing greyhounds.* (Marshall et al, 2002)

Vitamin C, vitamin E, and multivitamin supplement use and stomach cancer mortality in the Cancer Prevention Study II cohort (Jacobs, Connell, McCullough et al, 2002) (#1,045,923)

Supplementation with antioxidant vitamins has been associated with decreased risk of stomach cancer or regression of precancerous lesions in high-risk areas of China and Colombia. We examined the association between stomach cancer mortality and regular use (> or =15 times per month) of individual vitamin C supplements, individual vitamin E supplements, and multivitamins among **1,045,923 United States adults in the Cancer Prevention Study II (CPS-II) cohort.** CPS-II participants completed a questionnaire at enrollment in 1982 and were followed for mortality through 1998. During follow-up, there were 1,725 stomach cancer deaths (1,127 in men and 598 in women). After adjustment for multiple potential stomach cancer risk factors, **vitamin C use at enrollment was associated with reduced risk of stomach cancer mortality** [rate ratio (RR), 0.83; 95% confidence interval (CI), 0.68-1.01]. However, this reduction in risk was observed only among participants with short duration use at enrollment (RR, 0.68; 95% CI, 0.51-0.91 for <10 years of use; RR, 1.00; 95% CI, 0.73-1.38 for > or =10 years of use). **There was no association between stomach cancer mortality and regular use of vitamin E or multivitamins,** regardless of duration of use. Our results suggest that **the use of vitamin C, vitamin E, or multivitamin supplements may not substantially reduce risk of stomach cancer mortality in North American populations in which stomach cancer rates are relatively low.** Our results do not rule out effects of vitamin supplementation in areas in which stomach cancer rates are high and stomach cancer etiology may differ. (Jacobs, Connell, McCullough et al, 2002)

Effect of daily vitamin E and multivitamin-mineral supplementation on acute respiratory tract infections in elderly persons: a randomized controlled trial (Graat et al, 2002) (#652) Immune response in elderly individuals has been reported to improve after micronutrient supplementation. However, efficacy trials evaluating infectious diseases as outcomes are scarce and inconclusive. OBJECTIVE: To investigate the effect of daily multivitamin-mineral and vitamin E supplementation on incidence and severity of acute respiratory tract infections in elderly individuals. DESIGN: A randomized, double blind, placebo-controlled, 2 x 2 factorial trial. SETTING AND PARTICIPANTS: A total of **652 noninstitutionalized individuals** aged 60 years or older enrolled from 2 community-based sampling strategies in the Wageningen area of the Netherlands, conducted from 1998 to 2000. At baseline, 6% of participants had suboptimal ascorbic acid and 1.3% had suboptimal alpha-tocopherol plasma concentration. INTERVENTION: Physiological doses of multivitamin-minerals, 200 mg of vitamin E, both, or placebo. MAIN OUTCOME MEASURES: Incidence and severity of self-reported acute respiratory tract infections at 15 months, as assessed by a nurse (telephone contact), home visits, and microbiological and serological testing in subsets of patients. RESULTS: During a median observation period of 441 days, 443 (68%) of 652 participants recorded 1024 respiratory tract infection episodes. The incidence rate ratio of acute respiratory tract infection for multivitamin-mineral supplementation was 0.95 (95% confidence interval, 0.75-1.15; P =.58) and for vitamin E supplementation, 1.12 (95% confidence interval, 0.88-1.25; P =.21). **Severity of infections was not influenced by multivitamin-mineral supplementation.** *For vitamin E vs no vitamin E, severity was worse*: median (interquartile range) for illness-duration was 19 (9-37) vs 14 (6-29) days, P =.02; number of symptoms, 6 (3-8) vs 4 (3-8), P =.03; presence of fever, 36.7% vs 25.2%, P =.009; and restriction of activity, 52.3% vs 41.1%, P =.02. CONCLUSIONS: **Neither daily multivitamin-mineral supplementation at physiological dose nor 200 mg of vitamin E showed a favorable effect on incidence and severity of acute respiratory tract infections in well-nourished noninstitutionalized elderly individuals.** *Instead we observed adverse effects of vitamin E on illness severity*. (Graat et al, 2002)

Vitamin E and C supplements and risk of dementia (Laurin, Foley, 2002)

A controlled trial of vitamin E supplementation among patients with AD found delayed time to institutionalization, but no specific effect on cognitive function. In contrast to the previous analysis from the Honolulu-Asia Aging Study (HAAS), based on prevalent cases, we did not find a significant association of vitamin E or vitamin C supplement use and incident dementia. Our results are based on incident cases and a longer period between the 1988 report of supplement use and assessment of dementia. Our data suggest that **supplemental intake of both vitamins E and C does not alter the risk for dementia**. (Laurin, Foley, 2002)

2003

The antioxidants--vitamin C, vitamin E, selenium, and carotenoids (Johnson et al, 2003)

This is the second in a series of articles reviewing the recent revisions of the Recommended Dietary Allowances (RDA) and the resulting Dietary Reference Intakes (DRI). In April of 2000, the Food and Nutrition Board of the National Academy of Sciences released Dietary Reference Intakes for Vitamin C, Vitamin E, Selenium, and Carotenoids. **The central premise of the report did not perpetuate the prevailing popular thought that large doses of antioxidants will prevent chronic diseases**.

Instead **the panel concluded that at this time, insufficient scientific evidence exists to sustain claims that ingesting megadoses of dietary antioxidants** can prevent certain chronic illnesses such as cardiovascular disease or cancer. In some instances recommended nutrient levels were reduced from the previous report in 1989; e.g., for the first time upper tolerable levels of ingestion (UL) were established **to prevent the harmful effects of over consumption of essential nutrients, such as vitamin C, vitamin E, and selenium.** Although dietary recommendations do exist for vitamin A, **the panel did not set recommendations for beta-carotene or the other carotenoids** due to lack of sufficient research to support recommended intakes or upper tolerable levels of intake. However, **the panel advises the public to avoid intakes of provitamin A compounds, such as the numerous carotenoids, beyond the levels required to prevent vitamin A deficiency.** Changes were also made with regard to estimating the amount of provitamin A carotenoids required to make a unit of retinal. The revised estimate suggests a twofold higher conversion rate than previously believed. Although this comprehensive report on the dietary reference intakes for vitamin C, vitamin E, selenium, and the carotenoids did not decisively confirm the role of antioxidants for the prevention of chronic diseases in humans, many research studies have generated new data to support this concept. Additional research is needed to define the attributes of antioxidants as studies progress from in vitro and animal studies to human nutrition. (Johnson et al, 2003) Department of Food and Beverage Management, University of Nevada, Las Vegas, USA.

Lycopene increases urokinase receptor and fails to inhibit growth or connexin expression in a metastatically passaged prostate cancer cell line: a brief communication (Forbes et al, 2003)

The carotenoid lycopene, found in tomatoes, has been associated with decreasing prostate cancer risk. Potential mechanisms for this risk reduction include lycopene's status as a potent antioxidant, its inhibitory effect on cell proliferation, and its ability to increase intercellular gap junctional communication. Presently, **in the United States, almost 200,000 men are diagnosed with prostate cancer and approximately 30,000 succumb to its metastatic effects.** Therefore, novel treatment strategies are needed for patients who currently have the disease, especially those in advanced, i.e., metastatic status. In this study, we sought to determine if lycopene's inhibitory properties on premalignancy could be extended to advanced prostate cancer by assessing effects on a cell line derived through metastatic passage, the **PC-3MM2.** We report that in this cell line, *lycopene has a potentially unwanted effect of upregulating expression of the urokinase plasminogen activator receptor and facilitating invasion while failing to significantly inhibit proliferation or to induce detectable levels of the gap junctional protein connexin 43 expression.* Our results indicate that **some caution should be taken with regard to use of lycopene to treat potentially advanced and metastatic prostate cancers.** (Forbes et al, 2003)

Effects of vitamin E and C supplementation either alone or in combination on exercise-induced lipid peroxidation in trained cyclists (Bryant et al, 2003) (#7)

Seven trained male cyclists (age 22.3 +/- 2 years) participated in 4 separate supplementation phases. They ingested 2 capsules per day containing the following treatments: placebo (placebo plus placebo); vitamin C (1 g per day vitamin C plus placebo); vitamin C and E (1 g per day vitamin C plus 200 IU per kg vitamin E); and vitamin E (400 IU per kg vitamin E plus placebo). The treatment order (placebo, vitamin C, vitamin C and E, and vitamin E) was the same for all subjects. Performance trials consisting of a 60-minute steady state ride (SSR) and a 30-minute performance ride (PR) on Cybex 100 Metabolic cycles were performed after each trial. Workloads of 70% of the VO2max were set for the SSR and PR rides, with pedal rate maintained at 90 rpm (SSR) or self determined (PR). Blood samples (5 ml) were drawn pre- and postexercise and analyzed for malonaldehyde (MDA) and lactic acid. The results indicate that vitamin E treatment was more effective than vitamin C alone or vitamin C and E. Pre-exercise plasma levels of MDA in the vitamin E trial was 39% below the pre-exercise MDA levels of the placebo: 2.94 +/- 0.54 and 4.81 +/- 0.65 micromol per ml, respectively. Plasma MDA following exercise in the vitamin E group was also lower than teh placebo: 4.32 +/- 0.37 vs 7.89 +/- 1.0 micromol per ml, respectively. Vitamin C supplementation, on the other hand, elevated both the resting and exercise plasma levels of MDA. None of the supplemental phases had any significant effect on performance. In conclusion, the results indicate that 400 IU/day of vitamin E reduces membrane damage more effectively than vitamin C but does not enhance performance. Athletes are encouraged to include antioxidants, such as vitamin E and C, in their diet to counteract these detrimental effects of exercise. The data presented here suggests that 400 IU/day of vitamin E will provide adequate protection but supplementing the diet with 1 g per day of vitamin C may promote cellular damage. However **neither of these vitamins, either alone or in combination, will enhance exercise performance**. (Bryant et al, 2003)

Tolerability of NXY-059 at higher target concentrations in patients with acute stroke (Lees, 2003) (#134)

NXY-059 is a nitrone-based free radical-trapping agent in development for acute stroke. **In patients with acute stroke, NXY-059 is well tolerated at concentrations known to be associated with neuroprotection in animal models of transient cerebral ischemia; however, higher target concentrations appear necessary on the basis of animal models of permanent ischemia.** METHODS: This was a randomized, double-blind, placebo-controlled, parallel-group, dose-escalation, multicenter study that evaluated safety, tolerability, and plasma concentrations of 2 NXY-059 dosing regimens within 24 hours of acute stroke. NXY-059 was administered as either 915 mg over 1 hour followed by 420 mg/h for 71 hours or 1820 mg for 1 hour followed by 844 mg/h for 71 hours; plasma concentrations were monitored. Neurological and functional outcomes were recorded for up to 30 days. RESULTS: One hundred thirty-five patients were recruited, of whom 134 received study treatment and completed assessments (844 mg/h, n=39; 420 mg/h, n=48; placebo, n=47). Mean age was 69 years (range, 34 to 92 years), and baseline National Institutes of Health Stroke Scale score was 8.5 (SD, 6.6). **Serious adverse events occurred in 3, 17, and 13 patients, respectively, with deaths in 0, 4, and 3 patients and treatment discontinuations because of adverse events in 0, 1, and 3 patients. Good outcome, defined by modified Rankin Scale score of 0 or 1, was seen in 53%, 29% and 40%, respectively.** No safety concern was identified in analysis of body temperature, blood pressure, or other laboratory parameters. The unbound plasma concentration at steady state was 260+/-79 micromol/L, exceeding the target of 200 micromol/L in the high-dose group. CONCLUSIONS: NXY-059 was well tolerated in patients with an acute stroke at and above concentrations shown to be neuroprotective in an animal model when initiated 4 hours after onset of permanent focal ischemia. (Lees, 2003)

2004

Antioxidant supplementation prevents exercise-induced lipid peroxidation, but not inflammation, in ultra marathon runners. (Mastaloudis et al, 2004)

Evidence identifying the therapeutic influence of vitamin E and C supplementation on the preservation of muscle size following an injury ad surgery is limited in humans; however, **it was found to be ineffective** in preventing muscle damage following an ultra marathon (50 km) run in healthy participants, although the supplements did decrease markers of lipid peroxidation and DNA damage. (Mastaloudis et al, 2004)

Role of antioxidants in treatment of male infertility: an overview of the literature (Agarwal et al, 2004)

Seminal oxidative stress in the male reproductive tract is known to result in peroxidative damage of the sperm plasma membrane and loss of its DNA integrity. Normally, a balance exists between concentrations of reactive oxygen species and antioxidant scavenging systems. One of the rational strategies to counteract the oxidative stress is to increase the scavenging capacity of seminal plasma. Numerous studies have evaluated the efficacy of antioxidants in male infertility. In this review, the results of different studies conducted have been analysed, and the evidence available to date is provided. **It was found that although many clinical trials have demonstrated the beneficial effects of antioxidants in selected cases of male infertility, some studies failed to demonstrate the same benefit. The majority of the**

studies suffer from a lack of placebo-controlled, double-blind design, making it difficult to reach a definite conclusion. In addition, investigators have used different antioxidants in different combinations and dosages for varying durations. Pregnancy, the most relevant outcome parameter of fertility, was reported in only a few studies. Most studies failed to examine the effect of antioxidants on a specific group of infertile patients with high oxidative stress. Multicentre, double-blind studies with statistically accepted sample size are still needed to provide conclusive evidence on the benefit of antioxidants as a treatment modality for patients with male infertility. (Agarwal et al, 2004)

2005

Effects of atorvastatin and vitamin E on lipoproteins and oxidative stress in dialysis patients: a randomised-controlled trial. (Diepeveen et al, 2005) (#44)

The objective of this study was to examine the effects of treatment with atorvastatin, alpha-tocopherol and the combination of both, on lipoproteins and oxidative stress in dialysis patients. DESIGN AND SETTING: This double-blind randomised placebo-controlled trial was performed at the dialysis department of a non-university hospital. SUBJECTS, INTERVENTION AND MEASUREMENTS: A total of **44 clinically stable, non-diabetic patients on dialysis therapy** (23 on haemo- and 21 on peritoneal-dialysis) without manifest cardiovascular disease were included in this study. They were randomised for treatment during a period of 12 weeks with 40 mg atorvastatin + placebo alpha-tocopherol (group 1) once daily, 800 IU alpha-tocopherol + placebo atorvastatin once daily (group 2), 40 mg atorvastatin + 800 IU alpha-tocopherol once daily (group 3), or placebo atorvastatin + placebo alpha-tocopherol once daily (group 4). Assessment of lipid profile and oxidative stress was performed at the start of the study and after 12 weeks of treatment. RESULTS: Treatment with atorvastatin reduced total cholesterol, triglycerides (TG), low-density lipoprotein (LDL) cholesterol, apolipoprotein B (apoB) and levels of oxidized LDL (oxLDL) with 30-43%. It had no influence on LDL oxidizability. **Additional supplementation with alpha-tocopherol had no effect on lipid profile and oxLDL levels** but decreased in vitro LDL oxidizability. No side-effects were observed. CONCLUSIONS: Treatment with atorvastatin is effective in lowering plasma total cholesterol, TG, LDL, apoB and oxLDL in a population of stable dialysis patients and might therefore be an effective tool in improving the poor cardiovascular outcome in these patients. Supplementation of alpha-tocopherol to atorvastatin had beneficial effects on in vitro LDL oxidizability and might therefore be of additional value. Further research on the clinical effects of treatment with atorvastatin in combination with alpha-tocopherol is necessary. (Diepeveen et al, 2005)

The combination of vitamin C and grape-seed polyphenols increases blood pressure: a randomized, double-blind, placebo-controlled trial (Ward, Hodgson et al, 2005) (#69)

There is growing evidence that oxidative stress contributes to the pathogenesis of hypertension and endothelial dysfunction. Thus, dietary antioxidants may beneficially influence blood pressure (BP) and endothelial function by reducing oxidative stress. OBJECTIVE: To determine if vitamin C and polyphenols, alone or in combination, can lower BP, improve endothelial function and reduce oxidative stress in hypertensive individuals. DESIGN: A total of **69 treated hypertensive individuals** with a mean 24-h ambulatory systolic blood pressure > or = 125 mmHg participated in a randomized, double-blind, placebo-controlled, factorial trial. Following a 3-week washout, **participants received 500 mg/day vitamin C, 1000 mg/day grape-seed polyphenols, both vitamin C and polyphenols, or neither for 6 weeks**. At baseline and post-intervention, 24-h ambulatory BP, ultrasound-assessed endothelium-dependent and -independent vasodilation of the brachial artery, and markers of oxidative damage, (plasma and urinary F2-isoprostanes, oxidized low-density lipoproteins and plasma tocopherols), were measured. RESULTS: A significant interaction between grape-seed and vitamin C treatments for effects on BP was observed. **Vitamin C alone reduced systolic BP** versus placebo (-1.8 +/- 0.8 mmHg, P = 0.03), **while polyphenols did not** (-1.3 +/- 0.8 mmHg, P = 0.12). **However, *treatment with the combination of vitamin C and polyphenols increased systolic BP (4.8 +/- 0.9 mmHg versus placebo; 6.6 +/- 0.8 mmHg versus vitamin C; 6.1 +/- 0.9 mmHg versus polyphenols mmHg, each P < 0.0001) and diastolic BP* (2.7 +/- 0.6 mmHg, P < 0.0001 versus placebo; 1.5 +/- 0.6 mmHg, P = 0.016 versus vitamin C; 3.2 +/- 0.7 mmHg, P < 0.0001 versus polyphenols). Endothelium-dependent and -independent vasodilation, and markers of oxidative damage were not significantly altered**. CONCLUSION: Although the mechanism remains to be elucidated, *these results suggest caution for hypertensive subjects taking supplements containing combinations of vitamin C and polyphenols.* (Ward, Hodgson et al, 2005)

Effects of vitamins C and E on oxidative stress markers and endothelial function in patients with systemic lupus erythematosus: a double blind, placebo controlled pilot study (Tam et al, 2005) (#39 with SLE)

Patients with systemic lupus erythematosus (SLE) experience excess morbidity and mortality due to coronary artery disease (CAD) that cannot be fully explained by the classical CAD risk factors. Among emerging CAD risk factors, oxidative stress is currently being emphasized. We evaluated the effects of long-term antioxidant vitamins on markers of oxidative stress and antioxidant defense and endothelial function in **39 patients with SLE**. METHODS: Patients were randomized to receive either placebo or **vitamins (500 mg vitamin C and 800 IU vitamin E daily) for**

12 weeks. Markers of oxidative stress included malondialdehyde (MDA) and allantoin. Antioxidants measured included erythrocyte superoxide dismutase and glutathione peroxidase, plasma total antioxidant power (as FRAP value), and ascorbic acid and vitamin E concentrations. Endothelial function was assessed by flow-mediated dilatation (FMD) of the brachial artery and plasma concentration of von Willebrand factor (vWF) and plasminogen activator inhibitor type 1 (PAI-1). Primary outcome of the study included the change in lipid peroxidation as revealed by MDA levels. Secondary outcomes included changes in allantoin and antioxidant levels and change in endothelial function. RESULTS: **After treatment, plasma ascorbic acid and alpha-tocopherol concentrations were significantly ($p < 0.05$) increased only in the vitamin-treated group, associated with a significant decrease ($p < 0.05$) in plasma MDA.** Other oxidative stress markers and antioxidant levels remained unchanged in both groups. FMD and vWF and PAI-1 levels remained unchanged in both groups. CONCLUSION: **Combined administration of vitamins C and E was associated with decreased lipid peroxidation,** but **did not affect endothelial function in patients with SLE after 3 months of therapy.** (Tam et al, 2005)

Despite epidemiologic findings generally pointing toward an association between increased vitamin C and reduced oxidation and inflammation, **intervention trials assessing the effect of vitamin C supplementation on various markers of T2DM have yielded inconsistent results.** One randomized, crossover, double-blind intervention trial reported no improvement in fasting plasma glucose and no significant differences in levels of CRP, IL-6, IL-1 receptor agonist, or oxidized low-density lipoprotein (LDL) after supplementation with 3000 mg/day of vitamin C for 2 weeks in a group of 20 T2DM patients, compared to baseline levels. (Lu et al, 2005)

In general, inconsistent results from studies evaluating the effect of vitamin E on inflammation, oxidation, and T2DM risk may result partly from genetic differences between individuals that could lead to variations in response to micronutrient exposure.

Effect of alpha-tocopherol on the metabolic control and oxidative stress in female type 2 diabetics (Ble-Castillo et al, 2005) (#34)

In this study we evaluate the effects of alpha-tocopherol on the metabolic control and oxidative stress in female patients with type 2 diabetes mellitus. **Thirty-four** female type 2 diabetics 40-70 years old up to 14 years with diabetes, under medical treatment, were randomly divided in two groups. One group received placebo (Control group, n = 21) and the other received alpha-tocopherol (800 IU/day, n = 13) during 6 weeks. Blood samples were collected at the beginning and at the end of the study to measure malondialdehyde production, glycated hemoglobin, selenium dependent-glutathione peroxidase, Cu,Zn-superoxide dismutase in erythrocytes and total antioxidant status, glucose, lipid and lipoproteins in serum. Erythrocyte malondialdehyde decreased and serum-total antioxidant status increased after alpha-tocopherol treatment (P < 0.0001). However, *an unexpected increase on cholesterol levels and a reduced erythrocyte-Cu,Zn-superoxide dismutase activity was observed after alpha-tocopherol treatment. alpha-Tocopherol administration did not affect glucose, glycated hemoglobin, triacylglycerides, lipoprotein levels and serum malondialdehyde.* A minor oxidative stress was observed in female type 2 diabetic patients after alpha-tocopherol treatment inferred from the reduced levels of erythrocyte malondialdehyde and the increased values of total antioxidant status. On the other hand, **no beneficial changes were observed on glycemic control or lipid metabolism.** (Ble-Castillo et al, 2005)

Effect of ascorbic acid on microcirculation in patients with Type II diabetes: a randomized placebo-controlled cross-over study (Lu et al, 2005)

Manifestations of vascular disease, including microvascular changes, constitute the major part of the morbidity and mortality in diabetic patients. Oxidative stress has been suggested to play an important role in the vascular dysfunction of diabetic patients. Furthermore, epidemiological observations indicate a beneficial effect of an increased dietary intake of antioxidants. **The present study tested the hypothesis that the antioxidant ascorbic acid influences microcirculatory function in patients with Type II diabetes.** Patients with Type II diabetes were treated with 1 g of ascorbic acid three times a day for 2 weeks in a randomized placebo-controlled double-blind cross-over design. Microvascular reactivity was assessed by vital capillaroscopy and PRH (post-occlusive reactive hyperaemia). hs-CRP (high-sensitivity C-reactive protein), IL-6 (interleukin-6), IL-1ra (interleukin-1 receptor antagonist) and ox-LDL (oxidized low-density lipoprotein) were analysed. **The results showed no significant change in microvascular reactivity assessed after 2 weeks of ascorbic acid treatment.** TtP (time to peak) was 12.0+/-3.3 s before and 11.2+/-3.5 s after ascorbic acid (n=17). In comparison, TtP was 11.5+/-2.9 s before and 10.6+/-2.8 s after placebo (not significant). IL-1ra, IL-6, hs-CRP and ox-LDL did not change significantly after ascorbic acid, neither as absolute or relative values. In conclusion, in contrast with some studies reported previously, **we could not demonstrate an effect of continuous oral treatment with ascorbic acid on microvascular reactivity assessed at the level of individual capillaries.** Furthermore, **we found no indication of an effect on inflammatory cytokines or ox-LDL.** (Lu et al, 2005)

Cognitive performance in relation to vitamin status in healthy elderly German women-the effect of 6-month multivitamin supplementation (Wolters et al, 2005) (#220) Prior investigations have reported a link between poor status of antioxidants, folate, and cobalamin resulting in elevated total plasma homocysteine (tHcy) and methylmalonic acid (MMA) concentrations with an increased risk for reduced cognitive performance. The aim of the study was to evaluate the effect of a 6-month multivitamin supplementation on the cognitive performance of female seniors and to assess cognitive functioning in relation to vitamin status, tHcy, and MMA values at baseline. METHODS: The study was performed as a randomized placebo-controlled double-blind trial. **220 healthy, free-living women (aged 60-91 years) were included**. Blood drawings and cognitive tests were performed at the Institute of Food Science of the University of Hanover, Germany. Vitamin and cognitive status have been evaluated prior to and 6 months after supplementation. Plasma ascorbic acid, serum concentrations of alpha-tocopherol, beta-carotene, and coenzyme Q10, serum and erythrocyte folate as well as serum cobalamin, serum MMA, and plasma tHcy concentrations were measured. Activity coefficient of erythrocyte alpha aspartic aminotransferase was used as functional index for vitamin B(6) status. The cognitive performance was assessed by the Symbol Search test, a subtest of the Wechsler Adult Intelligence Scale (WAIS-III) and the pattern-recognition test. Intelligence as assessed by the 'Kurztest für Allgemeine Intelligenz' (KAI) was a further variable. RESULTS: **No significant differences in pattern-recognition and intelligence score were observed between vitamin and placebo group prior to and after multivitamin supplementation**. In the Symbol Search test, the vitamin group exhibited better test results than the placebo group at both measure points. One-way ANOVA showed a marginally significant linear trend between the baseline tHcy concentration and the pattern-recognition score (P = 0.051) in the total sample. Multiple backward regression revealed only a significant influence of the school graduation on baseline cognitive function test results. A general linear model showed that the changes in cognitive function scores could not be explained by the type of treatment or blood parameters. CONCLUSIONS: Our data indicate that **6 months supplementation of physiological dosages of antioxidants and B vitamins have no effect on cognitive performance in presumedly healthy and well-nourished female seniors**. An intervention period of only 6 months may be too short for improving cognitive performance in well-educated elderly women without dementia. (Wolters et al, 2005)

Astaxanthin supplementation

Six separate failed studies: (Bloomer et al, 2005) (Andersen et al, 2007) (Kupcinskas et al, 2008) (Astorg et al, 1997) (Park et al, 1999) (Black, 1998)

Astaxanthin supplementation does not attenuate muscle injury following eccentric exercise in resistance-trained men (Bloomer et al, 2005) (#20) An antioxidant study tested astaxanthin combined with the carotenoid lutein as a possible supplement for enhancing recovery from exercise . In this small trial, 20 bodybuilders were given either placebo or the carotenoid combination for three weeks. Participants then engaged in intense exercise. **The results failed to show that use of the astaxanthin/lutein combination reduced muscle soreness or signs of muscle injury**. (Bloomer et al, 2005)

Two studies failed to find astaxanthin significantly more effective than placebo for treating stomach irritation in people with dyspepsia (nonspecific stomach pain). (Andersen et al, 2007) (Kupcinskas et al, 2008)

In a study of chemically-induced hepatocarcinogenesis in rats, dietary astaxanthin had no effect on the development of preneoplastic liver foci while lycopene produced a significant reduction in foci. (Astorg et al, 1997)

Similarly, activation of *pim-1* gene expression (which is involved in regulating cell differentiation and apoptosis) was stimulated in lutein-fed but not in astaxanthin-fed mice. (Park et al, 1999)

Finally, **one *in vivo* dietary astaxanthin study has reported negative results; dietary supplementation with either β-carotene or astaxanthin exacerbated carcinogenic expression in the skin of hairless mice after UV irradiation.** (Black, 1998)

To date, there are no studies to indicate a relationship between systemic antioxidant or vitamin deficiency and male infertility. Silver et al, 2005 evaluated a cohort of fertile men and did not identify any relationships between dietary antioxidant intake (vitamins C, E or ß-carotene) and sperm DNA damage. (Silver et al, 2005).

I believe that this sums it up, in that there is no relationship between antioxidant supplement intake and prevention of DNA damage.

Effect of antioxidant intake on sperm chromatin stability in healthy non-smoking men (Silver et al, 2005) (#87)

Silver et al stated that oxidative stress is detrimental to sperm function and a significant factor in the etiology of male infertility. This report examines the association between dietary and supplementary intake of the antioxidants vitamin C, vitamin E, and beta-carotene and sperm chromatin integrity. **Eighty-seven healthy male volunteers** donated semen samples, completed food-frequency questionnaires, and provided information about their sociodemographic characteristics, medical and reproductive histories, and lifestyle habits. Sperm chromatin integrity was measured using the **DNA fragmentation index (DFI)** and related parameters, obtained from the sperm chromatin structure assay (SCSA). SCSA measures the susceptibility of sperm DNA to acid-induced denaturation in situ. After adjusting for age and duration of abstinence, **there was no dose-response association between any DNA fragmentation index (DFI) outcome and any antioxidant intake measure.** Non-dose-related associations were found between beta-carotene intake and both the standard deviation of DFI (SD DFI) and the percent of immature sperm. Participants with moderate, but not high, beta-carotene intake had an increase in SD DFI compared with participants with low intake (adjusted means 206.7 and 180.5, respectively; P = .03), as well as an increase in the percentage of immature sperm (adjusted means 6.9% and 5.0%, respectively; P = .04). If antioxidant intake in the range studied is indeed beneficial for fertility in healthy men, it does not appear to be mediated through the integrity of sperm chromatin. (Silver et al, 2005)

Nonetheless, it is possible that a subset of infertile men may be at risk for antioxidant deficiency, particularly, vitamin C deficiency. (Hampl et al, 2004) (Hampl JS, Taylor CA, Johnston CS. Vitamin C deficiency and depletion in the United States: the Third National Health and Nutrition Examination Survey, 1988 to 1994. Am J Public Health. 2004;94:870–5)

Moreover, infertile men with specific lifestyles may also be at risk for antioxidant or vitamin deficiency (e.g. smoking, increased alcohol intake, dieting). (Jacob, 1990)

High dose vitamin E therapy in amyotrophic lateral sclerosis as add-on therapy to riluzole: results of a placebo-controlled double-blind study (Graf et al, 2005) (#160)

Increasing evidence has suggested that oxidative stress may be involved in the pathogenesis of amyotrophic lateral sclerosis (ALS). The antioxidant vitamin E (alpha-tocopherol) has been shown to slow down the onset and progression of the paralysis in transgenic mice expressing a mutation in the superoxide dismutase gene found in certain forms of familial ALS. The current study, **a double blind, placebo-controlled, randomised, stratified, parallel-group clinical trial**, was designed to determine **whether vitamin E (5000 mg per day)** may be efficacious in slowing down disease progression when added to riluzole. METHODS: **160 patients** in 6 German centres with either probable or definite ALS (according to the El Escorial Criteria) and a disease duration of less than 5 years, treated with riluzole, were included in this study and were randomly assigned to receive either alpha-tocopherol (5000 mg per day) or placebo for 18 months. The Primary outcome measure was survival, calculating time to death, tracheostomy or permanent assisted ventilation, according to the WFN-Criteria of clinical trials. Secondary outcome measures were the rate of deterioration of function assessed by the modified Norris limb and bulbar scales, manual muscle testing (BMRC), spasticity scale, ventilatory function and the Sickness Impact Profile (SIP ALS/19). Patients were assessed at entry and every 4 months thereafter during the study period until month 16 and at a final visit at month 18. Vitamin E samples were taken for compliance check and Quality Control of the trial. For Safety, a physical examination was performed at baseline and then every visit until the treatment discontinuation at month 18. Height and weight were recorded at baseline and weight alone at the follow-up visits. A neurological examination as well as vital signs (heart rate and blood pressure), an ECG and VEP's were recorded at each visit. Furthermore, spontaneously reported adverse experiences and serious adverse events were documented and standard laboratory tests including liver function tests performed. For Statistical Analysis, the population to be considered for the primary outcome measure was an "intent-to-treat" (ITT) population which included all randomised patients who had received at least one treatment dose (n = 160 patients). For the secondary outcome measures, a two way analysis of variance was performed on a patient population that included all randomised patients who had at least one assessment after inclusion. RESULTS: Concerning the primary endpoint, **no significant difference between placebo and treatment group** could be detected either with the stratified Logrank or the Wilcoxon test. The functional assessments showed a marginal trend in favor of vitamin E, without reaching significance. CONCLUSION: **Neither the primary nor the secondary outcome measures could determine whether a megadose of vitamin E is efficacious in slowing disease progression in ALS as an add-on therapy to riluzol.** Larger or longer studies might be needed. However, administration of this megadose does not seem to have any significant side effects in this patient population. (Graf et al, 2005). **This is just one more of the diseases that predictions for antioxidant therapy have failed to reverse or cure.**

Cognitive performance in relation to vitamin status in healthy elderly German women-the effect of 6-month multivitamin supplementation (Wolters et al, 2005) (#220)

Prior investigations have reported a link between poor status of antioxidants, folate, and cobalamin resulting in elevated total plasma homocysteine (tHcy) and methylmalonic acid (MMA) concentrations with an increased risk for reduced cognitive performance. The aim of the study was to evaluate the effect of a 6-month multivitamin supplementation on the cognitive performance of female seniors and to assess cognitive functioning in relation to vitamin status, tHcy, and MMA values at baseline. METHODS: The study was performed as a randomized placebo-controlled double-blind trial. **220 healthy, free-living women (aged 60-91 years) were included.** Blood drawings and cognitive tests were performed at the Institute of Food Science of the University of Hanover, Germany. Vitamin and cognitive status have been evaluated prior to and 6 months after supplementation. Plasma ascorbic acid, serum concentrations of alpha-tocopherol, beta-carotene, and coenzyme Q10, serum and erythrocyte folate as well as serum cobalamin, serum MMA, and plasma tHcy concentrations were measured. Activity coefficient of erythrocyte alpha aspartic aminotransferase was used as functional index for vitamin B(6) status. The cognitive performance was assessed by the Symbol Search test, a subtest of the Wechsler Adult Intelligence Scale (WAIS-III) and the pattern-recognition test. Intelligence as assessed by the 'Kurztest für Allgemeine Intelligenz' (KAI) was a further variable. RESULTS: **No significant differences in pattern-recognition and intelligence score were**

observed between vitamin and placebo group prior to and after multivitamin supplementation. In the Symbol Search test, the vitamin group exhibited better test results than the placebo group at both measure points. One-way ANOVA showed a marginally significant linear trend between the baseline tHcy concentration and the pattern-recognition score (P = 0.051) in the total sample. Multiple backward regression revealed only a significant influence of the school graduation on baseline cognitive function test results. A general linear model showed that the changes in cognitive function scores could not be explained by the type of treatment or blood parameters. CONCLUSIONS: Our data indicate that **6 months supplementation of physiological dosages of antioxidants and B vitamins have no effect on cognitive performance in presumedly healthy and well-nourished female seniors.** An intervention period of only 6 months may be too short for improving cognitive performance in well-educated elderly women without dementia. (Wolters et al, 2005)

2006

Dietary supplements in a national survey: Prevalence of use and reports of adverse events (Timbo et al, 2006) (#)

To examine information collected from the 2002 Health and Diet Survey regarding the use dietary supplements and self-reported health problems that the survey participants believed were related to dietary supplements. METHODS: The US Food and Drug Administration sponsors a Health and Diet Survey to track trends of consumer awareness, attitudes, and practices related to health and diet issues. By telephone, the 2002 Health and Diet Survey staff interviewed English-speaking noninstitutionalized adults aged 18 years or older in households in the 50 states and District of Columbia. Survey respondents were queried as to whether or not they had taken a dietary supplement during the past year and if they had experienced any health problem that they attributed to supplement use. RESULTS: **Seventy-three percent of US noninstitutionalized adults aged 18 years or older who spoke English and resided in households with telephones used a *dietary supplement in the previous 12 months* and 4% of them had experienced an adverse event that they believed might be related to dietary supplement use. Eighty-five percent of supplement users reported taking multivitamins/multiminerals and 13.3% of adverse events reported were attributed to multivitamins/multiminerals.** A higher proportion of supplement users with adverse events than users without adverse events were concurrently taking supplements and prescription drugs or were taking supplements instead of prescription drug to treat or prevent a health condition. CONCLUSIONS: This self-reported data describes the prevalence of supplement use and related adverse events. **Multivitamins/multiminerals accounted for much of the supplements use and was attributed to a little more than 10% of the adverse events reported.** Food and nutrition-professionals and other health care professionals should take special care to learn about their patients' use of these products. (Timbo et al, 2006) **Epidemiology Team, Office of Scientific Analysis and Support, College Park, MD 20740, USA**.

Effects of vitamin E supplementation on oxidative stress at rest and after exercise to exhaustion in athletic students (Gaeini et al, 2006) (#20)

The purpose of this study is to determine the effect following exercise to exhaustion of vitamin E supplementation on oxidative stress in athletic students. METHODS: **Twenty male students voluntarily participated in the study and were randomly assigned (double blind) to either a vitamin E (daily dose of 450 mg of a-tocopherol for a period of 8 weeks)** or a placebo group (took capsules containing 450 mg of lactose for 8 weeks). Before and after 8 weeks blood samples were collected at rest and after exercise to exhaustion. Oxidative stress markers were malondialdehyde (MDA), carbonylated proteins (CP) and creatine kinase (CK). Also, the effect of vitamin E on ergometer cycling time, as an example of endurance performance, was evaluated. RESULTS: ANOVA and independent t-tests indicated that **vitamin E supplementation did not significantly change (P > 0.05) MDA, CP and CK values at rest, after exercise to exhaustion, and cycling time**, but plasma volume after exercise to exhaustion significantly decreased (P < 0.05). CONCLUSIONS: Although **vitamin E supplementation had no effect on exercise performance or capacity in athletic students**, further investigation is required using larger numbers of subjects and measures of vitamin E before unequivocal conclusion can be stated. (Gaeini et al, 2006)

Oral vitamin E supplementation on oxidative stress, vitamin and antioxidant status in intensely exercised horses (Williams, Carlucci, 2006) (#21)

REASONS FOR PERFORMING STUDY: **Vitamin E is the most commonly supplemented antioxidant in horses;** however, previous research is not conclusive as to the recommended level for exercising horses. OBJECTIVE: To evaluate the effects of 3 levels of vitamin E supplementation on oxidative stress and vitamin/antioxidant status in intensely exercised horses to determine the optimal level of vitamin E supplementation. METHODS: **Twelve unfit Standardbreds** were divided into 3 groups, supplemented orally with 0 (CON), 5000 (MOD), or 10,000 (HI) iu/day of DL-alpha-tocopheryl acetate. The 3 x 3 Latin square design consisted of three 4 week supplementation periods with 4 week wash out periods between. After each period, horses underwent a treadmill interval exercise test. Blood samples were collected and heart rate (HR) measured before, during and after exercise. Data were analysed using ANOVA with repeated measures in SAS. RESULTS: The CON group had lower HR throughout the test compared to the MOD and HI groups (P<0.05). There was an increase in plasma retinol (RET), beta-carotene (BC), red blood cell total glutathione and glutathione peroxidase with exercise (P<0.05), but all groups returned to baseline after 24 h.

Plasma alpha-tocopherol (TOC) increased from baseline with exercise (P<0.0001) in all groups; treatment differences were observed at 24 h (P<0.05). The HI and CON groups had lower BC compared to the MOD group (P = 0.05). CONCLUSIONS: **Horses supplemented with vitamin E, at nearly 10-times the 1989 NRC recommended level, did not experience lower oxidative stress compared to control horses. Additionally, lower plasma BC levels observed in the HI group, which may indicate that vitamin E has an inhibitory effect on BC metabolism.** POTENTIAL RELEVANCE: Supplementation above control levels is not more beneficial to oxidative stress and antioxidant status in intensely exercising horses; indeed, levels 10 times in excess may be detrimental to BC and should be avoided. (Williams, Carlucci, 2006)

Antioxidants did not prevent muscle damage in response to an ultramarathon run. (Mastaloudis et al, 2006) (#22) This study was conducted to determine if 6 wk of supplementation with vitamins E and C could alleviate exercise-induced muscle damage. We studied 22 runners during a 50-km ultramarathon. METHODS: Subjects were randomly assigned to one of two groups: (a) placebos (PL) or (b) antioxidants (AO) (1000 mg vitamin C and 300 mg RRR-alpha-tocopheryl acetate). Blood samples were obtained before supplementation (baseline), 24 h pre-, 12 h pre-, and 1 h pre-race; mid-race, post-race, 2 h post race, and for 6 d post-race. Plasma alpha-tocopherol (alpha-TOH), ascorbic acid (AA), and muscle damage markers (creatine kinase (CK) and lactate dehydrogenase (LDH)), as well as maximal voluntary contraction (MVC) of the hamstring and quadriceps were assessed. RESULTS: With supplementation, plasma alpha-TOH and AA increased in the AO but not the PL group. LDH and CK increased in response to the race; LDH peaked at post race and CK reached maximal values 2 h and 1 d post race; neither was affected by treatment. Adjusting for between-subject differences in baseline CK values revealed that men had higher levels of CK than did women throughout the study. Correcting CK values for lean body mass (kg) eliminated sex differences, but not changes over time. CK was significantly correlated (R = 0.52, P < 0.0001) with C-reactive protein, an acute phase response marker. MVC decreased 14-26% in all groups in response to the run. **Eccentric hamstring (EH) torque and concentric quadriceps (CQ) power exhibited the largest deficits, 26 and 24%, respectively, with no effect of treatment.** CQ recovered at a faster rate in women than in men. CONCLUSION: **Antioxidants appeared to have no effect on exercise-induced increases in muscle damage or recovery,** but important sex differences were observed. (Mastaloudis et al, 2006)

Fruit and vegetable juices and Alzheimer's disease: The Kame project. (Dai et al, 2006, the Kame Project) (#1,836)

Summary: A glass of fruit or vegetable juice 3 or more times weekly may fend off Alzheimer's disease, due to their polyphenol content, rather than vitamin antioxidants. **Introduction**: Oxidative damage is regarded today as one of the keys to the development of Alzheimer's. That's why many people take antioxidants in the hopes of delaying its onset. One of the targets of oxidative damage is the beta-amyloid peptide, and **hydrogen peroxide has been suggested as a possible mediator.** This has led to the use of polyphenols, which are described as being the most abundant dietary antioxidants, with stronger neuroprotection against hydrogen peroxide than antioxidant vitamins.

Polyphenols are usually found in the skin and peel of fruits and vegetables; when the produce is mechanically squeezed, the polyphenols pass into the juices. A study done in Japanese Americans, reported in the *American Journal of Medicine*, has explored the role of drinking juices in the development of Alzheimer's disease over a 9-year period.

What was done: The *Kame* project is part of a larger study of dementia in Japanese people living in Japan and the USA. The *Kame* cohort consists of participants aged 65 and older living in Washington State, USA. There were **1,836 subjects** who were free of dementia at enrollment in 1992-1994. At baseline the Cognitive Abilites Screening Instrument (CASI) was used to assess cognitive function; this was repeated every two years for a total of 4 times. A much broader neuropsychological exam was given to anyone scoring less than 87 out of 100 points on the CASI. Food-frequency questionnaires were completed by 87% of the participants at baseline; the questions used were appropriate for Asian populations. The usual dietary intake of nutrients, including calories, vitamins C and E, and beta-carotene were calculated for each person. Other baseline information included smoking, alcohol use, birthplace, education level, physical activity, usual eating preference (Asian or Western), and use of antioxidant vitamin supplements. The sense of smell was ascertained, and the apolipoprotein E (ApoE) gene status was determined. The participants were classified three times according to their intake of tea, wine, and juices (fruit and vegetable). Each classification used three categories, or 'tertiles': "less than once a week", "once or twice a week", and "at least 3 times a week". These tertiles were used to analyze the risks, or Hazards Ratios, of subjects in each category of developing Alzheimer's disease.

What was found: The average age at enrollment was 72; just over half of the subjects were women. One in five of them possessed an ApoE4 gene, which means they were at increased risk of developing Alzheimer's. Over the follow-up period (average duration 6.3 years) 81 cases of Alzheimer's disease were diagnosed; 63 of these had provided food frequency data at baseline, and were included in the analysis. Tea drinking, the most popular beverage in these studies, was not associated with Alzheimer's disease risk. Only a few participants drank wine, and although there may have been a trend towards a 'protective' effect of wine on the development of Alzheimer's, this was not statistically significant and so should be ignored. There was no association found for intake of vitamins E, C, or beta-carotene. After adjusting for factors that might bias the results, such as smoking, education, physical activity, and fat intake, it was found that those reporting drinking fruit or vegetable juice once or twice a week were 16% less likely to develop signs of Alzheimer's; this result was not statistically significant. But **those who drank juices three or more times a week were 76% less likely to develop the disease, a statistically significant finding.** The 'protective' effect of drinking juices was somewhat greater in those participants who were inactive, had a history of smoking, and who carried an ApoE4 gene.

What these results mean: This study shows that **Japanese Americans who drank fruit or vegetable juice 3 or more times a week were 76% less likely to develop the symptoms and signs of Alzheimer's in the next 6 years, compared with those who drank juices less than once a week.** Importantly, **there was no such association (decreased risk of AD) with the intake of vitamins C, E, or beta-carotene, although these are abundantly present in fruit and vegetable juices; other studies have also failed to find any effect of these substances on the development of Alzheimer's.**

This suggests that some other constituents were responsible for the benefit shown by the juices. The obvious candidates are polyphenols, such as quercetin, which are able to cross the blood-brain barrier and get to the brain, and which have a neuroprotective effect against hydrogen peroxide. (The major polyphenol in tea, catechin, is ineffective against hydrogen peroxide, which may explain why teas had no protective effect in this study.) The researchers say their results require confirmation in more studies, especially ones designed to detect which polyphenol is most effective, and which fruits and vegetables confer the greatest protection. In the meantime, while waiting for results, we suggest you include fruit and vegetable juices in your nutrition plan. They taste good, and carry numerous other health benefits, as well. (Dai et al, 2006, the Kame Project). **Dai's guess is that the responsible agents are polyphenols but there is no proof for this. It is merely wishful thinking to interject yet another antioxidant as the hero and protector.**

2007

Associations of antioxidant nutrients and oxidative DNA damage in healthy African-American and White adults (Watters JL, et al, 2007) (#164)

High antioxidant intake has been shown to reduce cancer risk and may also mitigate the effects of oxidative DNA damage, which is hypothesized to be causally linked to carcinogenesis. This study examined potential racial differences in (a) dietary intakes and plasma concentrations of vitamin C, vitamin E, and carotenoids and oxidative DNA damage and (b) associations between plasma antioxidants and oxidative DNA damage. Data were from a cross-sectional study of **164 generally healthy nonsmoking African-Americans and Whites in North Carolina**, ages

20 to 45 years, equally distributed by race and sex. Participants completed a demographic and health questionnaire, four 24-h dietary recalls, and a dietary supplement inventory; had height and weight measured; and provided a semifasting blood sample. **African-Americans had statistically significantly lower plasma concentrations of vitamin E, alpha-carotene, beta-carotene, and lutein + zeaxanthin than Whites, as well as lower self-reported intake of most antioxidants.**

Levels of oxidative DNA damage, measured using the alkaline comet assay, were lower in African-Americans than Whites. I believe that this is contrary to the FRT, in that lower levels of antioxidants should have been associated with higher levels of oxidative DNA damage, but just the opposite occurred.

An inverse association between lycopene and oxidative DNA damage (r = -0.20; P = 0.03) was found in the combined study population after adjusting for sex, age, body mass index, passive smoke exposure, physical activity, education, income, and alcohol intake. *There was also a positive association of vitamin E with oxidative DNA damage in the total population (r = 0.21; P = 0.02) and in African-American men (r = 0.63; P = 0.01) after adjusting for covariates.* This study is among the first to examine these associations in a sample of healthy adults with an adequate representation of African-Americans. (Watters JL, et al, 2007)

The effect of vitamin E on blood pressure in individuals with type 2 diabetes: a randomized, double-blind, placebo-controlled trial. (Ward, Wu et al, 2007) (#58)

Oxidative stress has been suggested to play a role in the development of diabetes, hypertension and vascular dysfunction. Vitamin E, a major lipid-soluble dietary antioxidant, has two major dietary forms, alpha-tocopherol and gamma-tocopherol. The potential importance of gamma-tocopherol has largely been overlooked. Our aim was to investigate the effect of alpha-tocopherol and gamma-tocopherol supplementation on 24-h ambulatory blood pressure (BP) and heart rate, vascular function and oxidative stress in individuals with type 2 diabetes. METHOD: **Fifty-eight individuals with type 2 diabetes were randomized in a double-blind, placebo-controlled trial.** Participants were randomized to a daily dose of 500 mg/day RRR-alpha-tocopherol, 500 mg/day mixed tocopherols (60% gamma-tocopherol) or placebo for 6 weeks. Primary endpoints were 24-h ambulatory BP and heart rate, endothelium-dependent and independent vasodilation and plasma and urinary F2-isoprostanes. RESULTS: *Treatment with alpha-tocopherol significantly increased systolic BP [7.0 (5.2, 8.8) mmHg, P < 0.0001], diastolic BP [5.3 (4.0, 6.5) mmHg, P < 0.0001], pulse pressure [1.8 (0.6, 3.0) mmHg, P < 0.005] and heart rate [2.0 (0.6, 3.3) bpm, P < 0.005] versus placebo. Treatment with mixed tocopherols significantly increased systolic BP [6.8 (4.9, 8.6) mmHg, P < 0.0001], diastolic BP [3.6 (2.3,*

4.9) mmHg, P < 0.0001], pulse pressure [3.2 (2.0, 4.4) mmHg, P < 0.0001] and heart rate [1.8 (0.5, 3.2) bpm, P < 0.01] versus placebo. Treatment with alpha-tocopherol or mixed tocopherols significantly reduced plasma F2-isoprostanes versus placebo, but had no effect on urinary F2-isoprostanes. Endothelium-dependent and independent vasodilation was not affected by either treatment. CONCLUSION: *In contrast to our initial hypothesis, treatment with either alpha- or mixed toco-pherols significantly increased BP, pulse pressure and heart rate in individuals with type 2 diabetes.* (Ward, Wu et al, 2007)

The combination of vitamin C and grape-seed polyphenols increases blood pressure: a randomized, double-blind, placebo-controlled trial (Ward, Hodgson et al, 2007) (#69)

There is growing evidence that oxidative stress contributes to the pathogenesis of hypertension and endothelial dysfunction. Thus, dietary antioxidants may beneficially influence blood pressure (BP) and endothelial function by reducing oxidative stress. OBJECTIVE: To determine if vitamin C and polyphenols, alone or in combination, can lower BP, improve endothelial function and reduce oxidative stress in hypertensive individuals. DESIGN: A total of **69 treated hypertensive individuals** with a mean 24-h ambulatory systolic blood pressure > or = 125 mmHg participated in a randomized, double-blind, placebo-controlled, factorial trial. Following a 3-week washout, **participants received 500 mg/day vitamin C, 1000 mg/day grape-seed polyphenols, both vitamin C and polyphenols, or neither for 6 weeks.** At baseline and post-intervention, 24-h ambulatory BP, ultrasound-assessed endothelium-dependent and -independent vasodilation of the brachial artery, and markers of oxidative damage, (plasma and urinary F2-isoprostanes, oxidized low-density lipoproteins and plasma tocopherols), were measured. RESULTS: A significant interaction between grape-seed and vitamin C treatments for effects on BP was observed. **Vitamin C alone reduced systolic BP** versus placebo (-1.8 +/- 0.8 mmHg, P = 0.03), **while polyphenols did not** (-1.3 +/- 0.8 mmHg, P = 0.12). **However, *treatment with the combination of vitamin C and polyphenols increased systolic BP** (4.8 +/- 0.9 mmHg versus placebo; 6.6 +/- 0.8 mmHg versus vitamin C; 6.1 +/- 0.9 mmHg versus polyphenols mmHg, each P < 0.0001) and diastolic BP* (2.7 +/- 0.6 mmHg, P < 0.0001 versus placebo; 1.5 +/- 0.6 mmHg, P = 0.016 versus vitamin C; 3.2 +/- 0.7 mmHg, P < 0.0001 versus polyphenols). **Endothelium-dependent and -independent vasodilation, and markers of oxidative damage were not significantly altered.** CONCLUSION: Although the mechanism remains to be elucidated, *these results suggest caution for hypertensive subjects taking supplements containing combinations of vitamin C and polyphenols.* (Ward, Hodgson et al, 2007)

Effects of atorvastatin and vitamin C on forearm hyperemic blood flow, asymmetrical dimethylarginine levels and the inflammatory process in patients with type 2 diabetes mellitus (Tousoulis et al, 2007) (#41)

Forty one patients with type 2 DM and no evidence of macroangiopathy were recruited.

Tousoulis et al reported that treatment with 2000 mg/day for 4 weeks had no effect on levels of CRP, IL-6, TNF-α, or soluble vascular cell adhesion molecule-1 in 13 T2DM patients. Atorvastatin **(but not vitamin C)** improved endothelial function and decreased the expression of IL-6, TNF-α, CRP, sVCAM-1 and ADMA in patients with type 2 DM, while the decrease in ADMA was correlated with the decrease in TNF-α. (Tousoulis et al, 2007)

Multivitamin use and risk of prostate cancer in the National Institutes of Health-AARP Diet and Health Study (Lawson et al, 2007) (#295,344 men) Multivitamin supplements are used by millions of Americans because of their potential health benefits, but the relationship between multivitamin use and prostate cancer is unclear. METHODS: We prospectively investigated the association between multivitamin use and risk of prostate cancer (localized, advanced, and fatal) in **295,344 men** enrolled in **the National Institutes of Health (NIH)-AARP Diet and Health Study** who were cancer free at enrollment in 1995 and 1996. During 5 years of follow-up, 10,241 participants were diagnosed with incident prostate cancer, including 8765 localized and 1476 advanced cancers. In a separate mortality analysis with 6 years of follow-up, 179 cases of fatal prostate cancer were ascertained. Multivitamin use was assessed at baseline as part of a self-administered, mailed food-frequency questionnaire. Relative risks (RRs) and 95% confidence intervals (CIs) were calculated by use of Cox proportional hazards regression, adjusted for established or suspected prostate cancer risk factors. RESULTS: No association was observed between multivitamin use and risk of localized prostate cancer. However, *we found an increased risk of advanced and fatal prostate cancers (RR = 1.32, 95% CI = 1.04 to 1.67 and RR = 1.98, 95% CI = 1.07 to 3.66, respectively) among men reporting excessive use of multivitamins (more than seven times per week) when compared with never users.* The incidence rates per 100,000 person-years for advanced and fatal prostate cancers for those who took a multivitamin more than seven times per week were 143.8 and 18.9, respectively, compared with 113.4 and 11.4 in never users. *The positive associations with excessive multivitamin use were strongest in men with a family history of prostate cancer or who took individual micronutrient supplements, including selenium, beta-carotene, or zinc.* CONCLUSION: These results suggest that regular multivitamin use is not associated with the risk of early or localized prostate cancer. The possibility that men taking high levels of multivitamins along with other supplements have increased risk of advanced and fatal prostate cancers is of concern and merits further evaluation. (Lawson et al, 2007)

Little Evidence That Lycopene Reduces Cancer Risk (Kavanaugh et al, 2007)

According to a review conducted by the U.S. Food and Drug Administration (FDA), there is "no credible evidence" that lycopene reduces the risk of cancers such as prostate cancer, and "very limited evidence" that tomato consumption reduces risk. The review was published in the *Journal of the National Cancer Institute.* (Kavanaugh et al, 2007)

Lycopene is a carotenoid found in tomatoes and other red fruits. Some studies have suggested that lycopene or lycopene-containing foods such as tomatoes may reduce the risk of certain types of cancer, particularly prostate cancer. Other studies, however, have failed to find a link. In response to groups who wanted to make claims about the cancer benefits of lycopene or tomatoes, the FDA conducted a review of the available scientific evidence. The main conclusions of the review were the following:

· **There is no credible evidence that lycopene reduces the risk of prostate, lung, colorectal, gastric, breast, ovarian, endometrial, or pancreatic cancer.**

· **There is very limited evidence that tomato consumption reduces the risk of prostate, ovarian, gastric, and pancreatic cancer.** (Kavanaugh et al, 2007)

Effect of multivitamin and multimineral supplementation on cognitive function in men and women aged 65 years and over: a randomised controlled trial (McNeill et al, 2007) (#910) Observational studies have frequently reported an association between cognitive function and nutrition in later life but randomised trials of B vitamins and antioxidant supplements have mostly found no beneficial effect. We examined the effect of daily supplementation with 11 vitamins and 5 minerals on cognitive function in older adults to assess the possibility that this could help to prevent cognitive decline. METHODS: The study was carried out as part of a randomised double blind placebo controlled trial of micronutrient supplementation based in six primary care health centres in North East Scotland. 910 men and women aged 65 years and over living in the community were recruited and randomised: 456 to active treatment and 454 to placebo. The active treatment consisted of a single tablet containing eleven vitamins and five minerals in amounts ranging from 50-210 % of the UK Reference Nutrient Intake or matching placebo tablet taken daily for 12 months. Digit span forward and verbal fluency tests, which assess immediate memory and executive functioning respectively, were conducted at the start and end of the intervention period. Risk of micronutrient deficiency at baseline was assessed by a simple risk questionnaire. RESULTS: **For digit span forward there was no evidence of an effect of supplements in all participants or in sub-groups defined by age or risk of deficiency.** For verbal fluency there was no evidence of a beneficial effect in the whole study population but there was weak evidence for a beneficial effect of supplementation in the two pre-specified subgroups: in those aged 75 years and over (n 290; mean difference between supplemented and placebo groups 2.8 (95% CI -0.6, 6.2) units) and in those at increased risk of micronutrient deficiency assessed by the risk questionnaire (n 260; mean difference between supplemented and placebo groups 2.5 (95% CI -1.0, 6.1) units). CONCLUSION: **The results provide no evidence for a beneficial effect of daily multivitamin and multimineral supplements on these domains of cognitive function in community-living people over 65 years**. However, the possibility of beneficial effects in older people and those at greater risk of nutritional deficiency deserves further attention. (McNeill et al, 2007)

2008

Why have antioxidants failed in clinical trials? (Steinhubl, 2008)

Antioxidant therapies have been evaluated in placebo-controlled trials involving tens of thousands of patients. Despite pathophysiologic, epidemiologic, and mechanistic data suggesting otherwise, these **clinical trial results have been, to date, mostly negative in the setting of chronic preventative therapy**. On the other hand, a much smaller number of trials involving handfuls of patients have been much more encouraging in terms of the acute benefit of antioxidants reflected by the data on N-acetylcysteine. However, **the seemingly overwhelmingly data not supporting a role for antioxidants in the chronic suppression of atherosclerosis must be kept in perspective.** Most antioxidant therapies that have been tested were not chosen because they were proved to be the best antioxidants, but rather because of their easy availability. An excellent example is vitamin E. Although easily available, it has many limitations as an antioxidant. In fact, in some studies, vitamin E has been shown to have some prooxidant effects. Another possible explanation for the lack of benefit in clinical trials is that **the trials have not lasted long enough**. It may be impossible to show the benefits of antioxidant therapy over several years if the therapy is trying to reverse the results of several decades of oxidative stress. **It is critical to remember that the lack of benefits seen in clinical trials to date does not disprove the central role of oxidative stress in atherosclerosis.** Rather, these results challenge us to evaluate optimal antioxidant therapies, the ideal study patients to study, and the appropriate trial duration. (Steinhubl, 2008)

Some folks just "can not handle the truth!"

Antioxidants do not help children with Down's syndrome develop (2008) (#156) An article in Science Daily in early 2008 said giving children with Down's syndrome antioxidants and nutrients does not help their condition improve at all, according to a study published today on bmj.com.

UK researchers studied the effect of giving such supplements to **156 babies under 7 months old with Down's syndrome over an 18-month period**. Down's syndrome is the most common genetic cause of learning disability in the UK affecting around 1 in 1,000 new born babies. Previous studies have investigated the possibility that giving folate, antioxidants, or both might improve the effects of Down's syndrome, particularly language and psychomotor development.

Although none have reported any significant effect, use of vitamin and mineral supplements is widespread in children with Down's syndrome in Europe and the USA due to marketing of commercial preparations claiming substantial benefits.

In this study, the babies, from several sites in England, were split into four groups. One group was given a daily dose of antioxidants, one folinic acid, one a combination of antioxidants and folinic acid, and one a placebo. All the supplements were given in a powder that could be mixed with food or drink. After 18 months, the children remaining in the study were assessed for their mental and cognitive development.

The researchers found that giving the supplements made no difference to the biochemical outcomes in the children and did not improve their language or psychomotor development.

This study provides no evidence to support the use of antioxidant or folinic acid supplements in children with Down's syndrome, conclude the authors. Parents who choose to give supplements to their children need to weigh their hope of unproved benefits against potential adverse effects from high dose, prolonged supplementation.

These findings are supported in an accompanying editorial, which states that **until evidence of any benefit of expensive vitamin supplements is available, they cannot be recommended.**

Effect of vitamin E supplementation with standard treatment on oxidant-antioxidant status in chronic obstructive pulmonary disease (Nadeem et al, 2008) (#24)

Chronic oxidant burden and depletion of endogenous antioxidants have been proposed to play a key role in the pathogenesis of chronic obstructive pulmonary disease (COPD). Exogenous antioxidants have potential therapeutic implications and their role has not been explored in COPD. The objective of this study was to investigate the effect of supplementation of standard treatment (inhaled long-acting beta(2) agonists, anticholinergics and corticosteroids) with **vitamin E** on oxidant-antioxidant balance in patients with COPD. METHODS: The study was carried out in the outpatient setting. Patients were divided into two groups: group A- placebo group (n=14), receiving only standard therapy, and group B- vitamin E-supplemented group (n=10), receiving 400 IU of vitamin E capsules twice daily in addition to standard therapy. Spirometry and clinical assessment were carried out at the start and completion of 8 wk treatment along with measurements of several biochemical parameters of oxidant-antioxidant status in plasma, leukocytes and red cells separated from venous blood. RESULTS: Leukocyte superoxide generation was decreased in both the groups. Vitamin E-supplemented group had significantly increased levels of plasma sulphydryls and red cell catalase while the placebo group had decreased levels of plasma nitrates and nitrites. **No significant differences were observed in red cell superoxide dismutase and glutathione peroxidase activities, total blood glutathione, and plasma total antioxidant capacity, lipid peroxides and glutathione peroxidase activity in either group. There was a similar degree of lung function and clinical improvement in both the groups.** INTERPRETATION & CONCLUSION: Our findings showed that **an 8 wk supplementation of standard treatment with 400 IU twice daily of vitamin E did not provide any additional clinical benefit although it augmented certain endogenous antioxidants in patients with COPD.** (Nadeem et al, 2008)

Effect of vitamin C supplementation on lipid peroxidation, muscle damage and inflammation after 30-min exercise at 75% VO2max (Nakhostin-Roohi et al, 2008) (#16)

Hypothetically, supplementation with the antioxidant vitamins C could alleviate exercise-induced lipid peroxidation. The purpose of this study was to evaluate the effect of vitamin C supplementation on exercise-induced lipid peroxidation, muscle damage and inflammation. METHODS: **Sixteen healthy untrained male volunteers** participated in a 30-min exercise at 75% Vo2max. Subjects were randomly assigned to one of two groups: 1) placebo and 2) vitamin C (VC: 1 000 mg vitamin C). Blood samples were obtained prior to supplementation (baseline), 2 h after supplementation (immediately pre-exercise), post-exercise, 2 and 24 h after exercise. Plasma levels of VC, total antioxidant capacity (TAC), creatine kinase (CK), malondealdehyde (MDA), total leukocytes, neutrophils, lymphocytes, interleukin-6 (IL-6) and cortisol were measured. RESULTS: Plasma vitamin C concentrations increased significantly in the VC in response to supplementation and exercise ($P<0.05$). TAC decreased significantly in Placebo group 24 h after exercise compared to pre-exercise ($P<0.05$). Although MDA levels were similar between groups at baseline, it increased significantly 2 h after exercise only in the Placebo group ($P<0.05$). CK increased immediately and 2 h after exercise in both groups and 24 h after exercise only in placebo group compared to pre-exercise ($P<0.05$). Markers of inflammation (total leukocyte counts, neutrophil counts and IL-6) were increased significantly in response to the exercise (P<0.05). In VC group, there was significant increase in lymphocyte counts immediately after exercise compared with pre-exercise (P<0.05). Serum cortisol concentrations significantly declined after supplementation compared with baseline (P<0.05) as well as declined 2 and 24 h after exercise compared with immediately after exercise in VC group (P<0.05). CONCLUSION: **VC supplementation prevented endurance exercise-induced lipid peroxidation and muscle damage but had no effect on inflammatory markers.** (Nakhostin-Roohi et al, 2008). **This study illustrates the unpredictability of the antioxidant vitamin C.**

Vitamins, minerals and race performance in ultra-endurance runners--Deutschlandlauf 2006 (Knechtle et al, 2008) (#20)

We investigated the effect of pre-race intake of vitamins and minerals, in the form of supplementation, before a multi-stage ultra-endurance run and their effect on race performance. At the Deutschlandlauf 2006 in Germany, where athletes had to run across Germany from the north (Kap Arkona-Rügen) to the south (Lörrach) over 1,200 km within 17 consecutive stages, **twenty male ultra runners** (46.2+/-9.6 years, 71.8+/-5.2 kg, 179+/-6 cm, BMI 22.5+/-1.9 kg/m2) completed a questionnaire about their intake of vitamin and mineral supplements in the four weeks before the race. Race performance of athletes with- and athletes without regular intake of these supplements were compared. In the four weeks before the run, nine runners (45%) ingested vitamin- and twelve athletes (60%) mineral supplements. **Athletes with an intake of vitamins (152.8+/-14.1 h versus 160.6+/-14.6 h, p>0.05) and minerals (151.6+/-14.5 h versus 165.3+/-10.8 h, p>0.05) finished the race no faster than athletes without an intake of vitamins and minerals.** We concluded that in the Deutschlandlauf 2006 of over 1,200 km within 17 consecutive stages, **athletes with a regular intake of vitamin and mineral supplements in the four weeks before the race finished the competition no faster than athletes without an intake of vitamins and minerals.** (Knechtle et al, 2008)

Results of a Randomized Clinical Trial of the Action of Several Doses of Lycopene in Localized Prostate Cancer: Administration Prior to Radical Prostatectomy (Kumar et al, 2008) (#45)

The purpose of this **Phase II randomized-controlled trial** was to evaluate the safety and effect of administering several doses of lycopene to men with clinically localized prostate cancer, on intermediate endpoint biomarkers implicated in prostate carcinogenesis. METHODS: **Forty-five eligible men with clinically localized prostate cancer were supplemented with 15, 30 or 45 mg of lycopene or no supplement** from biopsy to prostatectomy. Compliance to study agent, toxicity, changes in plasma lycopene, serum steroid hormones, PSA and tissue Ki-67 were analyzed from baseline to completion of intervention. RESULTS: **Forty-two of forty-five**

five subjects completed the intervention for approximately 30 days from the time of biopsy until prostatectomy. Plasma lycopene increased from baseline to post treatment in all treatment groups with greatest increase observed in the 45 mg lycopene-supplemented arm compared to the control arm without producing any toxicity. Overall, subjects with prostate cancer had lower baseline levels of plasma lycopene similar to those observed in previous studies in men with prostate cancer. **Serum free testosterone decreased with 30 mg lycopene supplementation** and **total estradiol increased significantly** with 30 mg and 45 mg supplementation from baseline to end of treatment, **with no significant increases in serum PSA or tissue Ki-67. These changes were not significant compared to the control arm for this sample size and duration of intervention.** CONCLUSIONS: **Although antioxidant properties of lycopene have been hypothesized to be primarily responsible for its beneficial effects,** our study suggests that **other mechanisms mediated by steroid hormones may also be involved.** (Kumar et al, 2008)

The association of folate, zinc and antioxidant intake with sperm aneuploidy in healthy non-smoking men (Young et al, 2008) (#89)

Little is known about the effect of paternal nutrition on aneuploidy in sperm. We investigated the association of normal dietary and supplement intake of folate, zinc and antioxidants (vitamin C, vitamin E and beta-carotene) with the frequency of aneuploidy in human sperm. METHODS: Sperm samples from **89 healthy, non-smoking men** from a non-clinical setting were analysed for aneuploidy using fluorescent in situ hybridization with probes for chromosomes X, Y and 21. Daily total intake (diet and supplements) for zinc, folate, vitamin C, vitamin E and beta-carotene was derived from a food frequency questionnaire. Potential confounders were obtained from a self-administered questionnaire. RESULTS: After adjusting for covariates, men with high folate intake (>75th percentile) had lower frequencies of sperm with disomies X, 21, sex nullisomy, and a lower aggregate measure of sperm aneuploidy (P <or= 0.04) compared with men with lower intake. In adjusted continuous analyses, total folate intake was inversely associated with aggregate sperm aneuploidy (-3.6% change/100 microg folate; 95% CI: -6.3, -0.8) and results were similar for disomies X, 21 and sex nullisomy. **No consistent associations were found between antioxidant or zinc intakes and sperm aneuploidy.** CONCLUSIONS: Men with high folate intake had lower overall frequencies of several types of aneuploid sperm. (Young et al, 2008)

Vitamin E fails in Alzheimer's disease and mild cognitive impairment 2008 (Isaac et al, 2008, CD002854)

Vitamin E is a dietary compound that functions as an antioxidant scavenging toxic free radicals. Evidence that free radicals may contribute to the pathological processes of cognitive impairment including Alzheimer's disease (AD) has led to interest in the use of Vitamin E in the treatment of Alzheimer's disease and Mild Cognitivie Impairment (MCI). OBJECTIVES: To assess the efficacy of Vitamin E in the treatment of Alzheimer's disease and prevention of progression of Mild Cognitive Impairment to Alzheimer's disease. SEARCH STRATEGY: **The Cochrane Dementia and Cognitive Improvement's Specialized Register** was searched on 8 January 2007 using the following terms: "Vitamin E", vitamin-E, alpha-tocopherol. The **CDCIG Registers** contains records from major health care databases and ongoing trial databases and is updated regularly. SELECTION CRITERIA: All unconfounded, double blind, randomized trials in which treatment with Vitamin E at any dose was compared with placebo for patients with Alzheimer's disease or Mild Cognitive Impairment. DATA COLLECTION AND ANALYSIS: Two reviewers independently applied the selection criteria and assessed study quality and extracted and analysed the data. For each outcome measure data were sought on every patient randomized. Where such data were not available an analysis of patients who completed treatment was conducted. MAIN RESULTS: Only 2 studies met the inclusion criteria. The primary outcome used in the AD study was survival time to the first of 4 endpoints: death, institutionalisation, loss of 2 out of 3 basic activities of daily living and severe dementia (defined as a global Clinical Dementia Rating of 3). The investigators reported the total numbers in each group who reached the primary endpoint within two years for participants completing the study ("completers"). There appeared to be some benefit from Vitamin E with fewer participants reaching endpoint - 58% (45/77) of completers compared with 74% (58/78) - a Peto odds ratio of 0.49, 95% confidence interval 0.25 to 0.96. However, more participants taking Vitamin E suffered a fall (12/77 compared with 4/78; odds ratio 3.07, 95% CI 1.09 to 8.62). It was not possible to interpret the reported results for specific endpoints or for secondary outcomes of cognition, dependence, behavioral disturbance and activities of daily living. The primary outcome used in the MCI study which had 769 participants (257 in the Vitamin E group and 259 in the placebo group; a third Donepezil group of 253 was not included in this review) was the time to progression from MCI to possible or probable AD. A total of 214 of the 769 participants had progression to dementia, with 212 being classified as having possible or probable AD. **There was no significant difference in the probability of progression from MCI to AD between the Vitamin E group and the placebo group.** There was no significant difference between the placebo group and the Vitamin E group in adverse events. Five subjects died in each group and 72 discontinued treatment in the Vitamin E group and 66 in the placebo group. AUTHORS' CONCLUSIONS: **There is no evidence of efficacy of Vitamin E in the prevention or treatment of people with AD or MCI.** More research is needed to identify the role of Vitamin E, if any, in the management of cognitive impairment. (Isaac et al, 2008, CD002854)

Ginkgo biloba for prevention of dementia. (DeKosky et al, 2008) (#3,069)

Ginkgo biloba is widely used for its potential effects on memory and cognition. To date, adequately powered clinical trials testing the effect of *G biloba* on dementia incidence are lacking. **Objective** To determine effectiveness of *G biloba* vs placebo in reducing the incidence of all-cause dementia and Alzheimer disease (AD) in elderly individuals with normal cognition and those with mild cognitive impairment (MCI). **Design, Setting, and Participants** Randomized, double-blind, placebo-controlled clinical trial conducted in 5 academic medical centers in the United States between 2000 and 2008 with a median follow-up of 6.1 years. Three thousand sixty-nine community volunteers aged 75 years or older with normal cognition (n = 2587) or MCI (n = 482) at study entry were assessed every 6 months for incident dementia. **Intervention** Twice-daily dose of 120-mg extract of *G biloba* (n = 1545) or placebo (n = 1524). **Main Outcome Measures** Incident dementia and AD determined by expert panel consensus. **Results** Five hundred twenty-three individuals developed dementia (246 receiving placebo and 277 receiving *G biloba*) with 92% of the dementia cases classified as possible or probable AD, or AD with evidence of vascular disease of the brain. Rates of dropout and loss to follow-up were low (6.3%), and the adverse effect profiles were similar for both groups. The overall dementia rate was 3.3 per 100 person-years in participants assigned to *G biloba* and 2.9 per 100 person-years in the placebo group. The hazard ratio (HR) for *G biloba* compared with placebo for all-cause dementia was 1.12 (95% confidence interval [CI], 0.94-1.33; P = .21) and for AD, 1.16 (95% CI, 0.97-1.39; P = .11). *G biloba* **also had no effect on the rate of progression to dementia in participants with MCI** (HR, 1.13; 95% CI, 0.85-1.50; P = .39). **Conclusions** In this study, *G biloba* **at 120 mg twice a day was not effective in reducing either the overall incidence rate of dementia or AD incidence in elderly individuals with normal cognition or those with MCI.** (DeKosky et al, 2008)

Antioxidants in central nervous system diseases: preclinical promise and translational challenges (Kamat et al, 2008)

Oxidative damage is allegedly strongly implicated in the pathogenesis of neurodegenerative diseases including Alzheimer's disease, amyotrophic lateral sclerosis, Huntington's disease, Parkinson's disease and stroke (brain ischemia/reperfusion injury).

The availability of transgenic and toxin-inducible models of these conditions has facilitated the preclinical evaluation of putative antioxidant agents ranging from prototypic natural antioxidants such as vitamin E (alpha-tocopherol) to sophisticated synthetic free radical traps and catalytic oxidants. **Literature review shows that antioxidant therapies have enjoyed general success in preclinical studies across disparate animal models, but little benefit in human intervention studies or clinical trials.**

Recent high-profile failures of vitamin E trials in Parkinson's disease, and nitrone therapies in stroke, have diminished enthusiasm to pursue antioxidant neuroprotectants in the clinic. The translational disappointment of antioxidants likely arises from a combination of factors including failure to understand the drug candidate's mechanism of action in relationship to human disease, and failure to conduct preclinical studies using concentration and time parameters relevant to the clinical setting. This review discusses the rationale for using antioxidants in the prophylaxis or mitigation of human neurodiseases, with a critical discussion regarding ways in which future preclinical studies may be adjusted to offer more predictive value in selecting agents for translation into human trials. (Kamat et al, 2008)

Vitamin E for Alzheimer's disease and mild cognitive impairment (Isaac et al, 2008 CD002854) (#769) Vitamin E is a dietary compound that functions as an antioxidant scavenging toxic free radicals. Evidence that free radicals may contribute to the pathological processes of cognitive impairment including Alzheimer's disease (AD) has led to interest in the use of Vitamin E in the treatment of Alzheimer's disease and Mild Cognitivie Impairment (MCI). OBJECTIVES: To assess the efficacy of Vitamin E in the treatment of Alzheimer's disease and prevention of progression of Mild Cognitive Impairment to Alzheimer's disease. SEARCH STRATEGY: The Cochrane Dementia and Cognitive Improvement's Specialized Register was searched on 8 January 2007 using the following terms: "Vitamin E", vitamin-E, alpha-tocopherol. The CDCIG Registers contains records from major health care databases and ongoing trial databases and is updated regularly. SELECTION CRITERIA: All unconfounded, double blind, randomized trials in which treatment with Vitamin E at any dose was compared with placebo for patients with Alzheimer's disease or Mild Cognitive Impairment. DATA COLLECTION AND ANALYSIS: Two reviewers independently applied the selection criteria and assessed study quality and extracted and analysed the data. For each outcome measure data were sought on every patient randomized. Where such data were not available an analysis of patients who completed treatment was conducted. MAIN RESULTS: Only 2 studies met the inclusion criteria. The primary outcome used in the AD study was survival time to the first of 4 endpoints: death, institutionalisation, loss of 2 out of 3 basic activities of daily living and severe dementia (defined as a global Clinical Dementia Rating of 3). The investigators reported the total numbers in each group who reached the primary endpoint within two years for participants completing the study ("completers"). There appeared to be some benefit from Vitamin E with fewer participants reaching endpoint - 58% (45/77) of completers compared with 74% (58/78) - a Peto odds ratio of 0.49, 95% confidence interval 0.25 to 0.96. However, more participants taking Vitamin E suffered a fall (12/77 compared with 4/78; odds ratio 3.07, 95% CI 1.09 to 8.62). It was not possible to interpret the reported results for specific endpoints or for secondary outcomes of cognition, dependence, behavioral disturbance and activities of daily living. The primary outcome used in the MCI study which had 769 participants (257 in the Vitamin E group and 259 in the placebo group; a third Donepezil group of 253 was not included in this review) was the time to progression from MCI to possible or probable AD. A total of 214 of the 769 participants had progression to dementia, with 212 being classified as having possible or probable AD. **There was no significant difference in the probability of progression from MCI to AD between the Vitamin E group and the placebo group.** There was no significant difference between the placebo group and the Vitamin E group in adverse events. Five subjects died in each group and 72 discontinued treatment in the Vitamin E group and 66 in the placebo group. AUTHORS' CONCLUSIONS: **There is no evidence of efficacy of Vitamin E in the prevention or treatment of people with AD or MCI.** More research is needed to identify the role of Vitamin E, if any, in the management of cognitive impairment. (Isaac et al, 2008 CD002854)

Does taking vitamin, mineral and fatty acid supplements prevent cognitive decline? A systematic review of randomized controlled trials (Jia et al, 2008) (#3,442)   Observational studies have shown associations between nutritional status and cognition in later life but evidence from intervention studies is unclear. The present study systematically reviewed the evidence on the effect of nutrient supplementation on cognitive function in people aged >or=65 years. METHODS: Databases including MEDLINE and EMBASE were searched up to 1 September 2006. Randomized controlled trials using at least one kind of vitamin, mineral or omega-3 fatty acid, evaluating standardized neuropsychological test(s), were included. There were no restrictions on participants' baseline nutritional status or cognitive function. Quality assessment and data abstraction were conducted by one author and checked by another. RESULTS: Of 4229 articles retrieved, 22 trials **(3442 participants)** were identified. Many were small, short duration and of poor methodology. Only 16 out of 122 cognitive tests were significantly different between groups. **A meta-analysis showed no significant effect of taking B vitamins or antioxidant vitamins on global cognitive function.**

There was insufficient evidence to evaluate the effect of omega-3 fatty acids on any cognitive domains.

CONCLUSION: **There was little evidence of a beneficial effect from taking B vitamins or antioxidant supplements on global cognitive function in later life.** Larger-scale randomized controlled trials of longer duration in selected age groups are needed. (Jia et al, 2008)

2009

A recent cross-sectional survey of healthy young adults of the Toronto Nutrigenomics and Health (TNH) Study reported that **one out of seven individuals is deficient in serum ascorbic acid.** (Cahill et al, 2009)

Oral antioxidants and cardiovascular health in the exercise-trained and untrained elderly: a radically different outcome (Wray, 2009) (#6)

Both antioxidant supplementation and exercise training have been identified as interventions which may reduce oxidative stress and thus improve cardiovascular health, but the interaction of these interventions on arterial BP (blood pressure) and vascular function has not been studied in older humans. Thus in **six older (71+/-2 years) mildly hypertensive men**, arterial BP was evaluated non-invasively at rest and during small muscle mass (knee-extensor) exercise with and without a pharmacological dose of oral antioxidants **(vitamins C and E, and alpha-lipoic acid).** The efficacy of the antioxidant intervention to decrease the plasma free radical concentration was verified via EPR (electron paramagnetic resonance) spectroscopy, while changes in endothelial function in response to exercise training and antioxidant administration were evaluated via FMD (flow-mediated vasodilation). Subjects were re-evaluated **after a 6-week aerobic exercise** training programme. Prior to training, acute antioxidant administration did not change resting arterial BP or FMD. Six weeks of knee-extensor exercise training reduced systolic BP (from 150+/-8 mmHg at pre-training to 138+/-3 mmHg at post-training) and diastolic BP (from 91+/-5 mmHg at pre-training to 79+/-3 mmHg at post-training), and improved FMD (1.5+/-1 to 4.9+/-1% for pre- and post-training respectively). **However, *antioxidant administration after exercise training negated these improvements, returning subjects to a hypertensive state and blunting training-induced improvements in FMD*.** In conclusion, **the paradoxical effects of these interventions suggest a need for caution when exercise and acute antioxidant supplementation are combined in elderly mildly hypertensive individuals.** (Wray et al, 2009)

Increased lipid peroxidation in trained men after 2 weeks of antioxidant supplementation (Lamprecht et al, 2009) (#8)

To assess the effects of an encapsulated antioxidant concentrate (EAC) and exercise on lipid peroxidation (LIPOX) and the plasma antioxidant enzyme glutathione peroxidase (Pl-GPx). METHODS: **Eight trained male cyclists** (VO2max > 55 ml x kg(-1) x min(-1)) participated in this randomized, placebo-controlled, double-blinded, crossover study and undertook 4 cycle-ergometer bouts: 2 moderate exercise bouts over 90 min at 45% of individual VO2max and 2 strenuous exercise bouts at 75% of individual VO2max for 30 min. The first 2 exercise tests--1 moderate and 1 strenuous-were conducted after 4 weeks wash-out and after 12 and 14 days of EAC (107 IU vitamin E, 450 mg vitamin C, 36 mg beta-carotene, 100 microg selenium) or placebo treatment. After another 4 weeks wash-out, participants were given the opposite capsule treatment and repeated the 2 exercise tests. Physical exercise training was equal across the whole study period, and nutrition was standardized by a menu plan the week before the tests. Blood was collected before exercise, immediately postexercise, and 30 min and 60 min after each test. Plasma samples were analyzed for LIPOX marker malondialdehyde (MDA) and the antioxidant enzyme pl-GPx. RESULTS: MDA concentrations were significantly increased after EAC supplementation at rest before exercise and after moderate exercise (p < .05). MDA concentrations showed no differences between treatments after strenuous exercise (p > .1). Pl-GPx concentrations decreased at all time points of measurement after EAC treatment (p < .05). CONCLUSIONS: **The EAC** induced an increase of **LIPOX** as indicated by **MDA** and decreased **pl-GPx** concentrations pre- and postexercise. (Lamprecht et al, 2009). **In this case, the antioxidants vitamins acted to stimulate prooxidant effects.**

Antioxidants do not prevent postexercise peroxidation and may delay muscle recovery (Teixeira et al, 2009) (#20)

This study aimed to determine the effects of 4 wk of antioxidants (AOX) supplementation on exercise-induced lipid peroxidation, muscle damage, and inflammation in kayakers. METHODS: **Subjects (n = 20)** were randomly assigned to receive a placebo (PLA) or an AOX capsule (AOX; 272 mg of alpha-tocopherol, 400 mg of vitamin C, 30 mg of beta-carotene, 2 mg of lutein, 400 mug of selenium, 30 mg of zinc, and 600 mg of magnesium). Blood samples were collected at rest and 15 min after a 1000-m kayak race, both before and after the supplementation period, for analysis of alpha-tocopherol, alpha-carotene, beta-carotene, lycopene, lutein plus zeaxanthin, vitamin C, uric acid, total AOX status (TAS), thiobarbituric reactive acid substances (TBARS) and interleukin-6 (IL-6) levels, and creatine kinase (CK), superoxide dismutase (SOD), glutathione reductase (Gr), and glutathione peroxidase (GPx) activities. RESULTS: With supplementation, plasma alpha-tocopherol ($P = 0.003$) and beta-carotene ($P = 0.007$) augmented significantly in the AOX group. IL-6 (exercise, $P = 0.039$), TBARS (exercise, $P < 0.001$), and uric acid (exercise, $P = 0.032$) increased significantly in response to the exercise regardless of treatment group. Cortisol level raised more from pre- to post-supplementation period in the PLA group (time x supplementation, $P = 0.002$). Although TAS declined after exercise before intervention, it increased above preexercise values after the 4-wk period in the AOX group (supplementation x time x exercise, $P = 0.034$). CK increased after exercise in both groups (exercise effect, $P < 0.001$) and decreased from week 0 to week 4 more markedly in the PLA group (supplementation x time, $P = 0.049$). CONCLUSIONS: **AOX supplementation does not offer protection against exercise-induced lipid peroxidation and inflammation** and *may hinder the recovery of muscle damage.* (Teixeira et al, 2009)

American College of Sports Medicine position stand. Nutrition and athletic performance - 2009 (Rodriguez et al, 2009)

It is the position of the American Dietetic Association, Dietitians of Canada, and the American College of Sports Medicine that physical activity, athletic performance, and recovery from exercise are enhanced by optimal nutrition. These organizations recommend appropriate selection of foods and fluids, timing of intake, and supplement choices for optimal health and exercise performance. This updated position paper couples a rigorous, systematic, evidence-based analysis of nutrition and performance-specific literature with current scientific data related to energy needs, assessment of body composition, strategies for weight change, nutrient and fluid needs, special nutrient needs during training and competition, the use of supplements and ergogenic aids, nutrition recommendations for vegetarian athletes, and the roles and responsibilities of the sports dietitian. Energy and macronutrient needs, especially carbohydrate and protein, must be met during times of high physical activity to maintain body weight, replenish glycogen stores, and provide adequate protein to build and repair tissue. Fat intake should be sufficient to provide the essential fatty acids and fat-soluble vitamins and to contribute energy for weight maintenance. Although exercise performance can be affected by body weight and composition, these physical measures should not be a criterion for sports performance and daily weigh-ins are discouraged. Adequate food and fluid should be consumed before, during, and after exercise to help maintain blood glucose concentration during exercise, maximize exercise performance, and improve recovery time. Athletes should be well hydrated before exercise and drink enough fluid during and after exercise to balance fluid losses. Sports beverages containing carbohydrates and electrolytes may be consumed before, during, and after exercise to help maintain blood glucose concentration, provide fuel for muscles, and decrease risk of dehydration and hyponatremia. **Vitamin and mineral supplements are not needed if adequate energy to maintain body weight is consumed from a variety of foods**. However, athletes who restrict energy intake, use severe weight-loss practices, eliminate one or more food groups from their diet, or consume unbalanced diets with low micronutrient density may require supplements. Because regulations specific to nutritional ergogenic aids are poorly enforced, they should be used with caution and only after careful product evaluation for safety, efficacy, potency, and legality. A qualified sports dietitian and, in particular, the Board Certified Specialist in Sports Dietetics in the United States, should provide individualized nutrition direction and advice after a comprehensive nutrition assessment. (Rodriguez et al, 2009)

Does antioxidant vitamin supplementation protect against muscle damage? (McGinley et al, 2009) The high forces undergone during repetitive eccentric, or lengthening, contractions place skeletal muscle under considerable stress, in particular if unaccustomed. Although muscle is highly adaptive, the responses to stress may not be optimally regulated by the body. Reactive oxygen species (ROS, EMODs) are one component of the stress response that may contribute to muscle damage after eccentric exercise. Antioxidants may in turn scavenge ROS, thereby preventing or attenuating muscle damage. **The antioxidant vitamins C (ascorbic acid) and E (tocopherol) are among the most commonly used sport supplements, and are often taken in large doses by athletes and other sportspersons because of their potential protective effect against muscle damage.** This review assesses studies that have investigated the effects of these two antioxidants, alone or in combination, on muscle damage and oxidative stress. Studies have used a variety of supplementation strategies, with variations in dosage, timing and duration of supplementation. Although there is some evidence to show that both antioxidants can reduce indices of oxidative stress, **there is little evidence to support a role for vitamin C and/or vitamin E in protecting against muscle damage. Indeed, antioxidant supplementation may actually interfere with the cellular signaling functions of ROS, thereby**

adversely affecting muscle performance. Furthermore, **recent studies have cast doubt on the benign effects of long-term, high-dosage antioxidant supplementation.** High doses of vitamin E, in particular, may increase all-cause mortality. **Although some equivocation remains in the extant literature regarding the beneficial effects of antioxidant vitamin supplementation on muscle damage, there is little evidence to support such a role. Since the potential for long-term harm does exist, the casual use of high doses of antioxidants by athletes and others should perhaps be curtailed.** (McGinley et al, 2009)

Acute exercise and oxidative stress: a 30 year history

The topic of exercise-induced oxidative stress has received considerable attention in recent years, with close to 300 original investigations published since the early work of Dillard and colleagues in 1978. **Single bouts of aerobic and anaerobic exercise can induce an acute state of oxidative stress.** This is indicated by an increased presence of oxidized molecules in a variety of tissues. Exercise mode, intensity, and duration, as well as the subject population tested, all can impact the extent of oxidation. Moreover, **the use of antioxidant supplements can impact the findings. Although a single bout of exercise often leads to an acute oxidative stress, in accordance with the principle of hormesis, such an increase appears necessary** to allow for an up-regulation in endogenous antioxidant defenses. This review presents a comprehensive summary of original investigations focused on exercise-induced oxidative stress. (Fisher-Willman, bloomer, 2009)

The mitochondrial theory of aging: Insight from transgenic and knockout mouse models (Youngmok et al. 2009)

A substantial body of evidence has accumulated over the past 35 years in support of a role for oxidative damage to the mitochondrial respiratory chain and mitochondrial DNA in the determination of mammalian lifespan. The goal of this review is to provide a concise summary of recent studies using transgenic and knockout mouse models with altered expression of mitochondrial antioxidant enzymes (MnSOD ($Sod2Tg$ and $Sod2^{+/-}$), thioredoxin 2 ($Trx2^{+/-}$), mitochondrial targeted catalase (mCAT) and mutant mice models that have been genetically manipulated to increase mitochondrial deletions or mutations ($Poly^{D257A/D257A}$ mutant mice) to examine the role of mitochondrial oxidative stress in aging. **The majority of studies using these strategies do not support a clear role for mitochondrial oxidative stress or a vicious cycle of oxidative damage in the determination of lifespan in mice and furthermore do not support the free radical theory of aging.** However, several key questions remain to be addressed and clearly more studies are required to fully understand the role of mitochondria in age-related disease and aging. (Youngmok et al. 2009)

Is there a benefit from lycopene supplementation in men with prostate cancer? A systematic review (Haseen et al, 2009) Lycopene has a chemopreventive effect against prostate cancer but its role in prostate cancer progression is unknown; many patients increase their intake of lycopene, although there are no evidence-based guidelines to suggest an effect. Our objective was to conduct a systematic review of literature to evaluate the association between lycopene intake and prostate cancer progression. MEDLINE, EMBASE CINAHL Plus, Web of Science, AMED and CENTRAL databases were systematically searched using terms for lycopene and prostate cancer progression to identify studies published before January 2009. Eight intervention studies were identified (five with no control group; one with an unmatched control group; and two randomized controlled trials (RCTs)). An inverse association was observed between lycopene intake and PSA levels in six studies. The rates of progression measured by bone scan in one RCT were lower in the intervention group. Lycopene resulted in lowering cancer-related symptoms (pain, urinary tract symptoms), and severe toxicity or intolerance was not evident. However, **the evidence available to date is insufficient to draw a firm conclusion with respect to lycopene supplementation in prostate cancer patients and larger RCTs are required in broader patient groups.** (Haseen et al, 2009)

Are the health attributes of lycopene related to its antioxidant function? (Erdman et al, 2009) A variety of epidemiological trials have suggested that higher intake of lycopene-containing foods (primarily tomato products) or blood lycopene concentrations are associated with decreased cardiovascular disease and prostate cancer risk. Of the carotenoids tested, lycopene has been demonstrated to be the most potent in vitro antioxidant leading many researchers to conclude that the antioxidant properties of lycopene are responsible for disease prevention. In our review of human and animal trials with lycopene, or lycopene-containing extracts, **there is limited support for the in vivo antioxidant function for lycopene. Moreover, tissue levels of lycopene appear to be too low to play a meaningful antioxidant role.** We conclude that there is an overall shortage of supportive evidence for the "antioxidant hypothesis" as lycopene's major in vivo mechanism of action. Our laboratory has postulated that **metabolic products of lycopene, the lycopenoids, may be responsible for some of lycopene's reported bioactivity (not its antioxidant character).** (Erdman et al, 2009)

Stroke: roles of B vitamins, homocysteine and antioxidants (Sanchez-Moreno et al, 2009)

In the present review concerning stroke, we evaluate the roles of B vitamins, - homocysteine and antioxidant vitamins. Stroke is a leading cause of death in developed countries. However, current therapeutic strategies for stroke have been largely unsuccessful. Several studies have reported important benefits on reducing the risk of stroke and improving the post-stroke-associated functional declines in patients who ate foods rich in micronutrients, including B vitamins and antioxidant vitamins E and C. Folic acid, vitamin B6 and vitamin B12 are all cofactors in homocysteine metabolism. Growing interest has been paid to hyperhomocysteinaemia as a risk factor for CVD. Hyperhomocysteinaemia has been linked to inadequate intake of vitamins, particularly to B-group vitamins and therefore may be amenable to nutritional intervention. Hence, poor dietary intake of folate, vitamin B6 and vitamin B12 are associated with increased risk of stroke. Elevated consumption of fruits and vegetables appears to protect against stroke. Antioxidant nutrients have important roles in cell function and have been implicated in processes associated with ageing, including vascular, inflammatory and neurological damage. Plasma vitamin E and C concentrations may serve as a biological marker of lifestyle or other factors associated with reduced stroke risk and may be useful in identifying those at high risk of stroke. After reviewing the observational and intervention studies, **there is an incomplete understanding of mechanisms and some conflicting findings; therefore the available evidence is insufficient to recommend the routine use of B vitamins, vitamin E and vitamin C for the prevention of stroke.** A better understanding of mechanisms, along with well-designed controlled clinical trials will allow further progress in this area. (Sanchez-Moreno et al, 2009)

2010

Null activity of selenium and vitamin E as cancer chemopreventive agents in the rat prostate (McCormick et al, 2010)

To evaluate the potential efficacy of selenium and vitamin E as inhibitors of prostate carcinogenesis, four chemoprevention studies using a common protocol were done in a rat model of androgen-dependent prostate cancer. After stimulation of prostate epithelial cell proliferation by a sequential regimen of cyproterone acetate followed by testosterone propionate, male Wistar-Unilever rats received a single i.v. injection of N-methyl-N-nitrosourea (MNU) followed by chronic androgen stimulation via subcutaneous implantation of testosterone pellets. At 1 week post-MNU, groups of carcinogen-treated rats (39-44/group) were fed either a basal diet or a basal diet supplemented with l-selenomethionine (3 or 1.5 mg/kg diet; study 1), dl-alpha-tocopherol (vitamin E, 4,000 or 2,000 mg/kg diet; study 2), l-selenomethionine + vitamin E (3 + 2,000 mg/kg diet or 3 + 500 mg/kg diet; study 3), or selenized yeast (target selenium levels of 9 or 3 mg/kg diet; study 4). Each chemoprevention study was terminated at 13 months post-MNU, and prostate cancer incidence was determined by histopathologic evaluation. **No statistically significant reductions in prostate cancer incidence were identified in any group receiving dietary supplementation with selenium and/or vitamin E.**

These data do not support the hypotheses that selenium and vitamin E are potent cancer chemopreventive agents in the prostate, and when considered with the recent clinical data reported in the Selenium and Vitamin E Cancer Prevention Trial (SELECT), show the predictive nature of this animal model for human prostate cancer chemoprevention. (McCormick et al, 2010) Life Sciences Research, IIT Research Institute, 10 West 35th Street, Chicago, IL USA.

The Selenium and Vitamin E Cancer Prevention Trial (SELECT), using oral selenium and vitamin E supplementation in disease-free volunteers, was designed to test a prostate cancer chemoprevention hypothesis. SELECT was terminated early because of both safety concerns and negative data for the formulations and doses given.

Selenomethionine and alpha-tocopherol do not inhibit prostate carcinogenesis in the testosterone plus estradiol-treated NBL rat model (Ozten et al, 2010)

Previous studies with selenium and/or vitamin E in prostate carcinogenesis animal models have been negative, but these models may not involve oxidative stress mechanisms. In this study, we examined the potential of selenomethionine and alpha-tocopherol to modulate prostate cancer development in the testosterone plus estradiol-treated NBL rat, a model that does involve sex hormone-induced oxidative stress mechanisms and prostatic inflammation. One week following the implantation with hormone-filled Silastic implants, rats were fed diets containing l-selenomethionine (1.5 or 3.0 mg/kg), DL-alpha-tocopherol acetate (2,000 or 4,000 mg/kg), or a natural ingredient control diet (NIH-07). **The development of prostate carcinomas was not affected by dietary treatment with either agent.** Food intake, body weight, and mortality were also not affected. The high dose of selenomethionine reduced the severity of epithelial dysplasia in the lateral prostate that was not associated with inflammation, and alpha-tocopherol reduced in a dose-related fashion the incidence of marked inflammation and marked epithelial dysplasia in the lateral prostate, regardless of whether these lesions were associated with inflammation. *alpha-Tocopherol significantly increased the incidence of adenocarcinomas of the mammary glands at both dietary concentrations.*

Collectively, **our findings suggest that selenomethionine and alpha-tocopherol supplementation does not prevent prostate cancer in rats fed diets with nutritionally adequate levels of selenium and vitamin E.** Importantly, **the results of the current animal studies and those reported previously were fully predictive of the outcome of the Selenium and Vitamin E Cancer Prevention Trial.** (Ozten et al, 2010) Department of Pathology, University of Illinois at Chicago.

Systematic review on "vitamin E and prevention of colorectal cancer"
(Arain, Abdul Qadeer, 2010) (#94,069)

Colorectal cancers (CRC) are highly prevalent cancer all over the world and need appropriate and timely prevention and treatment. Since years it has been argued that antioxidant vitamins have a potential role in the prevention of several neoplasm including colorectal cancer though the answer remained controversial. Most of the observational studies in past have shown that Vitamin E has some protective effect in the primary prevention of colorectal cancer, however its exact role is not yet established. On the other hand recently conducted experimental studies have shown variable results regarding the role of vitamin E in preventing colorectal cancers. Thus this review was conducted to study the role of vitamin E in preventing colorectal neoplasm. This review study was conducted from September 2008 to February 2009. We searched multiple electronic sources including (PUBMED) MEDLINE, Cochrane Database for identifying existing Systematic Reviews, OVID data base and other library sources to identify relevant studies for this review. Data was collected using data extraction form. Meta analysis was performed in Review Manager version 4.3. **We identified four trials on vitamin E role for primary prevention of CRC, includes 94,069 participants (47029 in vitamin E Vs 47040 in placebo), aged 40 years or above, who were randomized to vitamin E supplement versus placebo.** The outcome measure in our review was incidence of colorectal cancer in the follow up period of 7 to 10 years. We found no sufficient evidence of vitamin E role for decreasing risk of CRC incidence (RR: 0.89, CI: 0.76, 1.05; p-value = 0.18). It has been identified in the review that **Vitamin E does not have protective role in the prevention of colorectal cancer.** Further studies on diverse population are required to determine the role vitamin E for the primary prevention of colorectal cancer. (Arain, Abdul Qadeer, 2010)

Semen quality and sperm DNA damage in relation to urinary bisphenol A among men from an infertility clinic (Meeker et al, 2010) (#190)

Bisphenol A (BPA) (an antioxidant) impairs spermatogenesis in animals, but human studies are lacking. We measured urinary BPA concentrations, semen quality, and sperm DNA damage (comet assay) in 190 men recruited through an infertility clinic. BPA was detected in 89% of samples, with a median (interquartile range [IQR]) concentration of 1.3 (0.8-2.5) ng/mL. Urinary BPA concentration was associated with slightly elevated, though not statistically significant, odds for below reference sperm concentration, motility, and morphology. When modeled as continuous dependent variables, an IQR increase in urinary BPA concentration was associated with declines in sperm concentration, motility, and morphology of 23% (95%CI -40%, -0.3%), 7.5% (-17%, +1.5%), and 13% (-26%, -0.1%), respectively, along with a 10% (0.03%, 19%) increase in sperm DNA damage measured as the percentage of DNA in comet tail. In conclusion, *urinary BPA may be associated with declined semen quality and increased sperm DNA damage*, but confirmatory studies are needed. (Meeker et al, 2010)

Antioxidant intake and risks of rheumatoid arthritis and systemic lupus erythematosus in women (Costenbader et al, 2010) (Nurses' Health Study and Nurses' Health Study II)

Antioxidants may protect against development of rheumatoid arthritis or systemic lupus erythematosus by combating oxidative stress. The authors identified and confirmed incident cases of rheumatoid arthritis and systemic lupus erythematosus among 184,643 US women followed in the **Nurses' Health Study and Nurses' Health Study II** cohorts in 1980-2004. Semiquantitative food frequency questionnaires assessed intakes of vitamins A, C, and E and alpha-carotene, beta-carotene, beta-cryptoxanthin, lycopene, lutein, and zeaxanthin from foods and supplements. The authors examined total antioxidant intake by calculating a "ferric-reducing ability of plasma" score, a new method for quantifying the total antioxidant effect of a food based on the reduction of ferric to ferrous iron by antioxidants. Cumulative updated total energy-adjusted dietary intakes were used. Associations between intake of each nutrient and incident rheumatoid arthritis and systemic lupus erythematosus were examined in age-adjusted and Cox proportional hazards models, adjusted for confounders. Results from the cohorts were pooled meta-analytically by using random-effects models. The authors identified 787 incident rheumatoid arthritis cases and 192 systemic lupus erythematosus cases for whom prospective dietary information was available. **In these large, prospective cohorts of women, antioxidant intake was not associated with the risk of developing either rheumatoid arthritis or systemic lupus erythematosus.** (Costenbader et al, 2010)

2011

Use of vitamin supplements and risk of total cancer and cardiovascular disease among the Japanese general population: a population-based survey (Hara et al, 2011) (#28,903 men and 33,726 women for a total of 62,629) Despite the popular use of vitamin supplements and several prospective cohort studies investigating their effect on cancer incidence and cardiovascular disease (CVD), scientific data supporting their benefits remain controversial. Inconsistent results may be partly explained by the fact that use of supplements is an inconsistent behavior in individuals. We examined whether vitamin supplement use patterns affect cancer and CVD risk in a population-based cohort study in Japan. METHODS: A total of 28,903 men and 33,726 women in **the Japan Public Health Center-based Prospective Study cohort**, who answered questions about vitamin supplement use in the first survey from 1990-1994 and the second survey from 1995-1998, were categorized into four groups (never use, past use, recent use, and consistent use) and followed to the end of 2006 for cancer and 2005 for CVD. Sex-specific hazard ratios (HRs) and 95% confidence intervals (95% CIs) were used to describe the relative risks of cancer and CVD associated with vitamin supplement use. RESULTS: During follow-up, 4501 cancer and 1858 CVD cases were identified. **Multivariate adjusted analysis revealed no association of any pattern of vitamin supplement use with the risk of cancer and CVD in men. In women, consistent use was associated with lower risk of CVD** (HR 0.60, 95% CI 0.41-0.89), *whereas past (HR 1.17, 95% CI 1.02-1.33) and recent use (HR 1.24, 95% CI 1.01-1.52) were associated with higher risk of cancer.* CONCLUSIONS: To our knowledge, this is the first prospective cohort study to examine simultaneously the associations between vitamin supplement use patterns and risk of cancer and CVD. **This prospective cohort study demonstrated that vitamin supplement use has little effect on the risk of cancer or CVD in men.** In women, however, consistent vitamin supplement use might reduce the risk of CVD. Elevated risk of cancer associated with past and recent use of vitamin supplements in women may be partly explained by preexisting diseases or unhealthy background, but we could not totally control for this in our study. (Hara et al, 2011)

The biological relevance of direct antioxidant effects of polyphenols for cardiovascular health in humans is not established (Hollman et al, 2011) Human studies provide evidence for beneficial effects of polyphenol-rich foods on cardiovascular health. The antioxidant activity of polyphenols potentially explains these effects, but is the antioxidant activity a reliable predictor for these effects? **An International Life Sciences Institute Europe working group addressed this question and explored the potential of antioxidant claims for polyphenols in relation to cardiovascular health by using the so-called Process for the Assessment of Scientific Support for Claims on Foods project criteria.** In this process, analytical aspects of polyphenols, their occurrence in foods, dietary intake, and bioavailability were reviewed. Human studies on polyphenols and cardiovascular health were reviewed together with methods for biomarkers of oxidative damage and total antioxidant capacity (TAC). In retrospective studies, F2-isoprostanes and oxidized LDL, the most reliable biomarkers of lipid peroxidation, and measures for TAC showed the expected differences between cardiovascular disease patients and healthy controls, **but prospective studies are lacking, and a causal relationship between these biomarkers and cardiovascular health could not be established.** Therefore, the physiological relevance of a potential change in these biomarkers is unclear. We found limited evidence that some types of polyphenol-rich products modify these biomarkers in humans. **A direct antioxidant effect of polyphenols in vivo is questionable,** however, because concentrations in blood are low compared with other antioxidants and extensive metabolism following ingestion lowers their antioxidant activity. Therefore, **the biological relevance of direct antioxidant effects of polyphenols for cardiovascular health could not be established. Overall, although some polyphenol-rich foods exert beneficial effects on some biomarkers of cardiovascular health, there is no evidence that this is caused by improvements in antioxidant function biomarkers (oxidative damage or antioxidant capacity).** (Hollman et al, 2011)

The effects of two different doses of antioxidant vitamin C supplementation on bioenergetics index in male college students (Jourkesh et al, 2011)

In order to study the effects of consumption of 2 regimes of vitamin C (500 and 1000 mg) on bioenergetics index (aerobic and anaerobic power) in **36 physical education college male students,** were selected **non-randomly** procedure and they were set in 3 groups. Average of age, weight, height and Fat percentage of subjects was (22.48 1.84) years, (64.93 7.84) kg (175.4 5.66) cm and (10.94 5.29) mm respectively. The period

considered for consumption of vitamin C by experimental groups, was a **3 weeks** period that in this period the first group consumed dose of (500 mg) vitamin C and second group (1000 m.g) vitamin C and third group (control group) consumed placebo. The tests which have been exerted in this research consist of: assessment of anaerobic power by RAST test. 2) Assessment of aerobic power by Cooper test. Result indicated that **there was not a significant ($p < 0.05$) difference between the 3 groups in anaerobic and anaerobic power**. Therefore, **they concluded that daily consumption of 500 or 1000 m.g vitamin C for a period of 3 week does not have any effect on the basis of improvement of anaerobic and aerobic power in male college students.** (Jourkesh et al, 2011)

Vitamin A may not prevent asthma

7-15-11 Despite the important role of vitamin A in lung development, researchers have found that **giving the nutrient to pregnant women or preschoolers in Nepal doesn't protect kids against asthma**.

But the findings don't mean vitamin A isn't important, especially in regions where vitamin deficiencies are common, according to the scientists.

Women taking vitamin supplements had a lower chance of dying during pregnancy, for instance. And **those who took vitamin A while pregnant had kids with larger lungs, which have been linked to better survival.**

"We're kind of narrowing down what the effect of vitamin A is," **said Dr. William Checkley, from Johns Hopkins University in Baltimore,** who worked on the study.

The lungs need vitamin A as they are developing and the nutrient is also involved in keeping lung tissue healthy over time, the researchers explain in **the European Respiratory Journal.**

In addition, **previous studies hinted that people with lower levels of vitamin A in their blood are more likely to have asthma. But those kinds of studies, called observational studies, can't tease out cause and effect**. Checkley and his colleagues wanted to see if by adding vitamin A to kids' or pregnant women's diets, they might lower the children's risk of asthma.

So the team followed up on two different trials that gave vitamin A or vitamin-free placebo pills to Nepalese women or kids.

The studies involved **more than 5,000 kids and young adults, age nine to 23**, who had gotten vitamin A or a placebo as preschoolers, or whose mothers had done so before and during pregnancy. All of them were living in an area of **rural Nepal where vitamin deficiency is common.**

Researchers asked all the kids if they had problems with wheezing or coughing or had ever had asthma. They also tested how well the kids' lungs were working using a device called a spirometer.

Between zero and two percent of the kids said they had had asthma at some point, and less than one percent currently did so -- with **no differences between the placebo and vitamin groups.**

There were no differences in how many kids reported wheezing or coughing in the two groups either, or in how well their lungs worked.

Still, Checkley said the findings might have looked different in another location.

"The effect of vitamin A may vary as to the setting," he told Reuters Health. "The prevalence (of asthma) was low in Nepal."

In the U.S., for example, nearly 10 percent of kids are diagnosed with the disease.

It's possible that in an urban area where asthma is more common to begin with, giving pregnant moms or kids vitamin A may better protect kids against asthma, Checkley said.

It's also not clear how the findings would apply to a population where vitamin A deficiency wasn't such a problem.

More than 300 million people worldwide have asthma, Checkley said, and increases in asthma rates have put researchers on a search for possible culprits. Pollution and allergies have been linked to asthma, and food and nutrition are other targets of investigation. **RMH Note: multiple vitamins have been shown to increase the risk of allergies and asthma in children!!**

"Obviously diet is still one of those questions -- is it important or not?" Checkley said. **Researchers are still wondering, "Can we prevent or reduce the risk of asthma by giving (vitamin A) supplements?"**

So far, his work suggests the answer is no -- at least in this group of kids, in one part of the world.

Vitamin A and retinoid derivatives for lung cancer: a systematic review and meta analysis (Fritz et al, 2011) (#248 studies)

Despite reported antiproliferative activity of vitamin A and its common use for cancer, there is no comprehensive synthesis of its safety and efficacy in lung cancers. To address this issue we conducted a systematic review of the safety and efficacy of vitamin A for the treatment and prevention of lung cancers. METHODS AND FINDINGS: Two independent reviewers searched six electronic databases from inception to July 2009 for clinical, observational, and preclinical evidence pertaining to the safety and efficacy of vitamin A and related retinoids for lung cancers. 248 studies were included for full review and analysis. Five RCTs assessed treatment of lung cancers, three assessed primary prevention, and three looked at secondary prevention of lung cancers. Five surrogate studies, 26 phase I/II, 32 observational, and 67 preclinical studies were also included. 107 studies were included for interactions between vitamin A and chemo- or radiation- therapy. Although some studies demonstrated benefits, **there was insufficient evidence overall to support the use of vitamin A or related retinoids for the treatment or prevention of lung cancers.** Retinyl palmitate combined with beta carotene increased risk of lung cancer in smokers in the large CARET trial. **Pooling of three studies pertaining to treatment and three studies on secondary prevention revealed no significant effects on response rate, second primary tumor, recurrence, 5-year survival, and mortality.** There was a small improvement in event free survival associated with vitamin A compared to controls, RR 1.24 (95% CI 1.13-1.35). The synthetic retinoid bexarotene increased survival significantly among a subset of patients in two RCTs (p<0.014, <0.087). CONCLUSIONS: **There is a lack of evidence to support the use of naturally occuring retinoids for the treatment and prevention of lung cancers.** The rexinoid bexarotene may hold promise for use among a subset of patients, and deserves further study. (Fritz et al, 2011)

Vitamins D, C, and E in the prevention of type 2 diabetes mellitus: modulation of inflammation and oxidative stress (Garcia-Bailo et al, 2011) (Garcia-Bailo B et al. Vitamins D, C, and E in the prevention of type 2 diabetes mellitus: modulation of inflammation and oxidative stress. Biologics. 2011; 5: 7–19)

The Insulin Resistance Atherosclerosis Study, a 5-year prospective study of nearly 900 nondiabetic adults, found that plasma concentrations of ɑ tocopherol offered a significant protective effect against T2DM (OR = 0.12, 95% CI: 0.02–0.68). In contrast, various epidemiologic studies and intervention trials (see below) reported **inconsistent findings**. For example, supplementation with 750 IU/day of mixed tocopherols for 6 weeks reduced plasma but not urinary F_2-isoprostanes, a marker of oxidative stress in vivo, in two different studies on subjects with T2DM. This level of supplementation did not alter the serum concentration of CRP, IL-6, TNF-ɑ, or MCP-1 in one study *and was associated with increased blood pressure and heart rate in another trial.* Data from the Women's Health Study, assessing women health at baseline, demonstrated that supplementation with 600 IU of ɑ tocopherol for 10 years on alternate days **had no significant benefit for T2DM**. However, in another trial of 15 diabetics and 10 control individuals, 4 months of daily supplementation with 1350 IU of ɑ tocopherol significantly improved plasma glucose levels, triglycerides, total cholesterol levels, LDL, and HbA_{1c}, **but did not improve the response of β cells to glucose or FFAs**. In a trial involving 34 Mexican diabetic women, daily supplementation with 800 IU of ɑ tocopherol for 6 weeks improved total antioxidant status and reduced MDA levels, **but had no effect on serum glucose, lipids, or HbA_{1c} levels**. Daily supplementation with 1600 IU of ɑ tocopherol for 10 weeks in a group of 21 diabetic men **had no effect on HbA_{1c}, fasting blood glucose, or glycated plasma protein concentrations**, but had a beneficial effect on LDL oxidation. (Garcia-Bailo et al, 2011)

Although the epidemiologic evidence suggests that vitamin C, whether as a supplement or as part of a diet rich in fruits and vegetables, beneficially affects inflammatory markers and disease risk, the **results of intervention trials in T2DM are conflicting**. Despite epidemiologic findings generally pointing toward an association between increased vitamin C and reduced oxidation and inflammation, intervention trials assessing **the effect of vitamin C supplementation on various markers of T2DM have yielded inconsistent results**. One randomized, crossover, double-blind intervention trial **reported no improvement in fasting plasma glucose and no significant differences in levels of CRP, IL-6, IL-1 receptor agonist, or oxidized low-density lipoprotein (LDL) after supplementation with 3000 mg/day of vitamin C for 2 weeks in a group of 20 T2DM patients**, compared to baseline levels. Chen and colleagues performed a randomized, controlled, double-blind intervention on a group of 32 diabetic subjects with inadequate levels of vitamin C and found **no significant changes in either fasting glucose or fasting insulin after intake of 800 mg/day of vitamin C for 4 weeks**. Furthermore, Tousoulis et al reported that treatment with 2000 mg/day for 4 weeks **had no effect on levels of CRP, IL-6, TNF-ɑ, or soluble vascular cell adhesion molecule-1 in 13 T2DM patients**. (Garcia-Bailo et al, 2011)

Multivitamin use and the risk of mortality and cancer incidence: the multiethnic cohort study (Park et al, 2011) (#182,099) Although multivitamin/mineral supplements are commonly used in the United States, the efficacy of these supplements in preventing chronic disease or premature death is unclear. To assess the relation of multivitamin use with mortality and cancer, the authors prospectively examined these associations among **182,099 participants** enrolled in the Multiethnic Cohort Study between 1993 and 1996 in Hawaii and California. During an average 11 years of follow-up, 28,851 deaths were identified. In Cox proportional hazards models controlling for tobacco use and other potential confounders, **no associations were found between multivitamin use and mortality from all causes (for users vs. nonusers: hazard ratio = 1.07, 95% confidence interval: 0.96, 1.19 for men; hazard ratio = 0.96, 95% confidence interval: 0.85, 1.09 for women), cardiovascular diseases, or cancer.** The findings did not vary across subgroups by ethnicity, age, body mass index, preexisting illness, single vitamin/mineral supplement use, hormone replacement therapy use, and smoking status. There also was no evidence indicating that multivitamin use was associated with risk of cancer, overall or at major sites, such as lung, colorectum, prostate, and breast. In conclusion, **there was no clear decrease or increase in mortality from all causes, cardiovascular disease, or cancer and in morbidity from overall or major cancers among multivitamin supplement users**. (Park et al, 2011)

Antioxidant therapy in male infertility: fact or fiction? (Zini, 2011)

Infertile men have higher levels of semen reactive oxygen species (ROS, EMODs) than do fertile men. High levels of semen ROS can cause sperm dysfunction, sperm DNA damage and reduced male reproductive potential. This observation has led clinicians to treat infertile men with antioxidant supplements. The purpose of this article is to discuss the rationale for antioxidant therapy in infertile men and to evaluate the data on the efficacy of dietary and in vitro antioxidant preparations on sperm function and DNA damage. To date, most clinical studies suggest that dietary antioxidant supplements are beneficial in terms of improving sperm function and DNA integrity. **However, the exact mechanism of action of dietary antioxidants and the optimal dietary supplement have not been established. Moreover, most of the clinical studies are small and few have evaluated pregnancy rates.** A beneficial effect of in vitro antioxidant supplements in protecting spermatozoa from exogenous oxidants has been demonstrated in most studies; **however, the effect of these antioxidants in protecting sperm from endogenous ROS, gentle sperm processing and cryopreservation has not been established conclusively.** (Zini, 2011)

Fish oils can block chemotherapy drugs

9-12-11 Fats found in fish oil supplements can stop chemotherapy drugs working, according to researchers. Writing in the journal **Cancer Cell, they advise**

cancer patients not to take the supplements. The two fatty acids involved, which are also produced by stem cells in the blood, lead to tumours becoming immune to treatment.

Cancer Research UK advised patients to ask their doctor whether they would be affected. Scientists in the Netherlands were investigating how tumours develop resistance to treatments.

Fat shield

Experiments on mice showed that stem cells in the blood responded to the widely-used cancer drug cisplatin. The cells started producing two fatty acids, known as **KHT and 16:4(n-3). These fatty acids begin a series of chemical reactions, which mean cancerous cells become resistant to chemotherapy.**

"We currently recommend that these products should not be used whilst people are undergoing chemotherapy" said Prof Emile Voest University Medical Centre Utrecht. **Using drugs to block the production of the fatty acids prevented this form of resistance which "significantly enhances the chemotherapy,"** the study says. However, researchers warned that these fatty acids were "abundantly present in commercially available fish oil products". **They showed that off-the-shelf fish oil supplements, given to mice, could stop chemotherapy working against some tumours.**

Prof Emile Voest, lead researcher at University Medical Centre Utrecht, said: "We show that the body itself secretes protective substances into the blood that are powerful enough to block the effect of chemotherapy. These substances can be found in some types of fish oil. Whilst waiting for the results of further research, we currently recommend that these products should not be used whilst people are undergoing chemotherapy."

Jessica Harris, health information manager for Cancer Research UK, said: "This interesting study suggests one possible option for stopping cancers becoming resistant to treatment, but it is at an early stage and much more research would be needed to develop ways to halt resistance.

"The results also suggest that fish oil preparations may reduce the effectiveness of chemotherapy drugs.

"Cancer patients who are taking or thinking of taking these supplements should talk to their doctors to find out whether they could affect their treatments."

Selenium and genistein

First, selenium

Selenium and genistein are considered to be antioxidants and I will include this tag specifically on them. Some of the following was excerpted from an excellent discussion on this subject by Jerome-Morais et al. (Jerome-Morais et al, 2011)

In humans, 25 selenoproteins have been identified and while their functions remain under investigation, many are involved in redox reactions and serve roles in maintaining cellular homeostasis. (Reeves, Hoffman, 2009)

The first and best-studied selenoprotein, the cytoplasmic **glutathione peroxidase (GPx-1), is a so-called "anti-oxidant enzyme."**

It has been found that *over expression of GPx-1 in transgenic mice results in glucose intolerance,* raising the possibility that GPx-1 can contribute to the risk of diabetes that might be associated with elevated selenium status. (McClung et al, 2004)

Also, *overexpression of GPx-1 can also inhibit apoptosis and therefore potentially attenuate the clearance of premalignant lesions.* (Hockenbery et al, 1993)

Polymorphisms in the human GPx-1 gene are associated with increased risk of cancer. (Zhuo, Diamond, 2009) *and may impose a requirement of higher selenium concentrations being needed to obtain maximal activity as compared with individuals that express the alternative allele.* (Zhuo et al, 2009)

Apparently healthy French women randomized to receive a multivitamin containing β-carotene, selenium, vitamins E and C, and zinc at nutritional doses for an average of 7.5 years had a significant elevation in melanoma skin cancer risk compared with the placebo group. (Hercberg et al, 2007)

Also, please remember that *an observational epidemiological study of 300,000 American Association of Retired Persons members showed that excessive use of multivitamins (more than seven times per week) was associated with increased risks of advanced and fatal prostate cancer, particularly when coupled with use of individual β-carotene, selenium, or zinc supplements.* (Lawson et al, 2007)

We must not forget the adverse effects associated with other antioxidants, such as *high-dose vitamin E supplementation was found to slightly increase the risk of all-cause mortality in a meta-analysis of 19 randomized controlled trials.* (Miller et al, 2005), *and was also linked to a higher risk of heart failure in individuals with existing disease.* (Lonn et al, 2005)

Additionally, *high-dose vitamin C and E supplements not only failed to decrease pre-eclampsia in at-risk pregnant women, but resulted in increased numbers of adverse events such as low birth weight and hypertension.* (Poston et al, 2006)

Caution over antioxidant supplement use should also extend to cancer patients and survivors, over 65% of whom report taking some kind of vitamin or mineral supplement, often without consulting their physician or beknowst to their doctor. (Velicer, Ulrich, 2008)

This may be a serious cause for concern, given that *antioxidant supplements may interfere with the specific intent of radiotherapy and chemotherapy or promote the growth of residual disease in these patients.* (Lawenda et al, 2008)

In 1957, Klaus Schwarz reported that **an unknown factor, referred to as "Factor 3" and later discovered to be selenium, protected rats from liver necrosis resulting from being fed a purified casein diet.** (Schwarz, Foltz, 1958)

In man, selenium deficiency has been linked with several diseases including a pediatric cardiomyopathy endemic to China called Keshan's disease, a disorder of skeletal growth associated with abnormal neurological development and hypothyroidism referred to as Myxedematous cretinism that occurs most often in Central Africa, and an osteoarthropathy endemic in low selenium and iodine areas of China. (Tan et al, 2002) (Zimmerman, Kohrle, 2002)

Animal studies have established that nontoxic, low-level supplementation of the diets of experimental animals with selenium is effective in reducing cancer incidenceand it does so in most tissues types and **selenium appeared to be protective against a wide variety of carcinogens in these models.** (El-Bayoumy, 1991)

Also, **an inverse association between selenium levels and the risk of several cancers had been reported in humans.** (Gromadzinska et al, 2008)

The data were most consistent for colon and prostate cancer. (Peters, Takata, 2008) (Clark et al, 1996) (Duffield-Lillicoe, et al, 2002, NPC Trial)

However, selenium has had a long history of fatal toxicities. *Thousands of animals were killed by selenium over-dose and experienced adverse events associated with high-level selenium intake, referred to as selenosis.* **This has also been reported in humans, most often in regions of the world where there is very high levels of selenium in the soil and consequently, in the plants grown in that soil.** (Yang et al, 1983)

But, *the most shocking example of selenium toxicity in recent years occurred in 2008, when an outbreak of selenosis affecting 201 individuals* in nine different states in the United States was reported and attributed to extremely high doses from mis-labeled supplement pills. (MacFarquhar et al, 2010)

There exists a considerable literature indicating both cytotoxic and genotoxic effects of selenium when cells in culture or animals are provided high doses, and consequences include enhanced mutagenesis, induction of chromosomal abnormalities such as micronuclei formation, as well as induction of cell-cycle arrest and apoptosis. (Valdiglesias, et al, 2009)

Additionally, *data from the beginning of the NPC Trial (Nutritional Prevention of Cancer Trial) through 1996 indicated a statistically significant increase of basal cell, and total nonmelanoma skin cancer in the supplementation arm.* (Duffield-Lillicoe, et al, 2002, NPC Trial)

Shockingly, **the increased risk of a new skin cancer was most pronounced among participants with the highest baseline concentrations of plasma selenium, with those in the highest tertile experiencing a 60% increase in risk associated with selenium supplementation.** (Duffield-Lillicoe, et al, 2002, NPC Trial)

Surprisingly, further anaylsis of the NPC trial data indicated a higher incidence of type 2 diabetes in the selenium-supplemented group. Additional examination of the data *indicated a statistically significant dose–response gradient with the greatest risk for type 2 diabetes occurring in the supplemented group within the highest tertile of baseline selenium levels.* (Stranges et al, 2007)

Unlike the NPC trial, men were provided selenium in the form of selenomethionine. *The Selenium and Vitamin E Cancer Prevention Trial was terminated ahead of schedule in 2008 for an apparent lack of efficacy of the supplements. Interestingly, an analysis of the collected data indicated a nonsignificant increase in the risk of diabetes in the group receiving selenium.* (Lippman et al, 2009)

Consistently, *the possibility that selenium might increase the risk of diabetes emerged as a result of two independent clinical supplementation trials, conducted in two different populations and with different forms of selenium, and has raised concerns over the possible risks of selenium supplementation.*

Again, we start to see the danger of antioxidant over dosing. *Both studies also indicated that there may be a threshold above which higher selenium levels are deleterious. With regard to the selenium-associated risk of type 2 diabetes, two studies of National Health and Nutrition Examination Survey (NHANES)* *data on US populations have demonstrated an increased prevalence of type 2 diabetes among those with the highest (≥147 µg/L in NHANES 2003–2004 and ≥137.66 ng/mL in NHANES III) versus lowest (<124 µg/L and <111.62 ng/mL, respectively) levels of serum selenium.* (Laclaustra et al, 2009) (Bleys et al, 2007)

Additionally, Bleys et al found *positive associations to adverse serum lipid profiles and arterial disease.* (Bleys et al, 2009), *which was consistent with the report of a similar analysis of British citizens.* (Stranges et al, 2009)

Bleys et al also reported on the relationship between serum selenium levels and **causes of death,** also using **NHANES** data, where they *reported a nonlinear association between serum selenium levels and deaths by all causes, and specifically those due to cancer.* Below a baseline serum concentration of 130 ng/mL, increased selenium levels were associated with a reduced risk of all-cause mortality and cancer-associated deaths. On the contrary, selenium had no effect between 130 and 150 ng/mL, and *above this level, there was evidence for increased risk of death from all-causes, including cancer.* (Bleys et al, 2008)

Here are more of the "dead bodies" the proponents of antioxidant supplements say do not exist.

Jerome-Morais et al report that the results from both epidemiology and supplementation trials raise caution that some could increase their risk of diabetes and cancer if they were to supplement their diets with selenium. (Jerome-Morais et al, 2011)

Now, for genistein

Soybeans are a rich source of isoflavones – polyphenolic compounds found primarily in legumes. Genistein exhibits several potentially anticarcinogenic functions: it has the highest antioxidant activity of any soy isoflavone. (Arora et al, 1998) (Ruiz-Larrea et al, 1997)

ER-α and ER-β are nuclear hormone receptors that undergo a conformational change on hormone binding, triggering a translocation of the receptor from the cytoplasm to the nucleus. Although 17β-estradiol – produced by the ovary and the major estrogen in humans – binds ER-α and -β with equal affinity, genistein preferentially binds ER-β, albeit less strongly than estrogen. **The relative estrogenic potency of genistein at ER-β is ~30-fold higher compared with that at ER-α.**

Although genistein appears to exert anti-estrogenic effects at ER-β, high concentrations of genistein can actually exert weak estrogenic effects at ER-α, at least *in vitro.* Notably, **a recent study demonstrated that genistein exposure induced**

different gene and protein expression patterns in the T47D human breast cancer cell line, depending on the ER phenotype and the ratio between the ER sub-types in the cells.

Some studies have indicated that genistein may reduce the risk of breast cancer but **several studies have found no association between blood or urine genistein concentrations and breast cancer risk**. (Ward et al, 2008) (Grace et al, 2004) (Piller et al, 2006) (den Tonkelaar et al, 2001)

Reportedly, **genistein also has anti-tumorigenic efficacy as determined using animal models of cancer,** can **be selectively cytotoxic to neoplastic and pre-neoplastic cells grown in culture,** and **may inhibit metastasis as evidenced by its ability to attenuate the adhesion and migration of prostate, breast, lung, and pancreatic cancer cell lines *in vitro*.**

Genistein and isoflavone risks

There are concern of *genotoxicity associated with higher levels of genistein exposure* that are typically not achievable through dietary intake, with most of these data obtained from *in vitro* experiments using cells in culture. For example, *genistein exposure of L5178Y mouse lymphoma cells at concentrations less than 100 nM induced micronuclei formation and mutagenesis at the thymidine kinase locus.* (Boos, Stopper, 2000) *and chronic exposure (3 months) of human MCF-10A cells induced genomic instability.* (Kim et al, 2008)

It has also been found that *genistein at higher concentrations could also result in DNA damage detectable by either the comet assay or the chromosomal aberrations in both cells in culture* (Pool-Zobel et al, 2000) (Michael et al, 2006) *and in human sperm and lymphocytes obtained from donors.* (Anderson et al, 1997) (Kulling et al, 1999)

These genotoxic effects have been attributed, at least in part, to the known role of genistein in inhibiting topoisomerase II. (Markovits et al, 1989)

Genistein may have *possible harmful effects on reproductive health. A wide range of reproductive biological and behavioral defects were observed in male rats fed a gen-istein supplemented diet* (Wisniewski et al, 2003) *and recent data have demonstrated a direct effect of genistein on Leydig cells.* (Hancock et al, 2009) (Sherrill et al, 2010)

Providing physiologically relevant doses of genistein (i.e. those achievable through dietary intake) neonatally resulted in a wide range of defects in the developing female reproductive system and this has been extensively reviewed by Jefferson et al.. (Jefferson et al, 2006)

Additional concerns about possible teratogenic effects of genistein have been raised in the studies using zebrafish. (Kim et al, 2009) (Sassi-Messai et al, 2009)

There is a serious concern as to whether genistein supplementation can have an adverse effect on cancer survival. An extensive and comprehensive review of the preclinical and clinical literature on both the benefits and the possible risks of genistein has been published by Tayor et al. (Taylor et al, 2009)

Although several reports have indicated that genistein could stimulate the growth of the ER$^+$ human breast cancer cell line MCF-7, *it was shown early on that genistein concentrations as low as 10–100 nM can be growth stimulatory* with higher concentrations of 20 µM being inhibitory, presumably due to toxicity. (Hsieh et al, 1998)

In that regard, *genistein supplementation enhanced mammary gland growth and tumor development of estrogen-dependent MCF7 cells in athymic mice in a dose-dependent manner* (Allred et al, 2001) *and when ovariectomized mice were treated with the chemical carcinogen 1-methyl-1-nitrosourea to induce mammary tumorigenesis*. (Allred et al, 2004)

Supplementation studies conducted in humans have raised the possibility that soy may promote breast cancer development.

In a trial that randomized women with benign or malignant breast disease to soy supplementation (60 g of soy containing 45 mg of isoflavones) or their normal diet daily for 2 wk, women receiving the soy supplements had increased serum genistein levels in comparison to women on a standard diet, and their histologically normal breast tissue exhibited enhanced breast epithelial cell proliferation and significantly increased progesterone receptor levels. (McMichael-Phillips et al, 1998)

In general, **the data suggest that short-term exposure to soy caused a weak estrogenic effect.**

An additional concern about the potential harm that might be done by genistein stems from data that it can stimulate proliferation of tamoxifen-sensitive cells (Ju et al, 2008) (Ju et al, 2002) (Limer et al, 2006) *and attenuate the anti-tumor activities of both tamoxifen* (Liu et al, 2005) *and the aromatase inhibitor letrozole in mouse models of breast cancer*. (Ju et al, 2008)

Consequently, *there remains some concern regarding genistein's possible geno-toxic, teratogenic, and proestrogenic activity at high concentrations, and there-fore its long-term safety as a dietary supplement.*

Genistein may have very different effects on healthy breast tissue as com-pared with breast cancers, and this may be further complicated by the ER status of the tumor. There is also a possibility of an interaction between genistein and common approaches to manage breast cancer (tamoxifen and letrozole) that reduce the efficacy of these drugs. In addition, it is impor-tant to consider attainable physiological doses of genistein in humans when assessing its safety. Serum levels of genistein from soy consumption or supplementation are typically below 5 μM, with many of the reports of growth stimulation of cells in culture involving concentrations ranging from 0.01 to 10 μM and the growth inhibitory and genotoxic effects occur at higher concentrations.

REFERENCES

(Abou-Seif et al, 2004) (Abou-Seif MA, Youssef AA. Evaluation of some biochemical changes in diabetic patients. Clin Chim Acta. 2004 Aug 16;346(2):161-70)

(Agarwal et al, 2004) (Agarwal A, et al, Role of antioxidants in treatment of male infertility: an overview of the literature. Reprod Biomed Online. 2004 Jun;8(6):616-27)

(Aisen et al, 2008) (Aisen PS et al. High-dose B vitamin supplements and cognitive decline in Alzheimer's disease. JAMA. 2008;300(15):1774-1783)

(Albanes et al, 1996) (Albanes, D., Heinonen, O. P., Taylor, P. R., Virtamo, J. et al., Alpha-tocopherol and beta-carotene supplements and lung cancer incidence in the alpha-tocopherol, beta-carotene cancer prevention study: effects of base-line characteristics and study compliance. J. Natl. Cancer Inst. 1996, 88, 1560–1570)

(Albanes, 1999) (Albanes, D., Beta-carotene and lung cancer: a case study. Am. J. Clin. Nutr. 1999, 69, 1345S–1350S)

(Allred et al, 2001) (Allred, C. D., Allred, K. F., Ju, Y. H., Virant, S. M., Helferich, W. G., Soy diets containing varying amounts of genistein stimulate growth of estrogen-dependent (MCF-7) tumors in a dose-dependent manner. Cancer Res. 2001, 61, 5045–5050)

(Allred et al, 2004) (Allred, C. D., Allred, K. F., Ju, Y. H., Clausen, L. M. et al., Dietary genistein results in larger MNU-induced, estrogen-dependent mammary tumors following ovariectomy of Sprague-Dawley rats. Carcinogenesis 2004, 25, 211–218)

(Anderson et al, 1997) (Anderson, D., Dobrzynska, M. M., Basaran, N., Effect of various genotoxins and reproductive toxins in human lymphocytes and sperm in the Comet assay. Teratog. Carcinog. Mutagen. 1997, 17, 29–43)

(Andersen et al, 2007) (Andersen LP, Holck S, Kupcinskas L, et al. Gastric inflammatory markers and interleukins in patients with functional dyspepsia treated with astaxanthin. FEMS Immunol Med Microbiol. 2007 May 23)

(Arain, Abdul Qadeer, 2010) (Arain MA, Abdul Qadeer A. Systematic review on "vitamin E and prevention of colorectal cancer". Pak J Pharm Sci. 2010 Apr;23(2):125-30)

(Arendash et al, 2009) (Gary W Arendash, Takashi Mori, Chuanhai Cao, Malgorzata Mamcarz, Melissa Runfeldt, Alexander Dickson, Kavon Rezai-Zadeh, Jun Tan, Bruce A Citron, Xiaoyang Lin, Valentina Echeverria, and Huntington Potter. Caffeine Reverses Cognitive Impairment and Decreases Brain Amyloid-%u03B2 Levels in Aged Alzheimer's Disease Mice. Journal of Alzheimer's Disease, Volume 17:3 (July 2009)

(Arora et al, 1998) (Arora, A., Nair, M. G., Strasburg, G. M., Antioxidant activities of isoflavones and their biological metabolites in a liposomal system. Arch. Biochem. Biophys. 1998, 356, 133–141)

(Astorg et al, 1997) (Astorg, P. et al., Dietary lycopene decreases the initiation of liver preneoplastic foci by diethylnitrosamine in the rat, Nutr. Cancer, 29, 60, 1997)

(Atamna et al, 2007) (Atamna et al. Methylene blue delays cellular senescence and enhances key mitochondrial biochemical pathways. The FASEB Journal, 2007; 22 (3): 703 DOI: 10.1096/fj.07-9610com)

(ATBC group, 1994) (The Alpha-Tocopherol, Beta Carotene Cancer Prevention Study Group, The effect of vitamin E and beta carotene on the incidence of lung cancer and other cancers in male smokers. N. Engl. J. Med. 1994, 330, 1029–1035)

(Avenell et al, 2005) (Avenell A, Campbell MK, Cook JA, Hannaford PC, Kilonzo MM, McNeill G, Milne AC, Ramsay CR, Seymour DG, Stephen AI, Vale LD. Effect of multivitamin and multimineral supplements on morbidity from infections in older people (MAVIS trial): pragmatic, randomised, double blind, placebo controlled trial. BMJ. 2005;331:324–329)

(Bagis et al, 2005) (Bagis S, Tamer L, Sahin G, et al. Free radicals and antioxidants in primary fibromyalgia: an oxidative stress disorder? Rheumatol Int. 2005 Apr;25(3):188-90)

(Balasz, Brooksbank, 1985) (Balasz R., Brooksbank B.U.: Neurochemical approaches to the pathogenesis of Down's syndrome. J. Ment. Defic. Res. 1985, 29: 1-14)

(Balk et al, 2007) (Balk EM, Raman G, Tatsionis A, Chung M, Lau J, Rosenberg IH. Vitamin B6, B12 and folic acids supplementation and cognitive function: a systematic review of randomized trials. Arch Intern Med 2007;167:21–30)

(Baum et al, 2008) (Baum L, Lam CW, Cheung SK, Kwok T, Lui V, Tsoh J, Lam L, Leung V, Hui E, Ng C, Woo J, Chiu HF, Goggins WB, Zee BC, Cheng KF, Fong CY, Wong A, Mok H, Chow MS, Ho PC, Ip SP, Ho CS, Yu XW, Lai CY, Chan MH, Szeto S, Chan IH, Mok V. Six-month randomized, placebo-controlled, double-blind, pilot clinical trial of curcumin in patients with Alzheimer disease. J Clin Psychopharmacol. 2008;28:110–113)

(Bergamasco et al, 1994) (Bergamasco B, Scarzella L, La Commare P. Idebenone, a new drug in the treatment of cognitive impairment in patients with dementia of the Alzheimer type. Funct Neurol. 1994;9:161–168)

(Birks et al, 2007) (Birks J, Grimley Evans J. Ginkgo biloba for cognitive impairment and dementia. Cochrane Database Syst Rev 2007;2:CD00310)

(Bjelakovic et al, 2007, JAMA) (Bjelakovic G, Nikolova D, Gluud LL, Simonetti RG, Gluud C. Mortality in randomized trials of antioxidant supplements for primary and secondary prevention: systematic review and meta-analysis. JAMA. 2007;297:842–857) (Bjelakovic et al, 2008:CD007176)

(Bjelakovic et al, 2008) (Bjelakovic G, Nikolova D, Gluud LL, Simonetti RG, Gluud C. Antioxidant supplements for prevention of mortality in healthy participants and patients with various diseases. Cochrane Database Syst Rev. 2008:CD007176)

(Black, 1998) (Black, H.S., Radical interception by carotenoids and effects on UV carcinogenesis,

Nutr. Cancer, 31, 212, 1998)

(Ble-Castillo et al, 2005) (Ble-Castillo JL, Carmona-Diaz E, Mendez JD, et al. Effect of alpha-tocopherol on the metabolic control and oxidative stress in female type 2 diabetics. Biomed Pharmacother. 2005;59(6):290–295)

(Bleys et al, 2007) (Bleys, J., Navas-Acien, A., Guallar, E., Serum selenium and diabetes in US adults. Diabetes Care 2007, 30, 829–834)

(Bleys et al, 2008) (Bleys, J., Navas-Acien, A., Guallar, E., Serum selenium levels and all-cause, cancer, and cardiovascular mortality among US adults. Arch. Intern. Med. 2008, 168, 404–410)

(Bleys et al, 2009) (Bleys, J., Navas-Acien, A., Laclaustra, M., Pastor-Barriuso, R. et al., Serum selenium and peripheral arterial disease: results from the national health and nutrition examination survey, 2003–2004. Am. J. Epidemiol. 2009, 169, 996–1003)

(Blendon et al, 2001) (Blendon, R. J., DesRoches, C. M., Benson, J. M., Brodie, M., Altman, D. E., Americans' views on the use and regulation of dietary supplements. Arch. Intern. Med. 2001, 161, 805–810)

(Bloomer et al, 2005) (Bloomer RJ, Fry A, Schilling B, et al. Astaxanthin supplementation does not attenuate muscle injury following eccentric exercise in resistance-trained men. Int J Sport Nutr Exerc Metab . 2005;15:401-412)

(Boos, Stopper, 2000) (Boos, G., Stopper, H., Genotoxicity of several clinically used topoisomerase II inhibitors. Toxicol. Lett. 2000, 116, 7–16)

(Bower et al, 2003) (Bower JH, Maraganore DM, Peterson BJ, McDonnell SK, Ahlskog JE, Rocca WA. Head trauma preceding PD: a case-control study. Neurology.

2003;60:1610-1615)

(Brooksbank et al, 1983) (Brooksbank, B.W. & Balazs, R. Superoxide dismutase and lipoperoxidation in Down's syndrome fetal brain [letter]. Lancet 1, 881-882 (1983)

(Brooksbank, Balasz, 1984) (Brooksbank B.U., Balasz R.: Superoxide dismutase, glutathione peroxidase and lipoperoxidation in Down's syndrome fetal brain. Brain Res. 1984, 16: 37-44) (Balasz, Brooksbank, 1985)

(Brown, Fridovich, 1981) (Brown K., Fridovich I.: DNA strand scission by enzymatically generated oxygen radicals. Arch. Biochem. Biophys. 1981, 206: 414-420)

(Bryant et al, 2003) (Bryant RJ, et al. Effects of vitamin E and C supplementation either alone or in combination on exercise-induced lipid peroxidation in trained cyclists. J Strength Cond Res. 2003 Nov;17(4):792-800)

(Buchholz et al, 2008) (Buchholz K, et al. Interactions of methylene blue with human disulfide reductases and their orthologues from Plasmodium falciparum. Antimicrob Agents Chemother. 2008 Jan;52(1):183-91)

(Buchholz et al, July 2008) (Buchholz K, et al. Cytotoxic interactions of methylene blue with trypanosomatid-specific disulfide reductases and their dithiol products. Mol Biochem Parasitol. 2008 Jul;160(1):65-9)

(Bush, 2003) (Bush, A.I., The metallobiology of Alzheimer's disease. Trends Neurosci 26(4):207-14, 2003)

(Cahill et al, 2009) (Cahill L, Corey PN, El-Sohemy A. Vitamin C deficiency in a population of young Canadian adults. Am J Epidemiol. 2009;170(4):464–471)

(Cai et al, 2004) (Cai Q, Shu XO, Wen W, et al. Genetic polymorphism in the manganese superoxide dismutase gene, antioxidant intake, and breast cancer risk: results from the Shanghai Breast Cancer Study. Breast Cancer Res. 2004;6(6):R647-R55)

(Campbell, Gowran, 2007) (Campbell VA, Gowran A. Alzheimer's disease; taking the edge off with cannabinoids? Br J Pharmacol. 2007 Nov;152(5):655-62)

(Cao et al, 2009) (Chuanhai Cao, John R Cirrito, Xiaoyang Lin, Lilly Wang, Deborah K Verges, Alexander Dickson, Malgorzata Mamcarz, Chi Zhang, Takashi Mori, Gary W Arendash, David M Holzman, and Huntington Potter. Caffeine Suppresses Amyloid-%u03B2 Levels in Plasma and Brain of Alzheimer's Disease Transgenic Mice. Journal of Alzheimer's Disease, Volume 17:3 (July 2009)

(Cash et al, 2002) (Cash AD, Perry G, Ogawa O, Raina AK, Zhu X, Smith MA. Is Alzheimer's disease a mitochondrial disorder? Neuroscientist. 2002 Oct;8(5):489-96)

(Chan et al, 1987) (Chan P.H., Longar S., Fishman R.A.: Protective effects of liposome-entrapped superoxide-dismutase on post-traumatic brain edema. Ann. Neurol. 1987, 21: 540-547)

(Chance et al, 1979) (Chance B, Sies H, Boveris A. Hydroperoxide metabolism in mammalian organs. Physiol Rev 59:527–605, 1979)

(Chandra, 2001) (Chandra RK. Effect of vitamin and trace-element supplementation on cognitive function in elderly subjects. Nutrition. 2001;17:709–12)

(Chen, Buck, 2000) (Chen Y, Buck J. Cannabinoids protect cells form oxidative cell death: a receptor-independent mechanism. J Pharm Exp Ther. Vol. 293, No. 3. Pp 807-812)

(Chi et al, 2008) (Chi HJ, Kim JH, Ryu CS, Lee JY, Park JS, Chung DY, et al. Protective effect of antioxidant supplementation in sperm-preparation medium against oxidative stress in human spermatozoa. Hum Reprod. 2008;23:1023–8)

(Choi et al, 2005) (Choi J, Rees HD, Weintraub ST, et al. Oxidative modifications and aggregation of Cu,Zn-superoxide dismutase associated with Alzheimer and Parkinson diseases. J Biol Chem. 2005 Mar 25;280(12):11648-55)

(Christen, 2000) (Christen Y. Oxidative stress and Alzheimer disease. Am J Clin Nutr. 2000 Feb;71(2):621S-629S)

(Clark et al, 1996) (Clark, L. C., Combs, G. F. J., Turnbull, B. W., Slate, E. H. et al., Effects of selenium supplementation for cancer prevention in patients with carcinoma of the skin. A randomized controlled trial. J. Am. Med. Assoc. 1996, 276, 1957–1963)

(Clausen, 1984) (Clausen J.: Demential syndromes and the lipid metabolism. Acta Neurol. Scand. 1984, 70: 345-355)

(Cleaver, 1978) (Cleaver J.E.: DNA repair and its coupling to DNA replication in eukaryotic cells. Biochim. Biophys. Acta 1978, 516: 489-516) (Johnson et al, 1986)

(Cleaver, 1978) (Cleaver J.E.: DNA repair and its coupling to DNA replication in eukaryotic cells. Biochim. Biophys. Acta 1978, 516: 489-516)

(Cocchi, 1987) (Cocchi R.: Presenza di scavengers e incidenza di paralisi cerebrali infantili da prematurità e basso peso alla nascita in 381 soggetti Down allevati in famiglia. Giorn. Neurpsich. Età Evol. 1987, 7: 317-323)

(Cocchi et al, 1988) (Renato Cocchi, Giovanni Somenzine, Ferncesco Zerbi. The free radicals hypothesis in causing dementia: High probability refutation in Down's syndrome subjects. Italian Journal of Intellective Impairment 1 (2): 127-132. 1988)

(Cutler, 1984) (Cutler G.R.: Free radicals and aging. In: Roy A.K., Chatterjee B. (eds): Molecular basis of aging. Academic Press, New York, 1984)

(Cocchi, Branchesi, 1988) (Cocchi R., Branchesi R.: Non causal connection between cerebral palsy and squint outcomes in premature and/or low birthweight Down subjects. It. J. Intellect. Impair. 1988, 1: 141-144)

(Cockle et al, 2000) (Cockle SM, Haller J, Kimber S, Dawe RA, Hindmarch I. The influence of multivitamins on cognitive function and mood in the elderly. Aging and Mental Health. 2000;4:339–353)

(Costenbader et al, 2010) (Costenbader KH, Kang JH, Karlson EW. Antioxidant intake and risks of rheumatoid arthritis and systemic lupus erythematosus in women. Am J Epidemiol. 2010 Jul 15;172(2):205-16)

(Crosti et al, 1976) (Crosti N., Serra A., Rigo A., Vigliano P. : Dosage effect of SOD-1 gene in 21-trisomic cells. Hum. Genet. 1976, 31: 197-202)

(Cutler, 1985) (Cutler G.R.: Peroxide-producing potential of tissues. Inverse correlation with longevity of mammalian species. Proc. Natl. Acad. USA 1985, 82: 4798-4802)

(Dai et al, 2006, the Kame Project) (Q. Dai, AR. Borenstein , Y. Wu , et al., Fruit and vegetable juices and Alzheimer's disease: The Kame project. Am J Med, 2006, vol. 119, pp. 751-759)

(Dalton, Crapper, 1984) (Dalton A.J., Crapper McLachlan D.R.: Incidence of memory deterioration in aging persons with Down's syndrome. In: Berg J.M. (ed); Perspectives and progress in mental retardation. II. Biomedical aspects. University Park Press, Baltimore 1984: 55-62)

(de Haan et al, 1997) (de Haan, J., et al. Reactive Oxygen Species and Their Contribution to Pathology in Down Syndrome. Adv Pharmacol 1997;38:379-402)

(DeKosky et al, 2008) (DeKosky ST, et al, Ginkgo biloba for prevention of dementia. JAMA. 2008;300(19):2253-2262)

(den Tonkelaar et al, 2001) (den Tonkelaar, I., Keinan-Boker, L., Veer, P.V., Arts, C. J. et al., Urinary phytoestrogens and postmenopausal breast cancer risk. Cancer Epidemiol. Biomarkers Prev. 2001, 10, 223–228)

(Diepeveen et al, 2005) (Diepeveen SH, et al. Effects of atorvastatin and vitamin E on lipoproteins and oxidative stress in dialysis patients: a randomised-controlled trial. J Intern Med. 2005 May;257(5):438-45)

(Donnelley et al, 1999) (Donnelly ET, McClure N, Lewis SE. The effect of ascorbate and alpha-tocopherol supplementation in vitro on DNA integrity and hydrogen peroxide-induced DNA damage in human spermatozoa. Mutagenesis. 1999;14:505–12)

(Donnelly et al, 2000) (Donnelly ET, et al. Glutathione and hypotaurine in vitro: effects on human sperm motility, DNA integrity and production of reactive oxygen species. Mutagenesis. 2000 Jan;15(1):61-8)

(Doody et al, 2008) (Doody RS, Gavrilova SI, Sano M, Thomas RG, Aisen PS, Bachurin SO, Seely L, Hung D. Effect of dimebon on cognition, activities of daily living, behaviour, and global function in patients with mild-to-moderate Alzheimer's disease: a randomised, double-blind, placebo-controlled study. Lancet. 2008;372:207–215)

(Dröge, 2002) (Dröge W. Free radicals in the physiological control of cell function. Physiol Rev. 2002 Jan;82(1):47-95)

(Duffield-Lillicoe, et al, 2002, NPC Trial) (Duffield-Lillicoe, A., Reid, M., Turnbull, J., Combs, G. J. et al., Baseline characteristics and the effect of selenium supplementation on cancer incidence in a randomized clinical trial: a summary report of the Nutritional Prevention of Cancer Trial. Cancer Epidemiol. Biomarkers Prev. 2002, 11, 630–639)

(Dumont et al, 2010) (Dumont M, et al, Mitochondria and antioxidant targeted therapeutic strategies for Alzheimer's disease. J Alzheimer's Dis. 2010;20(Suppl 2):S633-S643)

(Durga et al, 2007) (Durga J, van Boxtel MPJ, Schouten EG, Kok FJ, Jolles J, Katan MB, Verhoef P. Effect of 3-year folic acid supplementation on cognitive function in older adults in the FACIT trial: a randomised, double blind, controlled trial. Lancet. 2007;369:208–16)

(Dwyer, Donoghue, 2010) (Dwyer J, Donoghue MD. Is risk of Alzheimer's disease a reason to use dietary supplements? Am J Clin Nutr. 2010 May; 91(5): 1155-1156)

(El-Bayoumy, 1991) (El-Bayoumy, K. (Ed.), The Role of Selenium in Cancer Prevention, J. B. Lippincott Co., Philadelphia 1991)

(Engelhart et al, 2002) (Engelhart MJ, Geerlings MI, Ruitenberg A, van Swieten JC, Hofman A, Witteman JC, Breteler MM. Dietary intake of antioxidants and risk of Alzheimer disease. JAMA. 2002;287:3223–3229)

(Erdman et al, 2009) (Erdman JW Jr, Ford NA, Lindshield BL. Are the health attributes of lycopene related to its antioxidant function? Arch Biochem Biophys. 2009 Mar 15;483(2):229-35)

(Erickson, Kramer, 2009) (Erickson K, Kramer AF. Aerobic exercise effects on cognitive and neural plasticity in older adults. Br J Sports Med 2009;43:22-24)

(Estevez et al, 1999) (Estevez, A.G. et al. Induction of nitric oxide-dependent apoptosis in motor neurons by zinc-deficient superoxide dismutase. Science 286: 2498-2500, 1999)

(Eubanks et al, 2006) (Eubanks LM. et al, A molecular link between the active component of marijuana and Alzheimer's disease pathology. Mol Pharm. 2006 Nov-Dec;3(6):773-7)

(Eussen et al, 2006) (Eussen SJ, De Groot LC, Joosten LW, et al. Effect of oral vitamin B12 with or without folic acid on cognitive function in older people with mild vitamin B12 deficiency a randomized placebo-controlled trial. Am J Clin Nutr 2006;84:361–70)

(Feaster et al, 1977) (Feaster U., Kwok L., Epstein C.: Dosage effect for superoxide dismutase-1 in nucleated cells aneuplid for chromosome 21. An. J. Human Genet. 1977, 29: 563-579)

(Fisher-Willman, bloomer, 2009) (Fisher-Wellman K, Bloomer RJ. Acute exercise and oxidative stress: a 30 year history. Dyn Med. 2009 Jan 13;8:1)

(Fletcher, 1907) (Fletcher, W., Rice and Beri-Beri: preliminary report on an experiment conducted at the Kuala Lampur lunatic asylum. *Lancet* 1907, 169, 1776–1779) (Lind, 1983)

(Floyd, 1999) (Floyd RA: Antioxidants, oxidative stress, and degenerative neurological disorders. Proc Soc Exp Biol Med 1999, 222(3):236-245)

(Floyd, Carney, 1992) (Floyd RA, Carney JM. Free radical damage to protein and DNA: Mechanisms involved and relevant observations on brain undergoing oxidative stress. Ann Neurol 32:S22–S27, 1992)

(Forbes et al, 2003) (Forbes K, Gillette K, Sehgal I. Lycopene increases urokinase receptor and fails to inhibit growth or connexin expression in a metastatically passaged prostate cancer cell line: a brief communication. Exp Biol Med (Maywood). 2003 Sep;228(8):967-71)

(Freeman et al, 1985) (Freeman B.A., Turrens J.F., Mina Z., Crapo J.D.: Modulation of oxidant lung injury by using liposome-entrapped superoxide dismutase and catalase. Fed. Proc. 1985, 44: 2591-2595)

(Freeman, Crapo, 1984) (Freeman B.A., Crapo J.D.: Biology of disease, free radicals and tissue injury. Lab.Invest.1982, 47: 412-426) (Slater T.F.: Free-radical mechanism in tissue injury. Biochem. J. 1984, 222: 1-15)

(Fridovich, Porter, 1981) (Fridovich I., Porter N.A.: Oxidation of arachidonic acid in micelles by superoxide and hydrogen peroxide. J. Biol. Chem. 1981, 256: 260-265)

(Fritz et al, 2011) (Fritz H, et al. Vitamin a and retinoid derivatives for lung cancer: a systematic review and meta analysis. PLoS One. 2011;6(6):e21107. Epub 2011 Jun 27)

(Gaeini et al, 2006) (Gaeini AA, Rahnama N, Hamedinia MR. Effects of vitamin E supplementation on oxidative stress at rest and after exercise to exhaustion in athletic students. J Sports Med Phys Fitness. 2006 Sep;46(3):458-61)

(Grace et al, 2004) (Grace, P. B., Taylor, J. I., Low, Y. L., Luben, R. N. et al., Phytoestrogen concentrations in serum and spot urine as biomarkers for dietary phytoestrogen intake and their relation to breast cancer risk in European prospective investigation of cancer and nutrition-norfolk. Cancer Epidemiol. Biomarkers Prev. 2004, 13, 698–708)

(Garcia-Bailo et al, 2011) (Garcia-Bailo B et al. Vitamins D, C, and E in the prevention of type 2 diabetes mellitus: modulation of inflammation and oxidative stress. Biologics. 2011; 5: 7–19)

(Graf et al, 2005) (Graf M et al. High dose vitamin E therapy in amyotrophic lateral sclerosis as add-on therapy to riluzole: results of a placebo-controlled double-blind study. J Neural Transm. 2005 May;112(5):649-60. Epub 2004 Oct 27)

(Graat et al, 2000) (Graat JM, Schouten EG, Kok FJ. Effedt of daily vitamin E and multi-vitamin-mineral supplementation on acute respiratory tract infections in elderly persons: a randomized controlled trial. JAMA. 2002 Aug 14;288(6):715-21)

(Grodstein et al, 2003) (Grodstein F, Chen J, Willett WC. High-dose antioxidant supplements and cognitive function in community-dwelling elderly women. Am J Clin Nutr. 2003;77:975–984)

(Gromadzinska et al, 2008) (Gromadzinska, J., Reszka, E., Bruzelius, K., Wasowicz, W., Akesson, B., Selenium and cancer: biomarkers of selenium status and molecular action of selenium supplements. Eur. J. Nutr. 2008, 47, 29–50)

(Guilloreau et al, 2007) (Guilloreau L, Combalbert S, Sournia-Saquet A, Mazarguil H, Faller P. Redox chemistry of copper-amyloid-beta: the generation of hydroxyl radical in the presence of ascorbate is linked to redox-potentials and aggregation state. Chembiochem. 2007 Jul 23;8(11):1317-25)

(Gulcln, 2008) (I≠lhami Gulcln.In vitro prooxidant effect of caffeine. Journal of Enzyme Inhibition and Medicinal Chemistry, Volume 23, Issue 1 February 2008 , pages 149 - 152)

(Gulesserian et al, 2001) (Gulesserian T, Seidl R, Hardmeier R, Cairns N, Lubec G., Superoxide dismutase SOD1, encoded on chromosome 21, but not SOD2 is overexpressed in brains of patients with Down syndrome. J Investig Med 2001 Jan;49(1):41-6)

(Guo et al, 2000) (Guo Z, Cupples LA, Kurz A, et al. Head injury and the risk of AD in the MIRAGE study. Neurology. 2000;54:1316-1323)

(Guskiewicz et al, 2005) (Guskiewicz KM, Marshall SW, Bailes J, et al. Association between recurrent concussion and late-life cognitive impairment in retired professional football players. Neurosurgery. 2005;57:719-726)

(Gutzmann et al, 1998) (Gutzmann H, Hadler D. Sustained efficacy and safety of idebenone in the treatment of Alzheimer's disease: update on a 2-year double-blind multicentre study. J Neural Transm Suppl. 1998;54:301–310)

(Gutzmann et al, 2002) (Gutzmann H, Kuhl KP, Hadler D, Rapp MA. Safety and efficacy of idebenone versus tacrine in patients with Alzheimer's disease: results of a randomized, double-blind, parallel-group multicenter study. Pharmacopsychiatry. 2002;35:12–18)

(Haan, 2003) (Mary N Haan. Dietary Intake of Antioxidants and Risk of Alzheimer Disease. American Journal of Clinical Nutrition, Vol. 77, No. 4, 762-763, April 2003)

(Hancock et al, 2009) (Hancock, K. D., Coleman, E. S., Tao, Y. X., Morrison, E. E. et al., Genistein decreases androgen biosynthesis in rat Leydig cells by interference with luteinizing hormone-dependent signaling. Toxicol. Lett. 2009, 184, 169–175)

(Hara et al, 2011 (Hara A, et al. Use of vitamin supplements and risk of total cancer and cardiovascular disease among the Japanese general population: a population-based survey. BMC Public Health. 2011 Jul 8;11:540)

(Harman, 1969) (Harman D.: Prolongation of life: Role of free radical reactions in aging. J. Am. Geriatr. Soc. 1969, 17: 721-735)

Harman, 1978) (Harman D.: Free radical theory of aging: Nutritional implications. Age 1978, 1: 143-150)

(Harman D.: The aging process. Proc, Natl. Acad. Sci. USA 1981, 78: 7124-7128)

(Haseen et al, 2009) (Haseen F, Cantwell MM, O'Sullivan JM, Murray LJ. Is there a benefit from lycopene supplementation in men with prostate cancer? A systematic review. Prostate Cancer Prostatic Dis. 2009;12(4):325-32)

(Hattori, 2004) (Hattori N. Etiology and pathogenesis of Parkinson's disease: from mitochondrial dysfunctions to familial Parkinson's disease. Rinsho Shinkeigaku. 2004 Apr;44(4-5):241-62)

(Heart Protection Study Collaborative Group MRC/BHF Heart Protection Study, 2002) (Heart Protection Study Collaborative Group MRC/BHF Heart Protection Study of antioxidant vitamin supplementation in 20536 high-risk individuals: a randomised placebo-controlled trial. Lancet. 2002;360:23–33)

(Hensley et al, 1998) (Hensley K, Pye QN, Maidt ML, Stewart CA, Robinson KA, Jaffrey F, Floyd RA. Interaction of α-phenyl-N-tert-butyl nitrone and alternative electron acceptors with complex I indicates a substrate reduction site upstream from the rotenone binding site. J Neurochem 71:2549–2557, 1998)

(Hercberg et al, 2007) (Hercberg, S., Ezzedine, K., Guinot, C., Preziosi, P. et al., Antioxidant supplementation increases the risk of skin cancers in women but not in men. J. Nutr. 2007, 137, 2098–2105)

(Hill et al, 2001) (Hill, R. C., Armstrong, D., Browne, R. W., Lewis, D. D., Scott, K. C., Sundstrom, D. & Harper, J. (2001) Chronic administration of high doses of vitamin E appear to slow racing greyhounds. FASEB J 15:A990)

(Hockenbery et al, 1993) (Hockenbery, D. M., Oltvai, Z. N., Yin, X. M., Milliman, C. L., Korsmeyer, S. J., Bcl-2 functions in an antioxidant pathway to prevent apoptosis. Cell 1993, 75, 241–251)

(Hof et al, 1992) (Hof PR, Bouras C, Buce L, et al. Differential distribution of neurofibrillary tangles in the cerebral cortex of dementia pugilistica and Alzheimer's disease cases. Acta Neuropathol. 1992;85:23-30)

(Hollman et al, 2011) (Hollman PC, Cassidy A, Comte B, Heinonen M. Richelle M, Richling E, Sarafini M, Scalbert A, Sies H, Vidry S. The biological relevance of direct antioxidant effects of polyphenols for cardiovascular health in humans is not established. J Nutr. 2011 May;141(5):989S-1009S. Epub 2011 Mar 30)

(Hooshmand et al, 2010) (Hooshmand B, Solomon A, Kårehold I, et al. Homocysteine and holotranscobalamin and the risk of Alzheimer disease. Neurology, 2010;75:1408-1414)

(Hsieh et al, 19980 (Hsieh, C.Y., Santell, R. C., Haslam, S. Z., Helferich, W. G., Estrogenic effects of genistein on the growth of estrogen receptor-positive human breast cancer (MCF-7) cells in vitro and in vivo. Cancer Res. 1998, 58, 3833–3838)

(Huang et al, 2006) (Huang HY, Caballero B, Chang S, et al. Multivitamin mineral supplements and prevention of chronic disease: executive summary. Am J Clin Nutr 2006;85(suppl):265S–9S)

(Hughes et al, 1998) (Hughes CM, Lewis SE, McKelvey-Martin VJ, Thompson W. The effects of antioxidant supplementation during Percoll preparation on human sperm DNA integrity. Hum Reprod. 1998;13:1240–7)

(Hughes et al, 2005) (Hughes S, Colantonio A, Santaguida PL, Paton T. Amantadine to enhance readiness for rehabilitation following severe traumatic brain injury. Brain Inj.

2005;19:1197-1206)

(Huret et al, 1987) (Huret, J. L et al. Down syndrome with duplication of a region of chromosome 21 containing the CuZn superoxide dismutase gene without detectable karyotypic abnormality. Hum. Genet. 75: 251-257, 1987)

(Isaac et al, 2008, CD002854) (Isaac MG, Quinn R, Tabet N. Vitamin E for Alzheimer's disease and mild cognitive impairment. Cochrane Database Syst Rev. 2008 Jul 16;(3):CD002854)

(Ito et al, 1986) (Ito N, Hirose M, Fukushima S, et al. Studies on antioxidants: Their carcinogenic and modifying effects on chemical carcinogenesis. Food and Chemical Toxicology. Vol. 35, Issues 10-11, Oct-Nov 1986, pp 1071-1082)

(Jack et al, 2008) (Jack CR, Jr, Petersen RC, Grundman M, Jin S, Gamst A, Ward CP, Sencakova D, Doody RS, Thal LJ. Longitudinal MRI findings from the vitamin E and donepezil treatment study for MCI. Neurobiol Aging. 2008;29:1285–1295)

(Jacob, 1990) (Jacob RA. Assessment of human vitamin C status. J Nutr. 1990;120(Suppl 11):1480–5)

(Jacobs, Connell, McCullough et al, 2002) (Jacobs EJ, Connell CJ, McCullough ML. et al. Vitamin C, vitamin E, and multivitamin supplement use and stomach cancer mortality in the Cancer Prevention Study II cohort. Cancer Epidemiol Biomarkers Prev. 2002 Jan;11(1):35-41)

(Jefferson et al, 2006) (Jefferson, W. N., Padilla-Banks, E., Newbold, R. R., Studies of the effects of neonatal exposure to genistein on the developing female reproductive system. J. AOAC Int. 2006, 89, 1189–1196)

(Jerome-Morais et al, 2011) (A. Jerome-Morais, A. M. Diamond, and M. E. Wright, "Dietary supplements and human health: for better or for worse?" *Molecular Nutrition and Food Research*, vol. 55, no. 1, pp. 122–135, 2011)

(Jezorowska et al, 1982) (Jezorowska A., Jacubowski L., Armatys A., Kaluzewski B.: Copper/zinc superoxide dismutase (SOD-1) in regular trisomy 21, trisomy 21 by translocation and mosaic trisomy 21. Clin. Genet. 1982, 22: 160-164)

(Jia et al, 2008) (Jia X, et al, Does taking vitamin, mineral and fatty acid supplements prevent cognitive decline? A systematic review of randomized controlled trials. J Hum Nutr Diet. 2008 Aug;21(4):317-36)

(Jiang et al, 2007) (Jiang D, Men L, Wang J, Zhang Y, Chickenyen S, Wang Y, Zhou F. Redox reactions of copper complexes formed with different beta-amyloid peptides and their neuropathological [correction of neuropathalogical] relevance. Biochemistry. 2007 Aug 14;46(32):9270-82)

(Johnson et al, 1986) (Johnson Jr J.E., Walford R., Harman D., Miquel J.: Free radicals, aging and degenerative diseases. Liss, New York 1986)

(Johnson et al, 2003) (Johnson LJ, Meacham SL, Kruskall LJ. The antioxidants--vitamin C, vitamin E, selenium, and carotenoids. J Agromedicine. 2003;9(1):65-82)

(Jourkesh et al, 2011) (Morteza Jourkesh, Iraj Sadri, mineh Sahranavard, li Ojagi, Mohammad Dehganpoori. The Effects of two different doses of Antioxidant Vitamin C supplementation on bioenergetics index in male college student. Journal of American Science 2011;7(6):852-858)

(Ju et al, 2002) (Ju, Y. H., Doerge, D. R., Allred, K. F., Allred, C. D., Helferich, W. G., Dietary genistein negates the inhibitory effect of tamoxifen on growth of estrogen-dependent human breast cancer (MCF-7) cells implanted in athymic mice. Cancer Res. 2002, 62, 2474–2477)

(Ju et al, 2008) (Ju, Y. H., Doerge, D. R., Woodling, K.A., Hartman, J.A. et al., Dietary genistein negates the inhibitory effect of letrozole on the growth of aromatase-expressing estrogen-dependent human breast cancer cells (MCF-7Ca) in vivo. Carcinogenesis 2008, 29, 2162–2168)

(Kamat et al, 2008) (Kamat CD, et al. Antioxidants in central nervous system diseases: preclinical promise and translational challenges. J Alzheimer's Dis. 2008 Nov;15(3):473-93)

(Kang et al, 2006) (Kang JH, Cook N, Manson J, Buring JE, Grodstein F. A randomized trial of vitamin E supplementation and cognitive function in women. Arch Intern Med. 2006;166:2462–2468)

(Katzman et al, 1996) (Katzman R, Galasko DR, Saitoh T, et al. Apolipoprotein-'4 and head trauma: synergistic or additive risks? Neurology. 1996;4:889-891)

(Kavanaugh et al, 2007) (Kavanaugh CJ, Trumbo PR, Ellwood KC. The U.S. Food and Drug Administration's evidence-based review for qualified health claims: tomatoes, lycopene, and cancer. Journal of the National Cancer Institute. 2007;99:1074-85)

(Kieburtz et al, 1994) (Kieburtz K, McDermott M, Como P, Growdon J, Brady J, Carter J, Huber S, Kanigan B, Landow E, Rudolph A, et al. The effect of deprenyl and tocopherol on cognitive performance in early untreated Parkinson's disease. Parkinson Study Group. Neurology. 1994;44:1756–1759)

(Kieburtz et al, 2010) (Kieburtz K, McDermott MP, Voss TS, Corey-Bloom J, Deuel LM, Dorsey ER, Factor S, Geschwind MD, Hodgeman K, Kayson E, Noonberg S, Pourfar M, Rabinowitz K, Ravina B, Sanchez-Ramos J, Seely L, Walker F, Feigin A. A randomized, placebo-controlled trial of latrepirdine in Huntington disease. Arch Neurol. 2010;67:154–160)

(Kim et al, 2008) (Kim, Y. M., Yang, S., Xu, W., Li, S., Yang, X., Continuous in vitro exposure to low-dose genistein induces genomic instability in breast epithelial cells. Cancer Genet. Cytogenet. 2008, 186, 78–84)

(Kim et al, 2009) (Kim, D. J., Seok, S. H., Baek, M. W., Lee, H. Y. et al., Developmental toxicity and brain aromatase induction by high genistein concentrations in zebrafish embryos. Toxicol. Mech. Methods 2009, 19, 251–256)

(Knechtle et al, 2008) (Knechtle B et al, Vitamins, minerals and race performance in ultra-endurance runners--Deutschlandlauf 2006. Asia Pac J Clin Nutr. 2008;17(2):194-8)

(Krauth-Siegel et al, 2008) (Krauth-Siegel RL, Comini MA. Redox control in trypanosomatids, parasitic protozoa with trypanothione-based thiol metabolism. mbiochim Biophys Acta. 2008 Nov;1780(11):1236-48)

(Kulling et al, 1999) (Kulling, S. E., Rosenberg, B., Jacobs, E., Metzler, M., The phytoestrogens coumoestrol and genistein induce structural chromosomal aberrations in cultured human peripheral blood lymphocytes. Arch. Toxicol. 1999, 73, 50–54)

(Kumar et al, 2008) (Kumar NB et al, Results of a Randomized Clinical Trial of the Action of Several Doses of Lycopene in Localized Prostate Cancer: Administration Prior to Radical Prostatectomy. Clin Med Urol. 2008 Apr 16;1:1-14)

(Kupcinskas et al, 2008) (Kupcinskas L, Lafolie P, Lignell A, et al. Efficacy of the natural antioxidant astaxanthin in the treatment of functional dyspepsia in patients with or without Helicobacter pylori infection: A prospective, randomized, double blind, and placebo-controlled study. Phytomedicine. 2008 May 6)

(Kwiecinski et al, 2001) (Kwieciński H, Janik P, Jamrozik Z, Opuchlik A. The effect of selegiline and vitamin E in the treatment of ALS: an open randomized clinical trials. Neurol Neurochir Pol. 2001;35(1 Suppl):101-6)

(Laclaustra et al, 2009) (Laclaustra, M., Navas-Acien, A., Stranges, S., Ordovas, J. M., Guallar, E., Serum selenium concentrations and diabetes in US adults: National Health and Nutrition Examination Survey (NHANES) 2003–2004. Environ. Health Perspect. 2009, 117, 1409–1413)

(Lamprecht et al, 2009) (Lamprecht M, et al. Increased lipid peroxidation in trained men after 2 weeks of antioxidant supplementation. Int J Sport Nutr Exerc Metab. 2009 Aug;19(4):385-99)

(Lannfelt et al, 2008) (Lannfelt L, Blennow K, Zetterberg H, Batsman S, Ames D, Harrison J, Masters CL, Targum S, Bush AI, Murdoch R, Wilson J, Ritchie CW. Safety, efficacy, and biomarker findings of PBT2 in targeting Abeta as a modifying therapy for Alzheimer's disease: a phase IIa, double-blind, randomised, placebo-controlled trial. Lancet Neurol. 2008;7:779–786)

(Larson et al, 2007) (Larson MJ, Kaufman DA, Schmalfuss IM, Perlstein WM. Performance monitoring, error processing, and evaluative control following severe TBI.

J Int Neuropsychol Soc. 2007;13:961-971)

(Laurin, Foley, 2002) (Laurin D, Foley DJ. Vitamin E and C supplements and risk of dementia. JAMA. 2002;288(18):2266-2268)

(Lawenda et al, 2008) (Lawenda, B. D., Kelly, K. M., Ladas, E. J., Sagar, S. M. et al., Should supplemental antioxidant administration be avoided during chemotherapy and radiation therapy? J. Natl. Cancer Inst. 2008, 100, 773–783)

(Lawson et al, 2007) (Lawson KA, Wright ME, Subar A, Mouw T, Hollenbeck A, Schatzkin A,. Leitzmann MF. Multivitamin use and risk of prostate cancer in the National Institutes of Health-AARP Diet and Health Study. J Natl Cancer Inst. 2007 May 16;99(10):754-64)

(Lees, 2003) (Lees KR, et al. Tolerability of NXY-059 at higher target concentrations in patients with acute stroke. Stroke 2003 Feb;34(2):482-7)

(Levin, 2005) (Levin, Edward D. Extracellular Superoxide Dismutase (EC-SOD) Quenches Free Radicals and Attenuates Age-Related Cognitive Decline: Opportunities for Novel Drug Development in Aging. Current Alzheimer Research, Volume 2, Number 2, April 2005 , pp. 191-196(6)

(Lim et al, 2001) (Lim GP, Chu T, Yang F, Beech W, Frautschy SA, Cole GM. The curry spice curcumin reduces oxidative damage and amyloid pathology in an Alzheimer transgenic mouse. J Neurosci. 2001;21:8370–8377)

(Lim et al, 2006) (Lim WS, Gammack JK, Van Niekerk JK, Dangour A. Omega 3 fatty acid for the prevention of dementia. Cochrane Database Syst Rev 2006;1:CD005379)

(Limer et al, 2006) (Limer, J. L., Parkes, A. T., Speirs, V., Differential response to phytoestrogens in endocrine sensitive and resistant breast cancer cells in vitro. Int. J. Cancer 2006, 119, 515–521)

(Lind, J., Nutrition classics. A treatise of the scurvy by James Lind, MDCCLIII. Nutr. Rev. 1983, 41, 155–157)

(Lippman et al, 2009) (Lippman, S. M., Klein, E. A., Goodman, P. J., Lucia, M. S. et al., Effect of selenium and vitamin E on risk of prostate cancer and other cancers: the Selenium and Vitamin E on risk of prostate cancer and other cancers: the Selenium and Vitamin E Cancer Prevention Trial (SELECT). J. Am. Med. Assoc. 2009, 301, 39–51)

(Liu et al, 2005) (Liu, B., Edgerton, S., Yang, X., Kim, A. et al., Low-dose dietary phytoestrogen abrogates tamoxifen-associated mammary tumor prevention. Cancer Res. 2005, 65, 879–886)

(Lonn, E., Bosch, J., Yusuf, S., Sheridan, P. et al., Effects of long-term vitamin E supplementation on cardiovascular events and cancer: a randomized controlled trial. J. Am. Med. Assoc. 2005, 293, 1338–1347)

(Lovell et al, 1995) (Lovell MA, Ehmann WD, Butler SM, Markesbery WR. Elevated thiobarbituric acid- reactive substances and antioxidant enzyme activity in the brain in Alzheimer's disease. Neurology 45: 1594-1601, 1995)

(Lu et al, 2005) (Lu Q, Bjorkhem I, Wretlind B, Diczfalusy U, Henriksson P, Freyschuss A. Effect of ascorbic acid on microcirculation in patients with type II diabetes: a randomized placebo-controlled cross-over study. Clin Sci (Lond) 2005;108(6):507–513)

(Luchsinger et al, 2003) (Luchsinger JA, Tang MX, Shea S, Mayeux R. Antioxidant vitamin intake and risk of Alzheimer disease. Arch Neurol. 2003;60:203–208)

(Luchsinger et al, 2004) (Luchsinger JA, Mayeux R. Dietary factors and Alzheimer's disease. Lancet Neurol. 2004;3:579–87)

(Lund-Olesen, 2000) (Lund-Olesen K. Etiology of multiple sclerosis: role of superoxide dismutase. Med Hypotheses. 2000 Feb;54(2):321-2)

(MacFarquhar et al, 2010) (MacFarquhar, J. K., Broussard, D. L., Melstrom, P., Hutchinson, R. et al., Acute selenium toxicity associated with a dietary supplement. Arch. Intern. Med. 2010, 170, 256–261)

(Malouf et al, 2008) (Malouf R, Grimley Evans J. Folic acid with or without vitamin B12 for the prevention and treatment of healthy elderly and demented people. Cochrane Database Syst Rev 2008;4:CD004514)

(Manju et al, 2002) (Manju V, Balasubramanian V, Nalini N. Oxidative stress and tumor markers in cervical cancer patients. J Biochem Mol Biol Biophys. 2002 Dec;6(6):387-90)

(Marccioni et al, 2001) (Maccioni RB, Muñoz JP, Barbeito L. The molecular bases of Alzheimer's disease and other neurodegenerative disorders. Arch Med Res. 2001 Sep-Oct;32(5):367-81)

(Markesbery, 1997) (Markesbery WR. Oxidative stress hypothesis in Alzheimer's disease. free Radic Biol Med. 1997;23(1):134-47)

(Markiund et al, 1985) (Markiund S.L., Adolfsson R., Gottfries C.G., Winblad B.: Superoxide dismutase isoenzymes in normal brains and in brains from patients with dementia of Alzheimer type. J. Neurol. Sci. 1985, 67: 319-325)

(Marklund et al, 1982) (Marklund SL, Westman NG, Lundgren E, Roos G. Copper- and zinc-containing superoxide dismutase, manganese-containing superoxide dismutase, catalase, and glutathione peroxidase in normal and neoplastic human cell lines and normal human tissues. Cancer Res 42:1955–1961, 1982)

(Markovits et al, 1989) (Markovits, J., Linassier, C., Fosse, P., Couprie, J. et al., Inhibitory effects of the tyrosine kinase inhibitor genistein on mammalian DNA topoisomerase II. Cancer Res. 1989, 49, 5111–5117)

(Marshall et al, 2002) (Marshall, RJ, Scott KC, Hill RC, et al, Supplemental vitamin C appears to slow racing Greyhounds. J. Nutr 2002;132:1616S-1621S)

(Masaki et al, 2000) (Masaki KH, Losonczy KG, Izmirlian G, Foley DJ, Ross GW, Petrovitch H, Havlik R, White LR. Association of vitamin E and C supplement use with cognitive function and dementia in elderly men. Neurology. 2000;54:1265–1272)

(Mastaloudis et al, 2001) (Mastaloudis A, Leonard SW, Traber MG. Oxidative stress in athletes during extreme endurance exercise. Free Radic Biol Med. 2001 Oct 1;31(7):911-22)

(Mastaloudis et al, 2004) (Mastaloudis A, Morrow JD, Hopkins DW, et al, Antioxidant supplementation prevents exercise-induced lipid peroxidation, but not inflammation, in ultra marathon runners. Free Radic Biol Med. 2004;36:1329-1341)

(Mastaloudis et al, 2006) (Mastaloudis A, et al, Antioxidants did not prevent muscle damage in response to an unltramarathon run. Med Sci Sports Exerc. 2006 Jan;38(1):72-80)

(Maxwell et al, 2005) (Maxwell CJ, Hicks MS, Hogan DB, Basran J, Ebly EM. Supplemental use of antioxidant vitamins and subsequent risk of cognitive decline and dementia. Dement Geriatr Cogn Disord. 2005;20:45–51)

(Mayeux et al, 1995) (Mayeux R, Ottman R, Maestre G, et al. Synergistic effects of traumatic head injury and apolipoprotein-epsilon 4 in patients with Alzheimer's disease.

Neurology. 1995;45:555-557)

(Mayne, 1996) (Mayne, S. T., Beta-carotene, carotenoids, and disease prevention in humans. FASEB J. 1996, 10, 690–701)

(McClung et al, 2004) (McClung, J. P., Roneker, C. A., Mu, W., Lisk, D. J. et al., Development of insulin resistance and obesity in mice overexpressing cellular glutathione peroxidase. Proc. Natl. Acad. Sci. USA 2004, 101, 8852–8857)

(McCormick et al, 2010) (McCormick DL, et al, Null activity of selenium and vitamin e as cancer chemopreventive agents in the rat prostate. Cancer Prev Res (Phila). 2010 Mar;3(3):381-92)

(McGinley et al, 2009) (McGinley C, Shafat A, Donnelly AE. Does antioxidant vitamin supplementation protect against muscle damage? Sports Med. 2009;39(12):1011-32)

(McIntosh et al, 1997) (McIntosh LJ, Trush MA, Troncoso JC. Increased susceptibility of Alzheimer's disease temporal cortex to oxygen free radical-mediated processes. Free Radic Biol Med. 1997;23(2):183-90)

(McLean et al, 1999) (C.A. McLean, R.A. Cherny, F.W. Fraser, S.J. Fuller, M.J. Smith, K. Beyreuther, A.I. Bush, C.L. Masters, Soluble pool of Abeta amyloid as a determinant of severity of neurodegeneration in Alzheimer's disease, Ann. Neurol. 46 (1999) 860-866)

(McMahon et al, 2006) (McMahon JA, Green TJ, Skeaff CM, Knight RG, Mann JI, Williams SM. A controlled trial of homocysteine lowering and cognitive performance. N Engl J Med. 2006;354:2764–72)

(McMichael-Phillips et al, 1998) (McMichael-Phillips, D. F., Harding, C., Morton, M., Roberts, S. A. et al., Effects of soy-protein supplementation on epithelial proliferation in the histologically normal human breast. Am. J Clin. Nutr. 1998, 68, 1431S–1435S)

(McNeill et al, 2007) (McNeill G, et al. Effect of multivitamin and multimineral supplementation on cognitive function in men and women aged 65 years and over: a randomised controlled trial. Nutr J. 2007 May 2;6:10)

(Mecocci et al, 2004) (Patrizia Mecocci, Usha MacGarvey, M. Flint Beal. Oxidative damage to mitochondrial DNA is increased in Alzheimer's disease. Annals of Neurology. 2004. Volume 36 Issue 5, Pages 747 - 751)

(Meeker et al, 2010) (Meeker JD, et al. Semen quality and sperm DNA damage in relation to urinary bisphenol A among men from an infertility clinic. Reprod Toxicol. 2010 Dec;30(4):532-9)

(Meguid, 2005) (Meguid MM. Retraction. Nutrition. 2005;21:286. doi: 10.1016/j.nut.2004.12.002)

(Mendelsohn et al, 1998) (Mendelsohn AB, Belle SH, Stoehr GP, Ganguli M. Use of antioxidant supplements and its association with cognitive function in a rural elderly cohort: the MoVIES Project. Monongahela Valley Independent Elders Survey. Am J Epidemiol. 1998;148:38–44)

(Michael et al, 2006) (Michael McClain, R., Wolz, E., Davidovich, A., Bausch, J., Genetic toxicity studies with genistein. Food Chem. Toxicol. 2006, 44, 42–55)

(Miller, 1974) (Miller E.: Dementia as an accelerated ageing of the nervous system: Some psychological and methodological considerations. Age Ageing 1974, 3: 197-202)

(Miller et al, 2005) (Miller ER, 3rd, Pastor-Barriuso R, Dalal D, Riemersma RA, Appel LJ, Guallar E. Meta-analysis: high-dosage vitamin E supplementation may increase all-cause mortality. Ann Intern Med. 2005;142:37–46)

(Miquel et al, 1977) (Miquel J., Oro J., Bensch K.G., Johnson J.E.: Lipofuscin; Fine-structural and biochemical studies. In: Pryor U.A. (ed): Free radicals in biology. Academic Press, New York 1977: 133-182)

(Moch, 1986) (Moch RW. Pathology of BHA- and BHT-induced lesions. Food and Chemical Toxicology. Vol. 24, Issues 10-11, Oct-Nov 1986, pp 1167-1169)

(Moreira et al, 2005) (Moreira PI, et al, A second look into the oxidant mechanisms in Alzheimer's disease. Curr Neurovasc Res. 2005 Apr;2(2):179-84)

(Morris et al, 1998) (Morris MC, Beckett LA, Scherr PA, Hebert LE, Bennett DA, Field TS, Evans DA. Vitamin E and vitamin C supplement use and risk of incident Alzheimer disease. Alzheimer Dis Assoc Disord. 1998;12:121–126)

(Morris et al, 2002) (Morris MC, Evans DA, Bienias JL, Tangney CC, Bennett DA, Aggarwal N, Wilson RS, Scherr PA. Dietary intake of antioxidant nutrients and the risk of incident Alzheimer disease in a biracial community study. JAMA. 2002;287:3230–3237)

(Mukai, Goldstein, 1976) (Mukai F.H., Goldstein B.D.: Mutagenicity of malondialdehyde, a decomposition product of peroxidized polyunsaturated fatty acids. Science 1976, 191: 868)

(Muller, 2004) (Müller S. Redox and antioxidant systems of the malaria parasite Plasmodium falciparum. Mol Microbiol. 2004 Sep;53(5):1291-305)

(Muth et al, 2000) (Muth ER, Laurent JM, Jasper P. The effect of bilberry nutritional supplementation on night visual acuity and contrast sensitivity. Altern Med Rev. 2000 Apr;5(2):164-73)

(Nadal et al, 2008) (Nadal RC, Rigby SE, Viles JH. Amyloid beta-Cu2+ complexes in both monomeric and fibrillar forms do not generate H2O2 catalytically but quench hydroxyl radicals. Biochemistry. 2008 Nov 4;47(44):11653-64. Epub 2008 Oct 11)

(Nadeem et al, 2008) (Nadeem A, Raj HG, Chhabra SK. Effect of vitamin E supplementation with standard treatment on oxidant-antioxidant status in chronic obstructive pulmonary disease. Indian J Med Res. 2008 Dec;128(6):705-11)

(Nahin et al, 2006) (Nahin RL, Fitzpatrick AL, Williamson JD, Burke GL, DeKosky ST, Furberg C.; GEM Study Investigators Use of herbal medicine and other dietary supplements in community dwelling older people: baseline data from the Ginkgo Evaluation of Memory Study. J Am Geriat Soc 2006;54:1725–35)

(Nakhostin-Roohi et al, 2008) (Nakhostin-Roohi et al, Effect of vitamin C supplementation on lipid peroxidation, muscle damage and inflammation after 30-min exercise at 75% VO2max. J Sports Med Phys Fitness. 2008 Jun;48(2):217-24)

(Navarro, Boveris, 2010) (Navarro A, Boveris A. Brain mitochondrial dysfunction in aging, neurodegeneration, and Parkinson's disease. Front Aging Neurosci. 2010 Sep 1;2. pii. 34)

(Neve et al, 1983) (Neve J., Sinet P.M., Molle L., Nicole A.: Selenium, zinc and copper in Down's syndrome (Trisomy 21): Blood levels and relations with glutathione peroxidase and superoxide dismutase. Clin. Chim. Acta 1983, 133: 209-214)

(Octave, 2005) (Octave JN. Alzheimer disease: cellular and molecular aspects. Bull Mem Acad R Med Belg. 2005;160(10-12):445-9)

(Olansky, Hayflick, 2004) (Position Statement on Human aging. S. Jay Olshansky, Ph.D. Leonard Hayflick, Ph.D. Bruce A. Carnes, Ph.D. Accessed 12-8-08. http://www.quackwatch.org/01QuackeryRelatedTopics/antiagingpp.html)

(O'Meara et al, 1997) (O'Meara ES, Kukull W, Sheppard L, et al. Head injury and risk of Alzheimer's disease by apolipoprotein E genotype. Am J Epidemiol. 1997;146:373-384)

(Omenn et al, 1996) (Omenn, G. S., Goodman, G. E., Thornquist, M. D., Balmes, J. et al., Effects of a combination of beta carotene and vitamin A on lung cancer and cardiovascular disease. N. Engl. J. Med. 1996, 334, 1150–1155)

(Omenn, 1998) (Omenn, G. S., Chemoprevention of lung cancer: the rise and demise of beta-carotene. Annu. Rev. Public Health 1998, 19, 73–99)

(Ough et al, 2004) (Ough M, Lewis A, Zhang Y, et al. Inhibition of cell growth by over-expression of manganese superoxide dismutase (MnSOD) in human pancreatic carcinoma. Free Radic Res. 2004 Nov;38(11):1223-33)

(Ozten et al, 2010) (Ozten N, Horton L,Lasano S, Bosland MC. Selenomethionine and alpha-tocopherol do not inhibit prostate carcinogenesis in the testosterone plus estradiol-treated NBL rat model. Cancer Prev Res (Phila). 2010 Mar;3(3):371-80)

(Palmer et al, 2009) (Palmer JC, Baig S, Kehoe PG, Love S: Endothelin-Converting Enzyme-2 is Increased in Alzheimer's Disease. Am J Pathol 2009, 174: 2672-2680)

(Pan et al, 2008) (Pan R, Qiu S, Lu DX, Dong J. Curcumin improves learning and memory ability and its neuroprotective mechanism in mice. Chin Med J (Engl). 2008;121(9):832-839)

(Paolisso etal, 1993) (Paolisso G, D'Amore A, Giugliano D, Ceriello A, Varricchio M, D'Onofrio F. Pharmacologic doses of vitamin E improve insulin action in healthy subjects and non-insulin-dependent diabetic patients. Am J Clin Nutr. 1993;57(5):650–656)

(Park et al, 1999) (Park, J.S. et al., Dietary lutein but not astaxanthin or β-carotene increases pim-1 gene expression in murine lymphocytes, Nutr. Cancer, 33, 206, 1999)

(Park et al, 2011) (Park SY et al. Multivitamin use and the risk of mortality and cancer incidence: the multiethnic cohort study. Am J Epidemiol. 2011 Apr 15;173(8):906-14)

(Parnetti et al, 1995) (Parnetti L,Ambrosoli L,Abate G,Azzini C, Balestreri R, Bartorelli L, Bordin A, Crepaldi G, Cristianini G, Cucinotta D, et al. Posatirelin for the treatment of late-onset Alzheimer's disease: a double-blind multicentre study vs citicoline and ascorbic acid. Acta Neurol Scand. 1995;92:135–140)

(Patterson et al, 2008) (Patterson C, Feightner JW, Garcia A, et al. Diagnosis and treatment of dementia: 1. Risk assessment and primary prevention of Alzheimer disease. CMAJ 2008;178:548-56)

(Peers et al, 2009) (Chris Peers, John P Boyle, Jason L Scragg. Hugh A Pearson. The Journal of Quality Research in Dementia, Issue 4 (lay summary) http://alzheimers.

org.uk/site/scripts/documents_info.php?documentID=383&pageNumber=2. Accessed 2-3-09.

(Perrig et al, 1997) (Perrig WJ, Perrig P, Stahelin H. The relation between antioxidants and memory performance in the old and very old. J Am Geriatr Soc 45: 718-724, 1997)

(Peters, Takata, 2008) (Peters, U., Takata, Y., Selenium and the prevention of prostate and colorectal cancer. Mol. Nutr. Food Res. 2008, 52, 1261–1272)

(Piller et al, 2006) (Piller, R., Chang-Claude, J., Linseisen, J., Plasma enterolactone and genistein and the risk of premenopausal breast cancer. Eur. J. Cancer Prev. 2006, 15, 225–232)

(Pool-Zobel et al, 2000) (Pool-Zobel, B. L., Adlercreutz, H., Glei, M., Liegibel, U. M. et al., Isoflavonoids and lignans have different potentials to modulate oxidative genetic damage in human colon cells. Carcinogenesis 2000, 21, 1247–1252)

(Poston et al, 2006) (Poston, L., Briley, A. L., Seed, P. T., Kelly, F. J., Shennan, A. H., Vitamin C and vitamin E in pregnant women at risk for pre-eclampsia (VIP trial): randomised placebo-controlled trial. Lancet 2006, 367, 1145–1154)

(Powers, Hamilton, 1999) (Powers SK, Hamilton K. Antioxidants and exercise. Clin Sports Med. 1999 Jul;18(3):525-36)

(Pratico, 2002) (Domenico Praticò. Alzheimer's disease and oxygen radicals: new insights.

Biochemical Pharmacology. Volume 63, Issue 4, 15 February 2002, Pages 563-567)

(Ramussen et al, 1995) (Rasmussen DX, Brandt J, Martin DB, Folstein MF. Head injury as a risk factor in Alzheimer's disease. Brain Injury. 1995;9:213-219)

33. (Schofield et al, 1997) (Schofield PW, Tang M, Marder K, et al. Alzheimer's disease after remote head injury: an incidence study. J Neurol Neurosurg Psychiatry. 1997;

37:1630-1633)

(Reaven et al, 1995) (Reaven PD, Herold DA, Barnett J, Edelman S. Effects of vitamin E on susceptibility of low-density lipoprotein and low-density lipoprotein subfractions to oxidation and on protein glycation in NIDDM. Diabetes Care. 1995;18(6):807–816)

(Reeves, Hoffman, 2009) (Reeves, M. A., Hoffmann, P. R., The human selenoproteome: recent insights into functions and regulation. Cell Mol. Life Sci. 2009, 66, 2457–2478)

(Ritchie et al, 2003) (Ritchie CW, Bush AI, Mackinnon A, Macfarlane S, Mastwyk M, MacGregor L, Kiers L, Cherny R, Li QX, Tammer A, Carrington D, Mavros C, Volitakis I, Xilinas M, Ames D, Davis S, Beyreuther K, Tanzi RE, Masters CL. Metal-protein attenuation with iodochlorhydroxyquin (clioquinol) targeting Abeta amyloid deposition and toxicity in Alzheimer disease: a pilot phase 2 clinical trial. Arch Neurol. 2003;60:1685–1691)

(Roberts et al, 1990) (Roberts GW, Allsop D, Bruton C. The occult aftermath of boxing. J Neurol Neurosurg Psychiatry. 1990;53:373-378)

(Rodriguez et al, 2009) (Rodriguez NR, Di Marco NM, Langley S. American Dietetic Association; Dietitians of Canada; American College of Sports Medicine, American College of Sports Medicine position stand. Nutrition and athletic performance. Med Sci Sports Exerc. 2009 Mar;41(3):709-31)

(Rosen et al, 1993) (Rosen, D. R. et al. Mutations in Cu/Zn superoxide dismutase gene are associated with familial amyotrophic lateral sclerosis. Nature 362: 59-62, 1993)

(Ruiz-Larrea et al, 1997) (Ruiz-Larrea, M. B., Mohan, A. R., Paganga, G., Miller, N. J. et al., Antioxidant activity of phytoestrogenic isoflavones. Free Radic. Res. 1997, 26, 63–70)

(Ryle, Thompson, 1984) (Ryle PR, Thomson AD. Nutrition and vitamins in alcoholism. Contemp Issues Clin Biochem. 1984;1:188–224)

(Sanchez-Moreno et al, 2009) (Sanchez-Moreno C, et al. Stroke: roles of B vitamins, homocysteine and antioxidants. Nutr Res Rev. 2009 Jun;22(1):49-67)

(Sano et al, 1997) (Sano M, Ernesto C, Thomas RG, Klauber MR, Schafer K, Grundman M, Woodbury P, Growdon J, Cotman CW, Pfeiffer E, Schneider LS, Thal LJ. A controlled trial of selegiline, alpha-tocopherol, or both as treatment for Alzheimer's disease. The Alzheimer's Disease Cooperative Study. N Engl J Med. 1997;336:1216–1222)

(Sanz et al, 2009) (C. Sanz, S. Andrieu, A. Sinclair, H. Hanaire, B. Vellas For the REAL. FR Study Group. Diabetes is associated with a slower rate of cognitive decline in Alzheimer disease. Neurology, Oct 2009; 73: 1359 – 1366)

(Sarafian, et al, 1999) (Sarafian TA, et al. Oxidative stress produced by marijuana smoke. Am. J. Respir. Cell Mol. Biol., Volume 20, Number 6, June 1999 1286-1293)

(Sassi-Messai et al, 2009) (Sassi-Messai, S., Gibert, Y., Bernard, L., Nishio, S. et al., The phytoestrogen genistein affects zebrafish development through two different pathways. PloS ONE 2009, 4, e4935)

(Schretlen et al, 2007) (Schretlen DS, et al. High-normal uric acid linked with mild cognitive impairment in the elderly. Neuropsychology 21: 136-140. January 2007)

(Schwarz, Sept. 2009) (Schwarz A. Dementia risk seen in players in NFL study. New York Times. September 29, 2009:A1)

(Schwarz, Oct. 2009) (Schwarz A. NFL's dementia study has flaws, experts say. New York Times. October 26, 2009)

(Schwarz, Foltz, 1958) (Schwarz, K., Foltz, C. M., Factor 3 activity of selenium compounds. J. Biol. Chem. 1958, 233, 245–251)

(Science and Sports, 2008) (Caffeine ingestion effects on oxidative stress in a steady-state test at $75\% V_{O2max}$. Science and Sports. Volume 23, Issue 2, April 2008, Pages 87-90)

(Scileppi et al, 1984) (Scileppi K.P., Blass J.P., Baker H.G.: Circulating vitamins in Alzheimer's dementia as compared to other dementias. J. Am. Geriatr. Soc. 1984, 32: 709-711)

(Sheng et al, 2007) (Sheng B, Cheng LF, Law CB, et al. Coexisting cerebral infarction in Alzheimer's disease is associated with fast dementia progression: applying the NINDS-ARIEN neuroimaging criteria in Alzheimer's disease with concomitant infarction. J Am Geriatr Soc 2007;55:918-22)

(Sherrill et al, 2010) (Sherrill, J. D., Sparks, M., Dennis, J., Mansour, M. et al., Developmental exposures of male rats to soy isoflavones impact leydig cell differentiation. Biol. Reprod. 2010, 83, 488–501)

(Shils, et al, 2006) (Shils, M. E., Shike, M., Ross, A. C., Caballero, B., Cousins, R. J. (Eds.), Modern Nutrition in Health and Disease, Lippincott Williams & Wilkins, Baltimore, MD 2006)

(Shoulson et al, 1993) (Shoulson I, Fahn S, Kieburtz K, Lang A, Langston JW, Olanow CW. Effects of tocopherol and deprenyl on the progression of disability in early Parkinson's disease. N Engl J Med 328:176–183, 1993)

(Shoulson, 1998) (Shoulson I. DATATOP: a decade of neuroprotective inquiry. Parkinson Study Group. Deprenyl And Tocopherol Antioxidative Therapy Of Parkinsonism. Ann Neurol. 1998;44:S160–166)

(Silver et al, 2005) (Silver EW, Eskenazi B, Evenson DP, Block G, Young S, Wyrobek AJ. Effect of antioxidant intake on sperm chromatin stability in healthy nonsmoking men. J Androl. 2005;26:550–6)

(Sinclair et al,1999) (Sinclair AJ, et al. Altered plasma antioxidant status in subjects with Alzheimer's disease and vascular dementia. International Journal of Geriatric Psychiatry.1999.Vol. 13. Issue 12, Pp. 840-845)

(Sinet et al, 1974) (Sinet P.M., Allard D., Lejeune J. Jerome H.: Augmentation de l'activité de la superoxide dismutase erythrocytaire dans la trisomie pour le chromosome 21. CR Acad. Sci. [D] (Paris) 1974, 278: 3267-3270)

(Sinet, 1975) (Sinet P.M.: Increase in glutathione peroxidase activity in erythrocytes from trisomy 21 subjects. Biochim. Biophys. Acta 1975, 67: 910-915)

(Singh et al, 1992) (Singh A, et al. Chronic multivitamin-mineral supplementation does not enhance physical performance. Medicine and Science in Sports and Exercise. 1992;24:726–32)

(Skullerud et al, 1960) (Skullerud K., Martstein S., Schrader H., Brundelet P.S., Jellun E.: The cerebral lesions in a patients with generalized glutathione deficiency and pyro-glutamic aciduria (5-oxo-prolinuria) Acta Neuropathol. 1960, 52: 235-238)

(Smith et al, 2007) (Smith DG, Cappai R, Barnham KJ. The redox chemistry of the Alzheimer's disease amyloid beta peptide. Biochem Biophys Acta. 2007 Aug;1768(8):1976-90)

(Song, 2006) (Weihong Song, Ph.D., professor, psychiatry, University of British Columbia, Vancouver, Canada; Ralph A. Nixon, M.D., Ph.D., professor, psychiatry and cell biology, New York University, and spokesman, Alzheimer's Association; Nov. 20-24, 2006, Proceedings of the National Academy of Sciences)

(Sonish et al, 2003) (Azam Sonish; Hadi Naghma; Khan Nizam Uddin; Hadi Sheikh Mumtaz. Antioxidant and prooxidant properties of caffeine, theobromine and xanthine. Medical science monitor : international medical journal of experimental and clinical research 2003;9(9):BR325-30)

(Srp Arh Celok Lek. 2008) ([Oxidative stress in human diseases]. [No authors listed] Srp Arh Celok Lek. 2008 May;136 Suppl 2:158-65)

(Steele et al, 2004) (Steele J et al. A Phase I safety study of hyperbaric oxygen therapy for ALS. Amyotroph Lateral Scler Other Motor Neuron Disord. 2004 Dec;5(4):250-4)

(Steinhubl, 2008) (Steinhubl SR. Why have antioxidants failed in clinical trials? Am J Cardiol. 2008 May 22;101(10A):14D-19D)

(Stott et al, 2005) (Stott DJ, MacIntosh G, Lowe GD, Rumley A, McMahon AD, Langhorne P, Campbell Tail R, O'Reilly DStJ, Spilg EG, MacDonald JB, MacFarlane PW, Westendorp RGJ. Randomised controlled trial of homocysteine lowering vitamin treatment in elderly people with vascular disease. Am J Clin Nutr. 2005;82:1320–6)

(Stranges et al, 2007) (Stranges, S., Marshall, J. R., Natarajan, R., Donahue, R. P. et al., Effects of long-term selenium supplementation on the incidence of type 2 diabetes: a randomized trial. Ann. Intern. Med. 2007, 147, 217–223)

(Stranges et al, 2009) (Stranges, S., Laclaustra, M., Ji, C., Cappuccio, F. P. et al., Higher selenium status is associated with adverse blood lipid profile in British adults. J. Nutr. 2009, 140, 81–87)

(Sulkava et al, 1986) (Sulkava R., Nordberg U.R., Erkinjuntti T., Westermark T.: Erythrocytes glutathione proxidase and superoxide dismutase in Alzheimer's disease and other dementias. Acta Neurol. Scand. 1986, 73: 487-489)

(Sun et al, 2006) (Sun X, He G, Qing H, et al. Hypoxia facilitates Alzheimer's disease pathogenesis by up-regulating BACE1 gene expression. Proc Natl Acad Sci USA 2006;49:18727-32)

(Sung et al, 2004) (Sung S, Yao Y, Uryu K, Yang H, Lee VM, Trojanowski JQ, Pratico D. Early vitamin E supplementation in young but not aged mice reduces Abeta levels and amyloid deposition in a transgenic model of Alzheimer's disease. FASEB J. 2004;18:323–325)

(Supplement Business Report, 2009) (2009 Supplement Business Report, Nutr. Bus. J., New Hope Natural Media, P. M. I. (Ed.), San Diego, CA 2009)

(Tam et al, 2005) (Tam et al, Effects of vitamins C and E on oxidative stress markers and endothelial function in patients with systemic lupus erythematosus: a double blind, placebo controlled pilot study. J Rheumatol. 2005 Feb;32(2):275-82)

(Tan et al, 2002) (Tan, J., Zhu, W., Wang, W., Li, R. et al., Selenium in soil and endemic diseases in China. Sci. Total Environ. 2002, 284, 227–235)

(Taylor et al, 2009) (Taylor, C. K., Levy, R. M., Elliott, J. C., Burnett, B. P., The effect of genistein aglycone on cancer and cancer risk: a review of in vitro, preclinical, and clinical studies. Nutr. Rev. 2009, 67, 398–415)

(Teixeira et al, 2009) (Teixeira VH et al. Antioxidants do not prevent postexercise peroxidation and may delay muscle recovery. Med Sci Sports Exerc. 2009 Sep;41(9):1752-60)

(Telford et al, 1992) (Telford R, et al. The effect of 7 to 8 months of vitamin/mineral supplementation on athletic performance. International Journal of Sport Nutrition. 1992;2:135–53)

(Thal et al, 2003) (Thal LJ, Grundman M, Berg J, Ernstrom K, Margolin R, Pfeiffer E, Weiner MF, Zamrini E, Thomas RG. Idebenone treatment fails to slow cognitive decline in Alzheimer's disease. Neurology. 2003;61:1498–1502)

(Tiidus, Houston, 1995) (Tiidus PM, Houston ME. Vitamin E status and response to exercise training. Sports Med. 1995 Jul;20(1):12-23)

(Timbo et al, 2006) (Timbo BB, et al, Dietary supplements in a national survey: Prevalence of use and reports of adverse events. J Am Diet Assoc. 2006 Dec;106(12):1966-74)

(Tousoulis et al, 2007) (Tousoulis D, Antoniades C, Vasiliadou C, et al. Effects of atorvastatin and vitamin C on forearm hyperemic blood flow, asymmentrical dimethylarginine levels and the inflammatory process in patients with type 2 diabetes mellitus. Heart. 2007;93(2):244–246)

(Tudor-Locke, 2010) (Tudor-Locke C. American Journal of Preventive Medicine, 2010;39:e13-e20)

(Turrens et al, 1984) (Turrens J.F., Crapo J.D., Freeman B.A,: Protection against oxygen toxicity by intravenous injection of liposome-entrapped catalase and superoxide dismutase. J. Clin. Ivest. 1984, 73: 87-95)

(Ueda, Ogata, 1978) (Ueda K, Ogata M. Levels of erythrocyte superoxide dismutase activity in Japanese people. Acta Med Okayama. 1978 Dec;32(6):393-7)

(Valdiglesias, et al, 2009) (Valdiglesias, V., Pasaro, E., Mendez, J., Laffon, B., In vitro evaluation of selenium genotoxic, cytotoxic, and protective effects: a review. Arch. Toxicol. 2009, 84, 337–351)

(Valko et al, 2007) (Valko M, Leibfritz D, Moncol J, Cronin MT, Mazur M, Telser J. Free radicals and antioxidants in normal physiological functions and human disease. Int J Biochem Cell Biol. 2007;39(1):44-84)

(Van den Heuvel et al, 2007) (Van den Heuvel C, Thornton E, Vink R. Traumatic brain injury and Alzheimer's disease: a review. In: Weber J, Maas A, eds. Progress in Brain Research. Vol. 161. 2007:303-316)

(van der Beek, 1985) (van der Beek EJ. Vitamins and endurance training. Food for running or faddish claims? Sports Med. 1985 May-Jun;2(3):175-97)

(Vatassery et al, 1998) (Vatassery GT, Fahn S, Kuskowski MA. Alpha tocopherol in CSF of subjects taking high-dose vitamin E in the DATATOP study. Parkinson Study Group. Neurology. 1998;50:1900–1902)

(Velicer, Ulrich, 2008) (Velicer, C. M., Ulrich, C. M., Vitamin and mineral supplement use among US adults after cancer diagnosis: a systematic review. J. Clin. Oncol. 2008, 26, 665–673)

(Votorica et al, 1984) (Vitorica J., Machado A., Sastrestegui J.: Age-dependent variations in peroxide-utilizing enzymes from rat brain mitochondria and cytoplasm. J. Neurochem. 1984, 42: 351-356)

(Vyth et al, 1996) (Vyth A, Timmer JG, Bossuyt PM, Louwerse ES, de Jong JM. Survival in patients with amyotrophic lateral sclerosis, treated with an array of antioxidants. J Neurol Sci. 1996 Aug;139 Suppl:99-103)

(Ward, Hodgson et al, 2005) (Ward NC, Hodgson JM, Croft KD, et al. The combination of vitamin C and grape-seed polyphenols increases blood pressure: a randomized, double-blind, placebo-controlled trial. J Hypertens. 2005 Feb;23(2):427-34)

(Ward, Hodgson et al, 2007) (Ward NC, Hodgson JM, Croft KD, et al. The combination of vitamin C and grape-seed polyphenols increases blood pressure: a randomized, double-blind, placebo-controlled trial. J Hypertens. 2005 Feb;23(2):427-34)

(Ward, Wu et al, 2007) (Ward NC, Wu JH, Clarke MW, et al, The effect of vitamin E on blood pressure in individuals with type 2 diabetes: a randomized, double-blind, placebo-controlled trial. J Hypertens. 2007 Jan;25(1):227-34)

(Ward et al, 2008) (Ward, H., Chapelais, G., Kuhnle, G. G., Luben, R. et al., Breast cancer risk in relation to urinary and serum biomarkers of phytoestrogen exposure in the European prospective into cancer-norfolk cohort study. Breast Cancer Res. 2008, 10, R32)

(Watters JL, et al, 2007) (Watters JL, et al, Associations of antioxidant nutrients and oxidative DNA damage in healthy African-American and White adults. Cancer Epidemiol Biomarkers Prev. 2007 Jul;16(7):1428-36)

(Weight et al, 1998) (Weight L, et al. Vitamin and mineral supplementation: Effect on the running performance of trained athletes. American Journal of Clinical Nutrition. 1998;47:192–95)

(Wengreen et al, 2007) (Wengreen HJ, Munger RG, Corcoran CD, Zandi P, Hayden KM, Fotuhi M, Skoog I, Norton MC, Tschanz J, Breitner JC, Welsh-Bohmer KA. Antioxidant intake and cognitive function of elderly men and women: the Cache County Study. J Nutr Health Aging. 2007;11:230–237)

(Weyer et al, 1997) (Weyer G, Babej-Dolle RM, Hadler D, Hofmann S, Herrmann WM. A controlled study of 2 doses of idebenone in the treatment of Alzheimer's disease. Neuropsychobiology. 1997;36:73–82)

(Williams, Carlucci, 2006) (Williams CA, Carlucci SA. Oral vitamin E supplementation on oxidative stress, vitamin and antioxidant status in intensely exercised horses. Equine Vet J Suppl. 2006 Aug;(36):617-21)

(Wisiewski, 1985) (Wisniewski H.M.: Alzheimer's disease in Down's syndrome. Neurol. 1985, 35: 957-961)

(Wisniewski et al, 2003) (Wisniewski, A. B., Klein, S. L., Lakshmanan, Y., Gearhart, J. P., Exposure to genistein during gestation and lactation demasculinizes the reproductive system in rats. J. Urol. 2003, 169, 1582–1586)

(Wolf, 1978) (Wolf, G., A historical note on the mode of administration of vitamin A for the cure of night blindness. Am. J. Clin. Nutr. 1978, 31, 290–292)

(Wolters et al, 2005) (Wolters M, et al. Cognitive performance in relation to vitamin status in healthy elderly German women-the effect of 6-month multivitamin supple-mentation. Prev Med. 2005 Jul;41(1):253-9)

(Wouters-Wesseling et al, 2005) (Wouters-Wesseling W, Wagenaar LW, Rozendaal M, Deijen JB, de Groot LC, Bindels JG, van Staveren WA. Effect of an enriched drink on cog-nitive function in frail elderly persons. J Gerontol A Biol Sci Med Sci. 2005;60:265–70)

(Wray et al, 2009) (Wray DW, et al, Oral antioxidants and cardiovascular health in the exercise-trained and untrained elderly: a radically different outcome. Clin Sci (Lond). 2009 Mar;116(5):433-41)

(Yaffe et al, 2004) (Yaffe K, Clemons TE, McBee WL, Lindblad AS. Impact of antioxidants, zinc, and copper on cognition in the elderly: a randomized, controlled trial. Neurology. 2004;63:1705–1707)

(Yang et al, 1983) (Yang, G., Wang, S., Zhou, R., Sun, S., Endemic selenium intoxication of humans in China. Am. J. Clin. Nutr. 1983, 37, 872–881)

(Yang et al, 2005) (Yang F, Lim GP, Begum AN, Ubeda OJ, Simmons MR, Ambegaokar SS, Chen PP, Kayed R, Glabe CG, Frautschy SA, Cole GM. Curcumin inhibits formation of amyloid beta oligomers and fibrils, binds plaques, and reduces amyloid in vivo. J Biol Chem. 2005;280:5892–5901)

(Young et al, 2008) (Young SS, et al. The association of folate, zinc and antioxidant intake with sperm aneuploidy in healthy non-smoking men. Hum Reprod. 2008 May;23(5):1014-22)

(Youngmok et al. 2009) (Youngmok C. Jang, Holly Van Remmen. The mitochondrial theory of aging: Insight from transgenic and knockout mouse models. Experimental Gerontology, Volume 44, Issue 4, April 2009, Pages 256-260)

(Zaleska, Floyd, 1985) (Zaleska MM, Floyd RA. Regional lipid peroxidation in rat brain in vitro: Possible role of endogenous iron. Neurochem Res 10:397–410, 1985)

(Zaleska et al, 1989) (Zaleska MM, Nagy K, Floyd RA. Iron-induced lipid peroxidation and inhibition of dopamine synthesis in striatum synaptosomes. Neurochemistry 14:597–605, 1989)

(Zandi et al, 2004) (Zandi PP, Anthony JC, Khachaturian AS, Stone SV, Gustafson D, Tschanz JT, Norton MC, Welsh-Bohmer KA, Breitner JC. Reduced risk of Alzheimer disease in users of antioxidant vitamin supplements: the Cache County Study. Arch Neurol. 2004;61:82–88)

(Zhuo, Diamond, 2009) (Zhuo, P., Diamond, A. M., Molecular mechanisms by which selenoproteins affect cancer risk and progression. Biochim. Biophys. Acta 2009, 790, 1546–1554)

(Zimmerman, Kohrle, 2002) (Zimmerman, M., Kohrle, J., The impact of iron and selenium deficiencies on iodine and thyroid metabolism: biochemistry and relevance to public health. Thyroid 2002, 12, 867–878)

(Zini, 2011) (Zini, Al-Hathal N. Antioxidant therapy in male infertility: fact or fiction? Asian J Androl 2011. May 13(3): 374-81)